ACKNOWLEDGMENTS

Thanks to A. Reza Farman-Farmaian for the photography, Wen-Ching Wu and Ramel Rones for general help, Michael Wiederhold for typesetting, and Sierra for the drawings and cover design. Thanks also to David Ripianzi, James O'Leary, Jr. and many other YMAA members for proofing the manuscript and for contributing many valuable suggestions and discussions. Special thanks to Alan Dougall for his editing and to my brother Yang Chin-Ming for his help in collecting information about the 250 year old man, Li Ching-Yuen. And a very special thanks to the artist Chow Leung Chen-Ying for her beautiful calligraphy on the front page of this book.

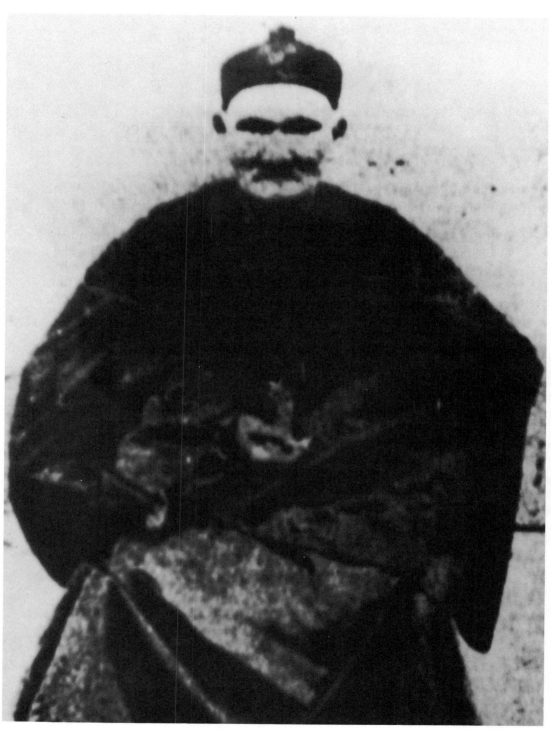

Li Ching-Yuen, the 250 Year Old Man
(Photo supplied by Internal Arts Magazine)

ABOUT LI CHING-YUEN

Li Ching-Yuen was born in 1678 A.D. (Ching Kang Shi 17th Year) in Chyi Jiang Hsien, Szechuan province. Later he immigrated to Kai Hsien, Chen's family field (Chen Jia Charng). He died in 1928 A.D. at the age of 250 years. When he was 71 years old (1749 A.D., Chyan Long 14th year), he joined the army of provincial Commander-in-Chief Yeuh Jong-Chyi. Most of his wives died early, so during the course of his life he married fourteen times.

Li was a herbalist, and skilled in Chi Kung and spent much of his life in the mountain ranges. In 1927 General Yang Sen invited Li to his residence in Wann Hsien, Szechuan province, where a picture was taken of him. Li died the next year when he returned from this trip.

After he died, General Yang investigated Li's background to determine the truth of his story, and later wrote a report about him entitled: "A Factual Account of the 250 Year-Old Good-Luck Man" (Er Bae Wuu Shyr Suey Ren Ruey Shyr Jih), which was published by the Chinese and Foreign Literature Storehouse (Jong Wai Wen Kuh), Taipei, Taiwan.

All of the information available indicates that the story is true. Li Ching-Yuen's legacy to us is the fact that it is possible for a human being to live more than 200 years if he or she knows how. Because of this we deeply believe that, if we humbly study and research, the day will come when everyone will live at least 200 years.

ABOUT THE AUTHOR

Dr. Yang Jwing-Ming, Ph.D.

Dr. Yang Jwing-Ming was born in Taiwan, Republic of China, in 1946. He started his Wushu (Kung Fu) training at the age of fifteen under the Shaolin White Crane (Pai Huo) Master Cheng Gin-Gsao. In thirteen years of study (1961-1974) under Master Cheng, Dr. Yang became an expert in White Crane defense and attack, which includes the use of both barehands and of various weapons such as saber, staff, spear, trident, and two short rods. With the same master he also studied White Crane Chin Na, massage, and herbal treatment. At the age of sixteen Dr. Yang began the study of Tai Chi Chuan (Yang Style) under Master Kao Tao. After learning from Master Kao, Dr. Yang continued his study and research of Tai Chi Chuan with several masters in Taipei. In Taipei he became qualified to teach Tai Chi. He has mastered the Tai Chi barehand sequence, pushing hands, the two-man fighting sequence, Tai Chi sword, Tai Chi saber, and internal power development.

When Dr. Yang was eighteen years old he entered Tamkang College in Taipei Hsien to study Physics. In college he began the study of traditional Shaolin Long Fist (Chang Chuan) with Master Li Mao-Ching at the Tamkang College Kuoshu Club (1964-1968), and eventually became an assistant instructor under Master Li. In 1971 he completed his M.S. degree in Physics at the National Taiwan University, and then served in the Chinese Air Force from 1971 to 1972. In the service, Dr. Yang taught Physics at the Junior Academy of the Chinese Air Force while also teaching Wushu. After being honorably discharged in 1972, he returned to Tamkang College to teach Physics and resume study under Master Li Mao-Ching. From Master Li, Dr. Yang learned Northern style Wushu, which includes both barehand (especially kicking) techniques and numerous weapons.

In 1974, Dr. Yang came to the United States to study Mechanical Engineering at Purdue University. At the request of a few students Dr. Yang began to teach Kung Fu, which resulted in the foundation of the Purdue University Chinese Kung Fu Research Club in the spring of 1975. While at Purdue, Dr. Yang also taught college-credited courses in Tai Chi Chuan. In May of 1978 he was awarded a Ph.D. in Mechanical Engineering by Purdue.

Currently, Dr. Yang and his family reside in Massachusetts. In January of 1984 he gave up his engineering career to devote more time to research, writing, and teaching at Yang's Martial Arts Association (YMAA) in Boston. The organization has continued to expand, and, as of July 1st 1989, YMAA has become just one division of Yang's Oriental Arts Association, Inc. (YOAA, Inc.).

In summary, Dr. Yang has been involved in Chinese Wushu (Kung Fu) for more than twenty years. During this time, he has spent thirteen years learning Shaolin White Crane (Pai Huo), Shaolin Long Fist

(Chang Chuan), and Tai Chi Chuan. Dr. Yang has more than twenty years of instructional experience: seven years in Taiwan, five years at Purdue University, two years in Houston, Texas, and seven years in Boston, Massachusetts.

Dr. Yang has published eleven other volumes on the martial arts and Chi Kung:

1. Shaolin Chin Na; Unique Publications, Inc., 1980.
2. Shaolin Long Fist Kung Fu; Unique Publications, Inc., 1981.
3. Yang Style Tai Chi Chuan; Unique Publications, Inc., 1981.
4. Introduction to Ancient Chinese Weapons; Unique Publications, Inc., 1985.
5. Chi Kung - Health and Martial Arts; Yang's Martial Arts Association (YMAA), 1985.
6. Northern Shaolin Sword; Yang's Martial Arts Association (YMAA), 1985.
7. Advanced Yang Style Tai Chi Chuan, Vol.1, *Tai Chi Theory and Tai Chi Jing*; Yang's Martial Arts Association (YMAA), 1986.
8. Advanced Yang Style Tai Chi Chuan, Vol.2, *Martial Applications*; Yang's Martial Arts Association (YMAA), 1986.
9. Analysis of Shaolin Chin Na, Yang's Martial Arts Association (YMAA), 1987.
10. The Eight Pieces of Brocade, Yang's Martial Arts Association (YMAA), 1988.
11. The Root of Chinese Chi Kung, *The Secrets of Chi Kung Training*; Yang's Martial Arts Association (YMAA), 1989.

Dr. Yang has also published the following videotapes:

1. Yang Style Tai Chi Chuan and Its Applications, Yang's Martial Arts Association (YMAA), 1984.
2. Shaolin Long Fist Kung Fu - Lien Bu Chuan and Its Applications, Yang's Martial Arts Association (YMAA), 1985.
3. Shaolin Long Fist Kung Fu - Gung Li Chuan and Its Applications, Yang's Martial Arts Association (YMAA), 1986.
4. Shaolin Chin Na, Yang's Martial Arts Association (YMAA), 1987.
5. Wai Dan Chi Kung, Vol. 1 - The Eight Pieces of Brocade, Yang s Martial Arts Association (YMAA), 1987.

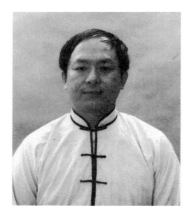

Dr. Yang Jwing-Ming

FOREWORD

Dr. Yang Jwing-Ming, Ph.D.

One of my dreams after I came to the USA in 1974 was to introduce traditional Chinese culture to the West. I believe that every culture in this world has its own independent, unique virtues which have already been tested, developed, and accepted over a long period of time. In ancient times, all of these different cultures and traditions were separated by the difficulty of travel and communication. Since travel and communication have become so convenient nowadays, I feel that the old separations should be bridged, and cultures should sincerely accept and learn from each other. If we share the experiences accumulated by the different human cultures, we will be able to remember the pain, the suffering, the hate, and the love, and we may be able to avoid making some of the same mistakes. We may even be able to help ourselves attain a higher standard of living both mentally, spiritually, and physically.

China has more than seven thousand years of history. The greatest contribution it can make to benefit the human race is to share the knowledge it has accumulated in the field of Chi. The study of Chi has contributed to the development of medicine, religion, martial arts, and methods for maintaining health and increasing longevity. Thousands of years of experience and experimentation have built up solid proof that this ancient medical and spiritual knowledge can help the human race.

In order to be content with life, you need to do more than just keep your physical body alive - you need to achieve mental and spiritual balance. The happiness comes from your feelings, not just from the enjoyment of material things. Looking at the Chinese and the American cultures, I see that people here consider the material sciences more important than the spiritual. The only place most people know of to find spiritual solace is in religious institutions. There are few people who can find comfort and mental balance within themselves. This is because Western culture has never placed much emphasis on researching the energy field which we have within ourselves, and so this spiritual inner science has never had a chance to develop.

China has been developing this inner energy science for thousands of years. China has been a pioneer in this field, but it is now time for the West to adopt this science: to see what it can learn from it, and what it can contribute to it. I deeply believe that Chi Kung is able to help people understand themselves better, reestablish their mental balance, and gain peace of mind.

Dr. Yang Jwing-Ming, Ph.D.

FOREWORD

Master Mantak Chia

There is a growing wave of popular interest in Chi Kung now, both in China and the rest of the world. To learn Chi Kung, the most important prerequisite is to have a qualified instructor. Unfortunately, masters who really know the full internal system of Chi development are few and far between.

Even if one finds an instructor who is qualified, receiving the instructions from him or her may be another matter. When I visited Taiwan in 1987, the going price for learning Bone Marrow Nei Kung (part of the Iron Shirt Chi Kung training) was about two thousand U.S. dollars for ten hours of instruction. Students were also required to take an oath of absolute secrecy, promising not to teach anyone else. Other masters required their students to serve them slavishly for years before imparting their secrets, and even then they would only teach a select few. After all of that, the master might still hold back some of the teachings for fear that the student might surpass him in knowledge and skill and usurp his position.

However, the world is quite different now. In the olden days, using Iron Shirt practice to strengthen the body so that it could withstand blows was regarded as a military secret of great value, and thus kept private. In the twentieth century with guns, planes and bombs, the need for this secrecy is outmoded. Now the deeper benefits of the training such as its ability to rejuvenate and energize the body and mind for health, spiritual development, and healing, must be emphasized. I feel it is now necessary to have full disclosure of these treasures to improve the energy and spiritual well-being of the world.

If Chinese masters have traditionally been secretive about teaching their Chinese students the true methods, they have been even more reluctant to teach foreigners. Fortunately, quite a few masters, including Dr. Yang Jwing-Ming and myself, have broken through this cultural barrier, and are offering to teach students who are sincerely interested in learning, regardless of nationality.

Dr. Yang has done considerable research, exploring the I Chin Ching (or Yi Gin Ching) and Iron Shirt Chi Kung within both historical and scientific contexts. Readers not fluent in the Chinese language will appreciate Dr. Yang's translations of the various ancient texts relating to these methods, and all readers should enjoy his breakdown and analysis of the different historical purposes of I Chin Ching and Iron Shirt among both the Taoists and the Buddhists.

Dr. Yang and I also share the view that it is essential to do our best to understand Chi Kung in the light of modern science, while still respecting the wisdom and research we have inherited from our own masters of the past. Chinese medical theory has a deep understanding

-XIof Chi and the energetic network of the body. As we combine this with the knowledge of Western anatomy, physiology and psychology, along with recent discoveries in bioelectricity, we will surely enjoy the best of both worlds.

Dr. Yang Jwing-Ming's book is a major contribution to the literature of Chinese Chi Kung. It is my hope that works such as this will continue to appear, so that the standards for Chi Kung practice around the world will not deteriorate behind a wall of secrecy, but will, through open sharing of our knowledge, rise to an unprecedented level of excellence.

Master Mantak Chia

PREFACE

Muscle/Tendon Changing (Yi Gin) and Marrow/Brain Washing (Shii Soei) Chi Kung have been known in China since the Liang dynasty (502 A.D.). However, they were kept secret, and only in the last fifty years has this knowledge gradually been revealed to the general public. Within a short period of time, these two arts have not only been widely adopted by Chi Kung practitioners, but they have also interested many Chinese medical scientists and bioscientists.

Muscle/Tendon Changing Chi Kung specializes in circulating Chi in the twelve primary Chi channels and the two major Chi vessels (Conception and Governing Vessels). The training will strengthen your physical body, including muscles and tendons, and maintain the smooth circulation of Chi in the primary channels and the internal organs, which is the key to maintaining health and slowing down the degeneration of the physical body.

Usually, after a practitioner becomes familiar with the Muscle/-Tendon Changing Chi Kung, he will enter the deeper field of Chi Kung training, that of Marrow/Brain Washing. This teaches the practitioner how to fill up the Chi in the "eight extraordinary Chi vessels." In Chinese medicine, the vessels are considered reservoirs of Chi, and they regulate the Chi in the body's primary Chi channels and organs. A strong and abundant store of Chi is the key to keeping your body healthy and extending your life. Theoretically, your body deteriorates as you age mainly because your blood loses its ability to feed and protect your body. The red and white blood cells are produced by your bone marrow, but as you grow older, the marrow becomes "dirty," and produces fewer and fewer useful blood cells. However, if you know how to "wash" the marrow, it will start, once again, to produce fresh, healthy blood. Your body will begin to rejuvenate itself, and restore itself to the glowing health of youth.

Most important of all, the practitioner of Marrow/Brain Washing Chi Kung is able to lead Chi to his brain to nourish it, and to raise up his spirit. To the Taoists and Buddhists, Marrow/Brain Washing Chi Kung is the path to reach the final goal of enlightenment or Buddhahood. Part of Marrow/Brain Washing involves stimulating the sexual organs. In their thoroughness, the ancient Chi Kung practitioners discovered that, in addition to providing hormones, the genitals are also a potent source of the Chi which is necessary for the training.

The contents of this volume are drawn from the many published documents that I have collected. Once I understood them, I filtered out the questionable parts and, based on my own knowledge, added some theory and commentary. Although I believe that this book provides an in-depth discussion of these two arts, there is one deficiency, namely that we only discuss the training for the male. There are two reasons for this. The first is that the available documents have very little information on women's training. The second is that as a male I do not have the necessary experience. I do believe, however, that it doesn't matter whether you are male or female, the training theory remains the same. Female readers who would like more information about these two arts may refer to the book: "Bone Marrow Chi Kung," by Mantak Chia and Maneewan Chia.

In the next few years, YMAA will continue to publish more volumes of its in-depth Chi Kung book series for those readers who wish to advance their Chi Kung knowledge and practice into a deeper level.

The complete series will consist of:

1. *THE ROOT OF CHINESE CHI KUNG* - The Secrets of Chi Kung Training (Published, 1989)
2. *MUSCLE/TENDON CHANGING AND MARROW/BRAIN WASHING CHI KUNG* - The Secret of Youth (Yi Gin Ching and Shii Soei Ching)
3. *CHI KUNG MASSAGE* - Chi Kung Tuei Na and Cavity Press for Healing (Chi Kung Ann Mo and Chi Kung Dien Shiuh)
4. *CHI KUNG AND HEALTH* - For Healing and Maintaining Health
5. *CHI KUNG AND MARTIAL ARTS* - The Key to Advanced Martial Arts Skill (Shaolin, Wuudang, Ermei, and others)
6. *BUDDHIST CHI KUNG* - Charn, The Root of Zen
7. *TAOIST CHI KUNG* (Dan Diing Tao Kung)
8. *TIBETAN CHI KUNG* (Mih Tzong Shen Kung)

The first volume, "The Root of Chinese Chi Kung" introduced the historical background and the different categories of Chi Kung, Chi Kung theory and principles, and the keys to Chi Kung training. That volume provided a map of the world of Chi Kung. We recommend that you read that book before any of the others.

In this second volume, "Muscle/Tendon Changing and Marrow/Brain Washing Chi Kung," Part One will introduce the general concepts of the two arts, Part Two will discuss both theory and training principles of the Muscle/Tendon Changing Chi Kung, and Part Three will discuss the theory and the training of Marrow/Brain Washing Chi Kung. Finally, Part Four will contain a list of the questions which remain in my mind, and the Conclusion to the book.

CONTENTS

PART ONE

GENERAL CONCEPTS

Chapter 1

Introduction

Before you start reading this book, you are advised to read the first volume of this series: "The Root of Chinese Chi Kung - The Secret of Chi Kung Training." It reviews the history of Chinese Chi Kung, explains important concepts and terminologies, and most importantly, gives you a foundation of knowledge of general Chi Kung principles and training theory. Without these roots, you might become confused and misunderstand this and subsequent YMAA Chi Kung books.

1-1. The Value of Tradition

Prior to this century, the understanding of nature was limited and technology was not yet well developed. Communication was not as convenient as today, and the human mind was not as open. People's thinking was restrained by the bondage of traditional, conservative beliefs. At that time, the ancient ways and writings which had been passed down were considered the absolute authorities in most areas. Anyone who strayed from the traditional ways was felt to be betraying society.

In this old, conservative community, accumulated "experience" was the source of knowledge, and was considered the most valuable treasure. Older people were generally respected by youngsters because of their experience. At that time, when something happened to a person, the first and most important thing was his emotional response to it. When these experiences were then explained by "wisdom" (wise thinking and judgement), knowledge increased. A person who had a great amount of experience and knowledge was then better able to sense and understand the "great nature," which includes, among other things, heavenly timing (seasonal changes), geomancy, and human relations. Such a person was respected as a wise man, a holy man, or a saint. "Human nature," which mainly originated from feelings and judgements through contact with nature and other human natures, was widely studied and researched. Philosophies were created. The accumulated experience led to traditions and societal rules, which formed the foundation of the culture.

You can see that tradition is the result of accumulated experiences filtered through human feelings. Different races have had different historical backgrounds and, therefore, have different traditions and rules. These traditions represent the characteristics of each race, which were developed through thousands of years.

In this century, modern science has developed and communication around the world has become very easy. Open minded youngsters have started to challenge the "traditional," and have re-entered the "experience" path of their ancestors. However, as they let go of the traditions they lose their bearings. Without experience to guide them they feel lost, and their lives seem to have no meaning. Because of this they suffer pain and confusion. In order to escape from this, they look to drugs and alcohol for temporary relief. These have become an ever-increasing problem, and I really believe that it is because we have ignored our culture and traditions in the last two decades.

As the material sciences have developed, material enjoyments have become people's main concern. They base their feelings and self-satisfaction on the enjoyment of material things. Tradition and accumulated human emotional experience have become the major source of a generation gap. Older people have lost the respect of the younger generation and become the lost group in this modern society. Human spiritual feelings and the appreciation of culture and fine, classic, creative arts have been downgraded.

Not until recently did our society start to realize the value of tradition and experience. This is especially true for the knowledge and experience which are based on spiritual feelings. This new society is beginning to understand that in order to have a happy life, you need not just material comfort, but also, and more importantly, spiritual cultivation in peace and calmness. Many people are starting to believe that the traditional practices of the ancient spiritual societies hold the key to solving many mental problems and improving our lives. Tradition and spiritual science are being re-evaluated. This tendency has become especially apparent in the last ten years with the increased cultural exchange between East and West. Finally, people are getting the chance to see how people in other parts of the globe deal with life's problems.

Chinese Chi Kung has started to bloom in the West. More and more, people are coming to believe that in addition to maintaining health and increasing longevity, Chi Kung can be one of the most effective ways to attain a peaceful, spiritual life.

Chi Kung is one of the greatest achievements of China. It was created from the accumulated experiences of countless generations by thousands of "wise men." These wise men, after learning the traditional knowledge, modified and added their own experiences to the practice. Finally, this treasure has reached our hands. Now, it is our responsibility to keep it and continue to develop it.

Many of the theories and training methods of Chi Kung were kept secret, and only recently made available to the general public. There are many reasons for this secrecy:

1. Every Chi Kung style considered its theory and methods to be precious treasures which offered something which could not be purchased with money - health and long life. Because this was so valuable, many masters did not want to share it.

2. Many Chi Kung training theories are hard to understand, and the practices dangerous if done incorrectly. Only advanced disciples have the necessary level of understanding, and few ever get to this level.
3. Many Chi Kung practitioners believed that the more you kept a mystery, the more valuable and precious it would be.
4. Some of the Chi Kung training, such as Marrow/Brain Washing, involves stimulation of the sexual organs. In the ancient, conservative society, this was considered immoral.

Many Chi Kung secrets were passed down only to a few students or to direct blood relatives. In religious Chi Kung, the limitations were even stricter. The religious exercises were passed down only to the priests. This was especially true for the Marrow/Brain Washing Chi Kung. In fact, these techniques were traditionally passed down to only a very few disciples who understood Chi Kung theory and had reached a high level of cultivation. This situation lasted until the beginning of this century, when it was gradually revealed to laymen. It was only during the last twenty years that many of the secret documents were made available to the public.

Nobody can deny that Western science which has been developed today is mainly focused on material development. Spiritual science has been downplayed. The major reason for this is simply that the spiritual energy world is harder to see and understand. This spiritual science is still in its formative stage. Recently, it was reported that even today's science understands probably only 10% of the functions of the human brain. You can see from this that, compared to the "great nature" which is still waiting for us to discover and understand it, science today is still in its infancy.

For these reasons, it is unwise to use today's infant science to judge the accumulated experience and phenomena of the past. I believe that as long as we respect the traditions and experience of the past, and continue our study and research, we will eventually be able to understand all of these natural phenomena scientifically.

Following this reasoning, traditional Chi Kung theory and training methods should remain the main source and authority for your training. The correct attitude in practicing Chi Kung is to respect and understand the past, and to also examine everything from a modern, scientific point of view. In this way you can improve upon the knowledge and experience of the past. The "secrets" should be opened to the public and should accept the questioning of modern science. A secret is a secret only if you do not know it. Once a secret is common knowledge, then it ceases to be a secret.

Many of you might be wondering: if people in ancient times had to invest at least fifty years of effort before they reached the higher levels of achievement, such as enlightenment, what chance do we have today to reach the same level? Very few people in our busy society can devote the time that the ancients did. The answer is that since the training theory used to be kept secret, it took most Chi Kung practitioners many years to learn and understand it. If we can first learn the theory and principles, and then train, we will start out on the correct path and avoid many many years of wondering and confusion. If you want to drive somewhere you have never been before, the best way is to check the map first to find the quickest route. However, if you get in your car with only a vague idea of where your destination is and how to get there, you may never reach it. It is said: "The Large Tao is no more than three or two sentences, when spoken and revealed, it is not worth more than half a penny."(*1) This means that the so-called secrets contain only some simple theories and principles. With the assistance of modern science, we might be able to find a path which shortens the training period.

Therefore, we should respect the past, and study and practice carefully. Whenever we are able to use modern science to explain something, we should dare to challenge the traditional beliefs and re-evaluate them. Only in this way will the ancient science be recognized and accepted in the present and future.

This volume will be divided into four parts. The first part, after introducing the general concepts, will survey the history of the Yi Gin Ching (Muscle/Tendon Changing Classic) and the Shii Soei Ching (Marrow/Brain Washing Classic). We will then discuss the training background of the two major religious sources of these two classics: Buddhism and Taoism. Since many documents originated with the Taoists, we will discuss the different Taoist approaches to Chi Kung in the third chapter. Finally, in order to help you understand the major keys to the entire training, the fourth chapter will review the general concepts of Kan (Water) and Lii (Fire), which will lead you to a deeper level of understanding of adjusting and balancing your Chi.

In the second part of this book, we will first discuss the theory and principles of Yi Gin Ching, and follow this with a detailed discussion of the traditional training methods. During the discussion, many documents will be translated and commented upon.

Shii Soei Ching theory, training principles and methods will be covered in the third part of the book. Naturally, the available documents will be translated and commented on. Finally, in the fourth part, I will list many of the questions I have about these two arts.

1-2. What are Yi Gin Ching and Shii Soei Ching?

It is extremely important that, before you read any further, you have a general understanding of the Yi Gin Ching and Shii Soei Ching, and of what kind of roles they can play in your health and longevity. This brief introduction will offer you a general idea of what you can expect and what will be involved. Parts Two and Three will discuss these subjects in greater depth.

Yi means "to change, to replace, or to alter," Gin means "muscles and tendons," and Ching means "classic or bible." Therefore, it is commonly translated as "Muscle Changing Classic," "Tendon Changing Classic," or "Muscle/Tendon Changing Classic." "Muscles and tendons" does not refer only to the literal muscles and tendons. It actually refers to all of the physical system which is related to the muscles and tendons, including the internal organs. The Yi Gin Ching describes Chi Kung theory and training methods which are able to improve your physical body, and change it from weak to strong. Naturally, these methods are also very effective in maintaining your physical health.

Shii means "to wash" or "to clean." Soei includes Guu Soei, which means "bone marrow," and Nao Soei, which refers to the brain - includ-

---

(*1). 大道不過三兩句，説破不値半文錢。

ing cerebrum, cerebellum, and medulla oblongata. Ching means "classic or bible." This work is commonly translated "Marrow Washing Classic," but "Marrow/Brain Washing Classic" is a more accurate translation. The first translation probably became popular because of a misunderstanding of the scope of the work, which had been kept secret for a long period of time. Also, the goal of "brain washing" is enlightenment or Buddhahood, which, in addition to being difficult to understand, is less interesting to laymen. It was not until recently, when many of the secret documents were made available to the general public, that a clearer and more complete picture of the training emerged. A correct translation shows that Shii Soei Ching training deals with the bone marrow and the brain. However, the training does not actually focus on the physical matter of the bone marrow and the brain. Instead, it emphasizes how you should take care of the Chi (energy) part of your body, and how to lead the Chi to the bone marrow and brain to nourish them and keep them functioning at an optimal level.

In order to give you a general understanding of how these two arts fit into the general picture of Chinese Chi Kung, we would like to summarize some important concepts which were discussed in the first volume of this series: "The Root of Chinese Chi Kung." First, we will discuss the concept of health, and then we will look at the different categories of Chi Kung which have been developed in China, and review their training goals. This will prepare you for an understanding of the role which the Yi Gin Ching and Shii Soei Ching play in Chinese Chi Kung society. Finally, we will list the differences between the Yi Gin Ching and Shii Soei Ching. Once you understand these basic concepts, you will be able to enter into an examination of the deeper aspects of Chi Kung without being confused by mystical "secrets."

1. What is Real Health?
A. Your body includes physical and mental parts. The physical body is considered to be Yang in Chinese Chi Kung, and the mental body, which is closely related to the Chi, thinking, and the spirit, is thought of as Yin. Only when these Yin and Yang parts of your body balance each other harmoniously do you have real health. In other words, to have true good health, you must have a strong physical body and a healthy Chi body and mind. When you have both, your spirit can be raised and your whole being will be vigorously alive.
B. In order to keep the physical part of your body strong, you must have smooth Chi circulation. Chi is the energy source for all of the body's activities. You also need to have healthy blood cells to carry nutrients and oxygen throughout the body. According to Chinese medicine, the blood cells need Chi to stay alive. However, blood cells have also been traditionally considered to be carriers of Chi. They distribute Chi throughout the body, and also act as a battery, storing excess Chi and releasing it when needed. You can see that if the blood cells are not healthy, they will not transport nutrients and oxygen efficiently, and they will also not be able to carry out the function of regulating the Chi.
C. In order to keep the mental part of your body healthy, you must learn how to keep your brain healthy. Your brain is the center of your thinking and the headquarters of the Chi. In order to keep your brain functioning properly, you must have plenty of Chi to

nourish it. When you have a healthy brain, your spirit of vitality can be raised.

D. In order to have smooth Chi circulation in your body, you must first understand the Chi circulatory system. Your body has twelve primary Chi channels which relate to twelve internal organs, and eight extraordinary vessels which store the Chi. The twelve primary Chi channels are sometimes compared to rivers which circulate the Chi to the organs to maintain their normal functioning, and the eight vessels are compared to reservoirs of Chi which regulate the Chi rivers. To have a healthy body and a long life, you must keep the Chi circulating smoothly in the twelve primary channels, and keep the Chi reservoirs full so that they can regulate the Chi rivers efficiently.

Many Chi Kung styles were created upon this foundation of knowledge, which is drawn from Chinese medical science. Each style has its own training goals. Generally speaking, the styles can be divided into four major categories.

2. Major Chi Kung Categories and Their Training Goals

A. Scholar Chi Kung. Styles in this category were developed by scholars, and their main purpose is maintaining health. They emphasize having an emotionally neutral, healthy mind and smooth Chi circulation.

B. Healing or Medical Chi Kung. This category was created mainly by Chinese medical doctors. Special exercises were created to emphasize the Chi circulation in specific channels in order to cure specific illnesses.

C. Martial Chi Kung. The goal of this category is to energize the physical and energy bodies to a more vigorous state so as to increase fighting ability. Most of the exercises in this category were created by Chi Kung practitioners who were martial artists.

D. Religious Chi Kung. This type of Chi Kung was developed mainly by Buddhist and Taoist monks. The original goal of religious Chi Kung was enlightenment or Buddhahood. Later, when the training techniques were revealed to laymen, it was discovered that this type of Chi Kung was very effective for longevity. Both training theory and methods are the hardest among all of the Chi Kung styles. This style emphasizes leading Chi to the marrow to keep it fresh and healthy and also to the brain to nourish it. In order to have an abundant supply of Chi for the training, not only must the Chi circulate smoothly in the twelve channels, but the Chi in the eight vessels must be full. For the monks, leading Chi to the brain to raise up the Shen is the key to enlightenment.

3. General Purposes of Yi Gin Ching and Shii Soei Ching

Before we discuss the purposes of each training, you should first know a few important points:

A. These two classics were a Buddhist creation, and were later developed continuously by both Buddhists and Taoists.

B. The original goal of training was enlightenment or Buddhahood. In order to reach this final goal, a practitioner needed first to have a strong physical body and an abundant supply of Chi. This Chi is led to the marrow and the brain to nourish them. Yi Gin Ching training is concerned with strengthening the physical body and building up the energy (Chi) body, while the Shii Soei Ching is concerned with using this Chi to nourish the bone marrow and to realize the goal of spiritual (Shen) cultivation.

C. Recently the training secrets were revealed to laymen and used mainly for health and longevity.

There is a section in the documents which talks about the general purposes of the Yi Gin Ching and Shii Soei Ching. We will translate it here for your reference. The Chinese version and the commentary will be offered in the second part of this book.

Yi Gin Kung Fu is able to change the tendons and shape, Shii Soei Kung Fu is able to change the marrow and Shen (spirit). (They are) especially capable of increasing spiritual bravery, spiritual power, spiritual wisdom, and spiritual intelligence. Its training methods, compared with the Taoist family's Liann Jieng (train Essence), Liann Chi (train Chi), and Liann Shen (train spirit), are repeatedly mutually related in many ways, and its Yi of practice (i.e., goal) is completely the same.

However, (the Buddhist approach is) trained from external, while elixir family (i.e., Taoist approach) is trained from internal. Cultivating life (i.e., the physical body) is the major support of cultivating the Tao, it is the ladder and the voyage to Buddhahood. It serves the same purpose as "methods" (of cultivation). Once (you have) achieved the goal, the life and the methods should all be given up; not hesitating is the important point.

Once you understand the general purpose of the Yi Gin Ching and Shii Soei Ching, you should further understand how each one fits into your total training.

4. The Purpose of the Yi Gin Ching

The main purpose of Yi Gin Ching training is to change the physical body from weak to strong and from sick to healthy. In order to reach this goal, the physical body must be stimulated and exercised, and the Chi in the energy body must be regulated. The main goals of the training are:

A. To open up the Chi channels and maintain the appropriate level of smooth Chi circulation in the twelve primary Chi channels. This maintains the health and proper functioning of the related organs. Smooth Chi circulation also makes it possible to greatly strengthen the physical body.

B. To fill up the Chi in the two main Chi reservoirs - the Conception and Governing Vessels (Ren Mei and Du Mei). The Conception Vessel is responsible for regulating the six Yin channels, while the Governing Vessel governs the six Yang channels. When an abundant supply of Chi is stored in these two vessels, the twelve primary channels can be regulated effectively.

C. To open the small Chi branches from the primary channels to the surface of the skin and maintain healthy conditions for the muscles and skin.

D. For those who also wish to train Shii Soei Ching and reach a higher level, Yi Gin Ching training is needed to build up the necessary level of Chi.

5. The Purpose of the Shii Soei Ching

The main purposes of Shii Soei Ching training are to use the abundant Chi generated from Yi Gin Ching training to wash the marrow, to nourish the brain, and to fill up the Chi in the other six vessels. The main goals of the training are:

A. To keep the Chi at an abundant level and continue to build up the Chi to a higher level from other sources. An abundant Chi supply is the key to successful marrow washing and nourishing of the brain for raising the spirit. Experience has shown that the genitals can be an important source of extra Chi. Therefore, one of the main goals of Shii Soei Ching training is learning how to increase the production of semen Essence and improving the efficiency of its conversion into Chi.

B. In order to keep an abundant supply of Chi, the fuel (Original Essence) must be conserved, protected, and firmed. Therefore, the second purpose of Shii Soei Ching is to regulate the usage of Original Essence.

C. Learning how to lead Chi to the marrow to keep the marrow fresh, and to lead Chi to the brain to raise up the spirit of vitality. Marrow is the factory which produces your red and white blood cells, when the marrow is fresh and clean the blood will be healthy. As this blood flows to every part of your body, it will slow down the degeneration of your cells. Practicing Shii Soei Ching can therefore slow down the aging process. When the brain has plenty of Chi to nourish it, you are able to maintain the normal functioning of your brain and also raise up the spirit of vitality. When the spirit is raised, the Chi in the body can be governed effectively.

D. For a sincere Buddhist or Taoist monk, the final goal of Shii Soei Ching is reaching enlightenment or Buddhahood. For them, the training purposes listed above are considered temporary. They are only steps in the process of building up their "spiritual baby" (Ling Tai) and nurturing it until it is independent and has eternal life.

From this brief summary, it is clear that the Yi Gin Ching and Shii Soei Ching can change both your physical and spiritual qualities and lead you to a higher level of physical and spiritual life. But to understand exactly how these two Chi Kung exercises help you to reach these goals, you must have a profound understanding of the relationship between your Chi, your physical body, and your spiritual body. Only then will you be able to grasp the keys of the training. At this point, you are encouraged to study the first book of YMAA's in-depth Chi Kung book series: "The Root of Chinese Chi Kung - The Secrets of Chi Kung Training."

1-3. How the Yi Gin Ching and Shii Soei Ching Have Affected Chinese Culture

Since the Yi Gin Ching and Shii Soei Ching were created about 550 A.D., they have significantly influenced the development of Chinese culture for more than 1400 years. Because the Yi Gin Ching has been taught to the public while the Shii Soei Ching has been kept more secret, the Yi Gin Ching should be credited with having more influence. We will look at their influence on three different fields: 1. religious society; 2. martial and political societies; and 3. medical society.

1. Religious Society:

A. Before these two classics were available, Buddhism and religious Taoism had existed for nearly 500 years in China. Within that period, though the philosophy of achieving Buddhahood or enlightenment was preached and methods of reaching it through meditation and spiritual cultivation were taught, they mainly emphasized the spiritual part of the cultivation and ignored the physical part of the training. Therefore, most of the monks had weak physical bodies and poor health. Naturally, their lives were short and very few of them actually reached the goal of their cultivation. It was not until these two classics were created by Da Mo that the monks had a more complete theory and more effective training methods that train both the physical and spiritual bodies. To the Chinese religious society, this was a revolution. These two classics provided the monks with an effective way to build up their health and extend their lives so they could continue their spiritual cultivation.

B. Da Mo is considered the original ancestor of Charn (Zen) Buddhist meditation in China. Charn meditation has influenced not only Chinese Buddhist society, but it has also significantly influenced the cultures of several Asian countries such as Japan and Korea. Charn meditation is part of the Yi Gin Ching and Shii Soei Ching training.

C. Because of Da Mo's training theories, Chinese Buddhism has split into two main groups with different theories of how to train to achieve Buddhahood. Though the Yi Gin Ching and Shii Soei Ching have been passed down within Buddhist society, many Buddhists have refused to use the methods. The main reason is that many of the monks do not believe that, when you are striving to become a Buddha, your physical body should be considered as important as your spiritual body. They believe that since the spiritual body is the one you cultivate to reach eternal life, why should you have to spend time training your physical body? Another important reason is that the Yi Gin Ching and Shii Soei Ching exercises were used at their original birthplace, the Shaolin Temple, to enhance fighting ability. Many monks believed that fighting and killing should be completely forbidden, and exercises that contributed to this were therefore evil. As a matter of fact, mainstream Buddhist society considered the Shaolin Temple unrighteous.

D. Since the Yi Gin Ching and Shii Soei Ching were introduced in China, their training theories have been combined with the theories of traditional Chinese medicine. For example, there are many places in the documents where the training theory and methods are explained according to Chinese medical Chi theory, especially the concepts of primary Chi channels and vessels. This combination has provided a better scientific and logical explanation of how to reach enlightenment or Buddhahood.

2. Martial and Political Societies:

A. Before the Yi Gin Ching was available, Chinese martial arts techniques and training were restricted to muscular strength. The Shaolin monks discovered that their power could be significantly increased through the Yi Gin Chi Kung exercises, and it gradually became part of the required training. Because of this, the entire Chinese martial society entered a new era and started to emphasize internal Chi training. The Shaolin

Temple was recognized as one of the highest authorities in Chinese martial arts. Now, Shaolin martial arts have not only spread widely in China but even throughout the world.

B. Many other martial styles were influenced by the Shaolin Temple and started to train internal strength. The first 100 years following the creation of the Yi Gin Ching saw the birth of several internal styles such as Sheau Jeou Tian (Small Nine Heaven) and Hou Tian Faa (Post-birth Techniques). It is believed that Tai Chi Chuan, which was created during the tenth century, was based on these two internal styles. Since then, many internal martial arts styles have been created, such as Ba Kua, Hsing Yi, and Liu Ho Ba Fa.

C. The most significant influence of the Yi Gin Ching and Shii Soei Ching on Chinese martial arts was probably the development of emotional qualities such as patience, endurance, perseverance, concentration, and discipline. In addition, morality was improved with such qualities as humility, respect, and loyalty being built up through the mental cultivation training. Through meditation and internal training, many martial artists could understand the real meaning of life and find their true nature. This understanding led to a re-evaluation and re-standardization of martial morality. Shaolin martial artists were commonly recognized as examples of righteousness.

D. Martial artists who trained the Yi Gin Ching and Shii Soei Ching often developed the highest levels of power. This was vitally important in ancient times before the advent of guns, when all of the fighting depended on the individual's strength and techniques. Those who reached the highest levels of fighting ability were respected as heroes and held up as models.

E. Because in ancient times skilled martial artists were the source of a nation's strength, they have often had a profound influence on politics. For example, it was Marshal Yeuh Fei who decided the destiny of the Song dynasty. He had learned Shaolin Kung Fu, and is credited with creating the internal martial style Hsing Yi Chuan as well as The Eight Pieces of Brocade, a popular Chi Kung set for health. The first emperor of the Chinese Tarng dynasty, Li Shyh-Min, was assisted by the Shaolin priests several times during the revolution which led to his assuming power. Later, emperor Li authorized the Shaolin temple to organize its own martial arts training system, which had previously been legally limited, and to maintain an army of priest-soldiers (Seng Bing). In addition, in order to express his appreciation he rewarded them with the right to eat meat and drink wine. However, this outraged other Buddhists, and they ejected the Shaolin Temple from the Chinese Buddhist community.

Another example is general Chi Jih-Guang, who significantly influenced the future of the Ming dynasty. The martial arts techniques in his books are said to be based on the Shaolin style. The most recent example of the close link between the martial and the political spheres was probably the disaster which happened directly to the Shaolin temple during the Ching dynasty. Primarily because Shaolin priests were involved in fighting against the Ching regime, the Shaolin temple was attacked and burned at least three times, and many martial priests were killed. Many priests escaped, and returned to secular life. However, they still wanted to resist the Ching emperor, and so they started teaching laymen their art and building up another fighting force.

The martial arts are not so important in today's world, but these two classics still have influence. Many young people still train them, and appreciate the challenge and discipline that they offer.

3. Medical Society:
A. Although many Chi Kung styles and exercises were created before the Yi Gin Ching and Shii Soei Ching, most of them only served to improve health and cure some illnesses. After Da Mo however, people began to realize that they could gain a significant increase in longevity through Yi Gin Ching and Shii Soei Ching training.

B. Since the Yi Gin Ching and Shii Soei Ching were introduced in China, many doctors and some martial artists have combined their training theories with traditional Chinese medicine. Out of this combination have come many different healing and health maintaining Chi Kung exercises which are more effective than the traditional healing Chi Kung exercises. For example, the famous Chi Kung set The Eight Pieces of Brocade was one of the fruits of this combination. Recently, many healing exercises for some types of cancer were created based on this combined theory.

1-4. The Value of the Yi Gin Ching and Shii Soei Ching in Today's World

You can see from the last section that the Yi Gin Ching and Shii Soei Ching have had a significant effect on Chinese culture. These two classics are the fruit of Chinese culture, and have been tasted for more than one thousand years. Now, the world is different. Ancient secrets are revealed. Different cultures from different races finally have a chance to look at each other. It is time for us to open our minds to other cultures and even adopt their good parts. These two classics have brought the Chinese people the great fortune of good health. I believe that if Western society can open its mind to study them, it will gain far more than anyone can predict. I would like to discuss this subject in three parts.

1. Religion:
With the improvement of communication since the beginning of this century, countries which used to close their gates to anything foreign have gradually opened. The exchange of culture, knowledge, and experiences has increased significantly in the last two decades. However, in the domain of religion, the situation remains the same as in the last century. Religious groups continue to build up walls to separate themselves from other religions, especially those from different cultures.

Because of this, the progress of religious education has stagnated or even gone backward. Fewer and fewer people believe in God or Buddha. The power of the religions which used to dominate and control morality in society has been weakening. More and more people have lost the feeling for and understanding of the meaning of life. The responsibility for the development of spiritual science has been taken over by non-religious groups. The main reason for this is simply that almost all religious preaching and education still remain at the pre-scientific stage. While science is rapidly advancing, and people are much better educated than ever, the old methods of study, research, and preaching have lost their power to persuade people. The old ideas of morality and the superstitious methods of persuasion no longer fit in our modern society.

Spiritual questions have always caused people a lot of confusion and doubt. I believe that the development of spiritual science has never been so important in human history. So many people today need a sense of direction for their lives, one which can be understood in the light of today's science. They need contemporary answers to contemporary questions. I sincerely believe that if all of the religions could open their minds, share their experiences, and study together, they would be able to find a modern way to regain people's belief and support, and continue to be the spiritual leaders of our society.

The Yi Gin Ching and Shii Soei Ching are only a small part of Chinese spiritual science. Both Buddhism and Taoism have had nearly two thousand years to study man's inner feelings and spiritual enlightenment. I believe that if the Western religions can open their minds, study them, and select the good parts to mix with their own, a new religious revolution can be expected.

2. Martial Arts:

Though traditional martial arts training is not as important as in ancient times, when an individual's power and fighting techniques were the decisive factors in battle, martial arts training still remains of value. It has many purposes today, the most common being the strengthening of the physical body and the maintenance of health. Though many other sports can serve the same purpose, Chinese martial arts are the product of thousands of years of experience, and the theory and philosophy are much deeper. Like Western classical music, the deeper you dig, the more depth you find. Another common use of the martial arts is for self-cultivation. This is so because their training is not just physical. In order to reach the higher levels of competence, you have to conquer yourself. One of the main reasons that parents send their children to martial arts schools is to learn self-discipline. Through the training, children learn responsibility, patience, perseverance, respect for culture and tradition, and most important of all, they develop the willpower which is so essential to achieve any kind of goal.

Another reason that many people study the martial arts is that they are looking for the meaning of life. The martial arts, like classical music and art, are profound because they developed out of an enormous accumulation of human experience. As you immerse yourself in the study of one of these arts, you are able to find the peace within yourself to analyze what is happening in your life. This is especially true for practitioners of the internal martial arts.

You can see that the Chinese martial arts today have become a sport, a form of self-cultivation, and a way to achieve a peaceful life. You can see why the internal spiritual arts have reached such a high level in the Chinese martial arts. Internal spiritual cultivation is part of the arts and cannot be separated from them. This has been the case in China since 500 A.D. Regardless of which martial style one studies in China, it must have both external techniques and internal Chi Kung power training.

However, when the Oriental martial arts were imported to the Western world, because of the traditional secrecy, the modern lifestyle, and the different cultural background, there was a separation between the training of the external techniques and the internal cultivation. This has made the arts and the training incomplete. Many Western martial artists have only learned the external training, and a large number only use the arts as a way to make money. The true meaning and content have been revised. Many people consider the Oriental martial arts to be simply fighting techniques, and they totally ignore the internal cultivation. This has caused the general public to despise and downgrade this highly elegant art. This situation was especially true during the 1960's.

This situation has only begun to change in the last ten years. With the increase of communication and cultural exchange between China and the Western world, the arts are finally beginning to be understood. More people understand acupuncture and Chi theory, and they have learned a new respect for the Chinese martial arts, especially for Tai Chi Chuan, which has spread to every corner of the world. It is now time for the Western martial arts community to change its point of view and study one step further. The internal aspect of the arts must be understood and combined with the external training. I predict that any martial style that doesn't start this now will be considered outdated in another ten or twenty years. The internal aspect of the oriental martial arts was kept secret, but now it has been revealed. Any martial artist who does not grasp this opportunity to learn is limiting his art to the external. The internal aspect of Chinese martial arts training will be discussed in the book: "Chi Kung and the Martial Arts" which will be published at a later date.

Yi Gin Ching and Shii Soei Ching Chi Kung are the foundation of the internal training in the martial arts. For example, "Iron Shirt" was a product of the Yi Gin Chi Kung. Internal "Light Kung Fu" was a result of the Shii Soei Ching training. Any martial artist who would like to enter the internal aspect of cultivation must first understand these two classics. You can see that because of the changes in the last ten years, the internal arts are moving up, and the external arts are moving down. I can easily predict that in the near future, any martial school that does not get involved in the internal aspect of training will find its business declining. When people look for a suitable master for themselves or their children, they must first determine how much each master really knows. Does he train only the external, or both external and internal? And what is his morality?

I believe that if there is a set of Chi Kung books available it will greatly help people to understand the mystery of Chi Kung and the internal arts, and stay on the right path. I hope to provide such a set with this series of books, and I sincerely hope that other people who are experienced in the internal arts will also publish their knowledge.

3. Medical Science:

Other than improving health, two of the most significant achievements which can be obtained from Yi Gin Ching and Shii Soei Ching training are longevity and a deeper spiritual life. Long life has been a major concern of mankind, and it is a major subject of modern medical research. Since the Yi Gin Ching and Shii Soei Ching offer proven theory and training methods, it would be wise for modern medicine to study and research them. Naturally, first modern science must reach an understanding of internal energy (Chi), which is still new to it. It is only in the last decade that Chi is beginning to be understood as bioenergy. Hopefully, modern science may be able to find quicker and easier ways to achieve the same results as the Yi Gin Ching and Shii Soei Ching.

In order to have a calm and peaceful mind, you must first have a healthy brain. This is achieved by leading Chi to nourish the brain. You next have to learn how to regulate your emotional mind and keep your mental center. This training can be a highly effective way to deal with mental problems which modern science cannot heal.

For a normal, healthy person, the training of these two classics is probably one of the most efficient ways to maintain and improve physical and mental health. They should be able to provide modern science with many useful ideas for research into longevity and mental illness.

1-5. How to Approach this Book

In order to accept the challenge of studying this old science, we must have a modern, scientific attitude. This is especially necessary for the Yi Gin Ching and Shii Soei Ching because of the mystery which has surrounded them. I would like to recommend some attitudes which will be very useful during your study.

1. No Prejudices. All cultures and traditions which have survived must have their benefits. Perhaps some of them do not fit into our modern world, but they still deserve our respect. Remember, if you get rid of your past, you have pulled out your root. Naturally, you should not be stubborn and claim that the traditional culture is absolutely right or claim that an alien culture must be better than the one you have grown up in. You should keep the good parts of the traditional and absorb the best of the alien.

2. Be Neutral in Your Judgement. You should consider every new statement you read from the viewpoint of both your emotional feelings and the judgement of your wisdom. You should always consider your emotions, but they should not dominate your judgement.

3. Be Scientific. Although there are many phenomena which still cannot be explained by modern science, you should always remember to judge events scientifically. This will lead to the development of new science. You should use modern equipment to test phenomena when possible.

4. Be Logical and Make Sense. When you read or study, in your mind you should always ask, "Is it logical and does it make sense?" When you keep these questions in mind, you will think and understand instead of believing blindly.

5. Respect Prior Experience. Prior experience which has been passed down is the root of research. You should always be sincere and respectful when you study the past. The past helps you to understand the present. By understanding the present, you will be able to create the future. The accumulation of experience is the best teacher. You should respect the past, be cautious about the present, and challenge the future.

China has more than 7000 years of culture, and it has brought forth many brilliant accomplishments. Chi Kung is only one of them. In all of human history, there has never been such open communication among different cultures as is happening in our time. It is our responsibility to encourage the general public to accept, study, and research other cultures. In this way, the human race will be able to use the good parts of other cultures to live in a more peaceful and meaningful way.

Chinese Chi Kung is part of traditional Chinese medical science. It has brought the Chinese thousands of years of calm, peace, and happiness. I believe that this brilliant part of Chinese culture will especially help Westerners in the spiritual part of their training. Further publications must be encouraged. Wide scale scholastic and scientific research must be conducted, especially by universities and medical organizations. In this way, we will be able to introduce this new culture to the Western world in a short time.

I predict that the study of Chinese medical science and internal, meditative Chi Kung will attain great results in the next decade. I invite you to join me and become a pioneer of this new field in the Western world.

1-6. About This Book

When you study this book, there are a few things which you should know.

1. The major part of this book is compiled from many documents acquired from many sources. These documents are explained or commented upon, based on my personal Chi Kung knowledge and experience. Therefore, during the course of study, you should remain open minded, and also refer to other related books. In this case, your mind will not be restricted to a small domain of Chi Kung study.

   The main sources of the documents used in this book are:

   A. "The Real Manuscript of Yi Gin Ching" (Jen Been Yi Gin Ching). This document was revealed by Mr. Jiang Jwu-Juang, having been passed down secretly by his ancestors. Later, the same document was found in a manuscript stored in the "Tower of Fragrance" (Harn Fen Lou), which is a Taoist organization. After these two versions were compared and edited, the document was published in the book "Chinese Shen Kung," Vol. 1, by Gong Jiann Lao Ren (which means "Humbly Studious Old Man).

   B. "The Real Meaning of the Chinese Shii Soei Kung" (Jong Gwo Shii Soei Kung Fu Jy Jen Dih). This document was published by Mr. Chyau Charng-Horng. Comparing this document with the last one, it is evident that even though some training methods are slightly different, the theory and the training principles remain the same.

   C. Other excerpts of documents which have been collected in the book: "Chinese Shen Kung," Vol. 1, by Gong Jiann Lao Ren. In the last fifteen years, in addition to the many books which reveal Chi Kung training secrets, there is a twenty-one volume Chi Kung series published by Gong Jiann Lao Ren. This name, which is clearly as pseudonym, means Humbly Studious Old Man. His real identity is unknown. All we know about him is that, since his family is rich, he was able to purchase or collect many documents, which he compiled and published. The above two sources are also listed in his first volume.

   D. Many other individual documents and exercises, such as the Wai Dan Grand Circulation exercises, which I learned from my masters or collected over the last twenty-four years.

2. The foundation of this book is those documents which were passed down from ancient times. Although, in my opinion, there are some minor errors or concepts which I do not agree with, the text of these documents remains the most important source of information for this book. Since there are numerous documents available now, and also because much of their contents are not related to the Yi Gin

Ching and Shii Soei Ching, only those parts which relate to these two classics will be translated and commented upon.

3. Though many documents are available, most of these documents were written hundreds of years ago, in the ancient style of writing, and they are very difficult to translate. Furthermore, they originated as Buddhist or Taoist treatises, and were only part of the training for monks who were trying to reach enlightenment. Since most of the Buddhist bibles or treatises are very deep philosophy, even in China there are not too many people who are able to understand the real meaning. In order to understand these documents perfectly, you must have a deep understanding of Buddhism and Taoism. This increases the difficulty of translation.

   Because of the cultural differences, when one tries to translate these verses into non-Chinese languages, it is extremely difficult to find equivalent words which would be understood by the reader. Many expressions would not make sense to the Westerner if translated literally. Often, a knowledge of the historical background is necessary. When you read these verses, especially in translation, you will have to do a lot of thinking, feeling, and pondering before you are able to sense the real and deep meaning. With this main difficulty in mind, I have attempted to convey as much of the original meaning of the Chinese as possible, based on my own Chi Kung experience and understanding. Although it is impossible to totally translate the original meaning, I feel that I have managed to express the majority of the important points. The translation has been made as close to the original Chinese as possible, including such things as double negatives and, sometimes, idiosyncratic sentence structure. Words which are understood but not actually written in the Chinese text have been included in parentheses. Also, some Chinese words are followed by the English in parentheses, e.g. Shen (Spirit). For reference, the original Chinese text is included after each translation.

4. The Yi Gin Ching and Shii Soei Ching are only part of the Chinese Chi Kung training, and compared to other Chinese Chi Kung practices, they are considered to be deep. Therefore, many of the terminologies or the discussions may confuse you. If you have this feeling, you should study the first book in this series: "The Root of Chinese Chi Kung." It will offer you a clear concept of Chi Kung and lead you to a better understanding of this and future books.

Chapter 2

Historical Survey

In volume 1 of this YMAA in-depth Chi Kung book series we reviewed the general history of Chinese Chi Kung. From there we know that religious Chi Kung was only one category among several. In this book we will survey only the history of the religious Chi Kung which is related to the Yi Gin Ching and Shii Soei Ching Chi Kung.

From all of the available documents, it is very clear that Yi Gin Ching and Shii Soei Ching Chi Kung originated within Buddhist society. Although Buddhism was already a major religion in China, most of its Chi Kung training and ways of reaching Buddhahood had always been kept secret. For more than one thousand years, only limited parts of the secret documents were revealed to laymen. As a matter of fact, most of the documents and historical surveys about Yi Gin and Shii Soei Chi Kung practices available today come from religious Taoism and the martial arts community, rather than the Buddhists.

Almost all of the documents credit the Buddhist Da Mo with the authorship of these two classics. Therefore, we will first review the history of Chinese Chi Kung and religion before Da Mo, and then we will talk about Da Mo, the Yi Gin Ching and Shii Soei Ching. In the third section we will discuss the influence of the Yi Gin Ching and Shii Soei Ching on Chinese society after Da Mo's death. Finally, we will translate some of the documents and stories which relate to Da Mo and these two classics.

2-1. Before Da Mo

Although Chi Kung in China can be traced back before the Shang dynasty (1766-1154 B.C.), historical documents written before the Eastern Han dynasty (c. 58 A.D.) are scarce today, and it is difficult to obtain detailed information, especially about training practices. From the limited publications we understand that there were two major types of Chi Kung training, and that there was almost no religious color to the training. One type was used by the Confucian and Taoist scholars, who used it primarily to maintain their health. The other type of Chi Kung was for medical purposes, using needles, massage, or healing Chi Kung exercises to adjust the Chi or cure illness. All of the training theory focused on following the natural way to improve and maintain health. Actively countering the effects of nature was considered impossible.

Later, during the Eastern Han dynasty (c. 58 A.D.), Buddhism was imported to China, as well as some of the Chi Kung practices which had been developed in India. Buddhism was created by an Indian prince named Guatama (558-478 B.C.). When he was 29 years old, he became dissatisfied with his comfortable and sheltered life and left his country. He went out into the world among the common people to experience the pain and suffering in their lives. Six years later, he suddenly apprehended the "Truth," and he started traveling around to spread his philosophy. Buddhism is a major religion based on the belief that Gautama, the Buddha (Sanskrit For Awakened One), achieved nirvana, or perfect bliss and freedom from the cycle of birth and death, and taught how to achieve this state. In order to reach this goal, a Buddhist monk must learn the way of spiritual cultivation, which is a high level of Chi Kung practice.

Because the Han emperors were sincere Buddhists, Buddhism became the main religion in China. Naturally, the monks learned some of the Buddhist spiritual meditation methods. However, because of transportation and communication difficulties, they did not learn the complete system. For example, it is said that before the Liang dynasty (500 A.D.), almost 500 years since Buddhism was imported to China, only two Indian priests had visited China to teach Buddhism. This means that for five hundred years Chinese Buddhist monks could only learn the philosophy and theory which could be passed down through written Buddhist scriptures. They learned little of the actual cultivation and training methods, because most of these must be taught directly by an experienced master.

Because of this, after five hundred years of derivation and deduction the Chinese monks had established a way of reaching Buddhahood which was different from that of the Indian priests. The monks believed that the goal of Buddhahood could be accomplished simply through spiritual cultivation. However, according to the available documents this over-emphasis on spiritual cultivation resulted in their ignoring their physical bodies. They considered the physical body of only temporary use because it served as a ladder to reach Buddhahood. They even scoffed that the physical body was only a "Chow Pyi Nang," which means "notorious skin bag." They believed that since it was the spirit which would reach Buddhahood, why should they spend time training the physical body? Therefore, still meditation was emphasized and physical exercise was ignored. Naturally, most of the monks were weak and unhealthy. This problem was aggravated by an unnutritional, protein-deficient diet. This inaccurate approach to cultivation was not changed until Da Mo arrived in China.

Another religion, religious Taoism, also developed in this same time period. Religious Taoism was created by a Taoist scholar named Chang Tao-Ling, who combined the traditional scholarly Taoist philosophy with Buddhist cultivation theory and created "religious Taoism" (Tao Jiaw). Traditional scholarly Taoism was created by Lao Tzyy (Li Erh) in the 6th century B.C. He wrote a book titled "Tao Te Ching" (Classic on Morality) which discussed natural human morality. Later, his follower Juang Jou in the Warring States Period wrote a book called "Juang Tzyy." Scholarly Taoism studied the human spirit and nature but, according to the available documents, it was not considered a religion.

Before the creation of religious Taoism, scholarly Taoism had already been around for nearly seven hundred years. Naturally, the scholars' meditative Chi Kung methods had already reached a high level. After Buddhism was combined with scholarly Taoism, though some scholar meditation methods might have been modified, the physical Chi Kung exercises developed were still ignored. It is believed that the only physical Chi Kung exercises developed were part of medical Chi Kung, and were created mainly by physicians. You can see from this analysis that before Da Mo, both Buddhists and Taoists emphasized spiritual cultivation and ignored the physical Chi Kung training.

Now that you have a general idea of the historical background of Buddhism and Taoism, let us discuss the Buddhist Shaolin temple. This temple became very important because it was the place where Da Mo created his two classics, and where he is buried.

According to the available documents, the original Shaolin temple (Figure 2-1) was built in 495 A.D. (Wey Shiaw Wen Dih 19th year) on

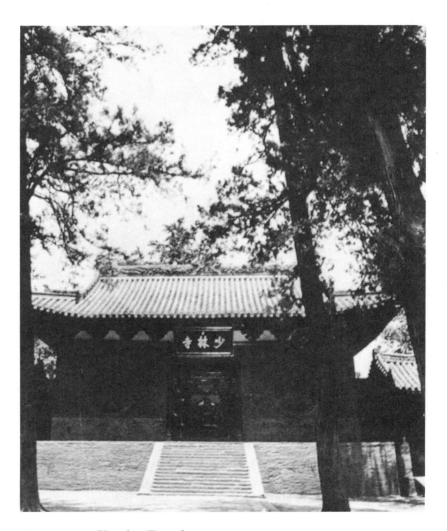

Figure 2-1. Shaolin Temple

Shao Shyh Mountain, Deng Feng Hsien, Henan province, by the order of Emperor Wey. The temple was built for an Indian Buddhist priest named Pao Jaco for the purpose of preaching and worship. In Chinese history, it is believed that Pao Jaco was the first Buddhist monk to come to China to preach. He was commonly called "Happy Buddha" (Mi Leh For)(Figure 2-2). At that time, Buddhism was at the peak of its popularity and prosperity. It was said that at that time there were thirteen thousand Buddhist temples and more than one hundred thousands monks. However, not long after this time the religion came under severe criticism from the scholars, and in a short 30 years it lost a great deal of its influence and popularity. When Da Mo came to China in 527 A.D. (Wey Shiaw Ming Dih, Shiaw Chang 3rd year), Buddhism's stock was quite low.

2-2. Da Mo, the Yi Gin Ching and Shii Soei Ching

Da Mo (Figure 2-3), whose last name was Sardili and who was also known as Bodhidarma, was once a prince of a small tribe in southern India. He was of the Mahayana school of Buddhism, and was considered by many to have been a bodhisattva, or an enlightened being who had renounced nirvana in order to save others. From the fragments of historical records it is believed he was born about 483 A.D. At that time, India was considered a spiritual center by the Chinese, since it was the source of Buddhism, which was still very influential in China. Many of the Chinese emperors either sent priests to India to study Buddhism and bring back scriptures, or else they invited Indian priests to come to China to preach. It is believed that Da Mo was the second Indian priest to be invited to China.

Da Mo was invited to China to preach by Emperor Liang in 527 A.D. (Liang Wuu Dih, Dah Torng first year or Wey Shiaw Ming Dih, Shiaw

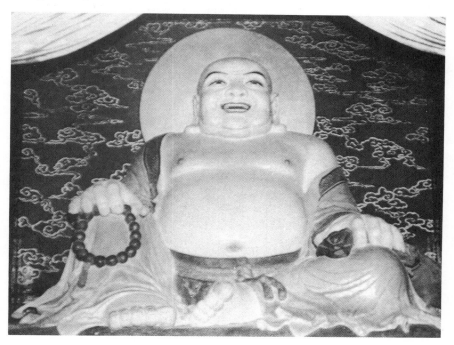

Figure 2-2. Happy Budda (Mi Leh For)

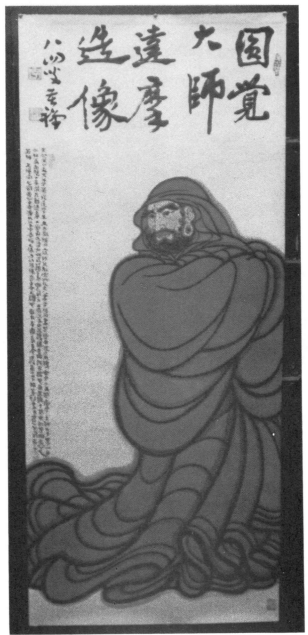

Figure 2-3. Da Mo

Chang 3rd year). When the emperor decided he did not like Da Mo's Buddhist theory, the monk withdrew to the Shaolin Temple. When Da Mo arrived, he saw that the priests were weak and sickly, so he shut himself away to ponder the problem (Figure 2-4). When he emerged after nine years of seclusion he wrote two books: "Yi Gin Ching" (Muscle/Tendon Changing Classic) and "Shii Soei Ching" (Marrow/Brain Washing Classic).

The Yi Gin Ching taught the priests how to gain health and change their physical bodies from weak to strong. After the priests practiced the Yi Gin Ching exercises, they found that not only did they improve their

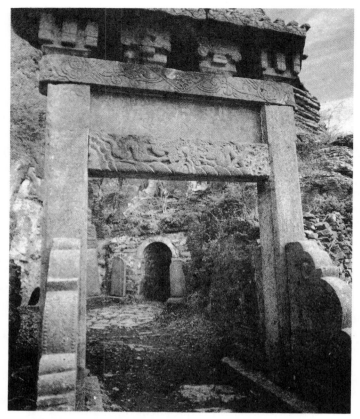

Figure 2-4. Entrance to the Cave where Da Mo Meditated for Nine Years

health, but they also greatly increased their strength. When this training was integrated into the martial arts forms, it increased the effectiveness of their techniques. This change marked one more step in the growth of the Chinese martial arts: martial Chi Kung.

The Shii Soei Ching taught the priests how to use Chi to clean the bone marrow and strengthen the blood and immune system, as well as how to energize the brain, which helped them to attain Buddhahood. Because the Shii Soei Ching was hard to understand and practice, the training methods were passed down secretly to only a very few disciples in each generation.

Because of the lack of historical documents about Da Mo, nobody really knows what kind of person he was. However, there is a poem written by Lu Yu, a famous poet of the Southern Song dynasty (1131-1162), which described Da Mo's personal philosophy. It said:

Others are revolted, I am unmoved.
Gripped by desires, I am unmoved.
Hearing the wisdom of sages, I am unmoved.
I move only in my own way.

宗陸游為達磨詩

亦不觀惡而生嫌，亦不觀善而勤措。亦不捨智而近愚，亦不拋迷而就悟。達大道今過量，通佛心今出度。不與凡聖同經，超然名之曰祖。

Naturally, we cannot judge him from this poem, especially since it was written more than 500 years after his death. The teaching philosophy which has traditionally been attributed to him is: "Jiaw Wai Bye Chwan, Buh Lih Wen Tzyh, Jyr Jyy Ren Hsin, Jiann Shing Cherng For"(*1) (Do not pass on to people outside of our religion, words should not be written down, point directly to the person's mind, to see and cultivate the personality, humanity, and become a Buddha.) His teaching philosophy seems to coincide with the poem by Lu Yu. Da Mo was a stubborn, conceited, and wise man.

As previously explained, before Da Mo, the main training method for reaching Buddhahood in China was only spiritual cultivation through meditation. The complete training methods used in India were not passed down to the Chinese Buddhists. This situation lasted until Da Mo's two classics became available. There is a couplet in the Shaolin Temple which says: "In the West Heaven (i.e., India) for twenty-eight ancestors, came to East Land (i.e., China) to begin at Shaolin."(*2). This means that Da Mo was the twenty-ninth generation of Charn Buddhism in India, and when he came to Shaolin he became the first ancestor of Chinese Charn Buddhism.

You can see that before Da Mo, the Chinese had not even learned Charn Buddhism. Furthermore, if Da Mo was the twenty-ninth generation of Charn Buddhism in India, then Charn meditation had already been studied and developed in India for quite some time. It is reasonable to assume that his two classics were written based on his knowledge of Charn Buddhism. To Chinese Buddhists, his two classics were revolutionary, and provided them with a new way of achieving Buddhahood. Like other revolutionary ideas, it encountered strong resistance from Chinese Buddhists. Naturally, the main resistance came from the traditional Buddhists who had developed their own system of cultivation over the last 500 years.

The major difference between these two classics and the traditional Chinese method was Da Mo's emphasis that the training of the physical body was just as important as the spiritual cultivation. Without a strong and healthy body, the final goal of spiritual cultivation was hard to reach. Though his new training theory was resisted by many Buddhists, many others believed his theory and started to train. The Shaolin temple became a center for teaching his theories, and soon after his death they had spread to every corner of China. His Charn meditation was exported to Japan, where it became known as Zen.

Despite the popularity of his methods, however, many priests still insisted on using the traditional methods of cultivation. When the Shaolin temple applied Da Mo's Chi Kung training to fighting techniques, the new theories gained more opponents among the traditionalists. Although it was often necessary to defend oneself during that violent period, there were many priests who were against the martial training. They believed that as Buddhist priests they should avoid all violence.

(*1). 教外別傳，不立文字，直指人心，見性成佛。

(*2). 在西天二十八祖，過東土初開少林。

2-3. After Da Mo

In the first chapter we discussed the significant influence which Da Mo's Yi Gin Ching and Shii Soei Ching exerted on Chinese culture. Here we would like to take a deeper look at how Da Mo's Yi Gin Ching and Shii Soei Ching have influenced Chinese religious and martial arts societies.

Da Mo is considered the ancestor of Charn Tzong, the Zen sect of Buddhism. It was said that when Da Mo died in 539 A.D., he passed his Charn Buddhist philosophy and his Shii Soei Ching techniques to his best and most trusted disciple, Huoy Kee. Huoy Kee's name as a layman was Jih Guang. He was a scholar who gave up his normal life and became a priest in order to conquer himself. Huoy Kee passed the Buddhist philosophy on to Seng Tsann. It then went to Tao Shinn, Horng Zen, and Huoy Neng. These five and Da Mo are called the Six Ancestors of Charn (Charn Tzong Liow Tzuu). Later, Chinese Buddhists honored another monk, Shen Huey of the Tarng dynasty of Kai Yuan (713-742 A.D.), and subsequently referred to the Seven Ancestors of Charn (Charn Tzong Chii Tzuu).

Sitting Charn meditation, which is part of the Shii Soei Ching enlightenment training, is able to bring you to the highest level of spiritual cultivation. We read that Da Mo's Yi Gin Ching was taught in the Shaolin temple, and Shii Soei Ching was passed down to Huoy Kee. However, according to my understanding of the available documents, these two classics must both be trained in order to reach the final goal of Buddhahood. Surprisingly, however, there is almost no Yi Gin Ching training in Chinese Charn and Japanese Zen Buddhism. Also, it is very curious that Shii Soei Ching was not generally trained in the Shaolin temple. As a matter of fact, we have found more Taoist and martial arts documents than we have Buddhist documents about the training of these two classics. Therefore, it would be very interesting to analyze what happened in these societies after Da Mo's death.

First, we must analyze the early structure of religious Taoism. Religious Taoism was neither the purely traditional, conservative scholar Taoism, nor the pure Buddhism imported from India, but it began as a combination of the philosophy and theories of both. If we look at the historical background of that time, we can see an important point. At that time, China was the strongest country is Asia, and its culture was the most advanced. It is incredible that China would be so open as to absorb Buddhism into its culture, especially at a time when Chinese society was so conservative and its people were all so proud of their long history. If the Han emperor were not so open-minded, the spread of Buddhism in China would probably have been delayed for several centuries.

Religious Taoism was born during this period. It not only kept the good parts of the traditional Taoist philosophy, but it also absorbed useful parts of Buddhist culture and their methods of spiritual cultivation which were imported from India. Over the years they have kept this open-mindedness, and have never hesitated to learn useful things from other styles.

Next, let us take a look at the fundamental theory and philosophy of Taoism. Taoism emphasized the "Tao" (the way), which means the way of nature. They believed that "what will happen will happen." It was pointless to obey a tradition or doctrine, but it was equally pointless to rebel against it. Taoist monks did not have all the rules that the Buddhists did. They did not have to cut their hair like the Buddhists, and they were allowed alcohol and meat. They were even allowed to have sex and marry, which the Buddhists were absolutely forbidden to do. This tendency of the Taoists to be more openminded than the Buddhists carried over into how they worked for enlightenment.

There is another important fact. Since the Taoists and Buddhists shared essentially the same goal and had many practices and philosophies in common, both worshiped the same Buddha and followed the same philosophy in many ways, Taoist and Buddhist monks often studied together and became close friends. In China it is often said that "For Tao Yi Jia,"(*3) which means "Buddhism and Taoism are one family." Before Da Mo, the Taoists already knew many of the Buddhist methods of cultivation. After Da Mo's death, they naturally were able to acquire his new secret methods of Chi cultivation. Eventually, in addition to the traditional Taoist texts, the Taoist libraries also had a considerable number of Buddhist training documents.

Because of Da Mo's Yi Gin Ching, Shaolin priests got heavily involved in martial arts training. At that time it was necessary for the defense of temple property. This marked the beginning of a new era for Chinese martial arts: from the concentration on external techniques they moved into the cultivation of internal Chi Kung, or spiritual power.

Naturally, after a few hundred years, many of the Yi Gin Ching techniques were also learned by Taoists. During the Song dynasty (960 A.D.), Tai Chi Chuan, an internal martial art which emphasizes Chi development, was created in Wuudang Mountain. Since then, Wuudang mountain has become the center of Taoism and the internal martial arts. Naturally, the Shaolin temple has always been considered the authority on the external martial styles.

Today, many people mistakenly believe that the Shaolin martial arts do not have internal Chi Kung training, while the internal martial arts do not emphasize the practice of external techniques. They don't realize that internal Chi Kung training originated in the Shaolin temple, and it was always an important part of the training there. Furthermore, if an internal martial artist has strong internal power but he does not have good fighting techniques, he will be defeated. Traditionally, therefore, Shaolin training has been from external to internal, while Wuudang training is from internal to external. Only when you have learned both internal and external may you say that you have completed Chinese martial arts training.

For many years it was generally believed that the training methods for Shii Soei Ching Chi Kung had been lost. However, a change came during the Ching dynasty (1644-1912 A.D). During that period, many Buddhist and Taoist monks got involved in politics, fighting to overthrow the Ching dynasty. In retaliation, the main Shaolin temple and several branches (such as those at Fujian Chyuan Jou and Hebei Horng Long), were attacked and burned several times by Ching soldiers. Many priests escaped and started teaching the martial techniques to laymen to continue the fight. Some laymen also secretly learned many of the Yi Gin Ching and some Shii Soei Ching Chi Kung training methods.

In the last twenty years, due to the convenience of modern transportation and communication, people are more open minded than ever. Many

---

(*3). 佛道一家。

of the secrets have been published, and are opening up a new era of Chi Kung study. However, because of the years of secrecy, the information is coming out in random bits and pieces, and is incomplete.

2-4. Stories

In the fourteen hundred years since Da Mo's death, many people have claimed to have the secrets of Yi Gin Ching and Shii Soei Ching training, including Buddhist monks, Taoist priests, and martial artists. However, nobody really knew who had the "original" secrets passed down by Da Mo. Many of the documents that are available to us have a preface or foreword explaining how the author obtained the original secrets. It is interesting to read them. Since nobody actually knows what is true, you should simply treat them like stories.

The following three forewords were written by three different people who owned the same document at different times. This document was then released to the public by the Harn Fen Lou (Tower of Fragrance), a Taoist organization. As a matter of fact, this document has the most complete theory and training methods, and a large portion of the Yi Gin Ching discussed in this book is based on it.

A. Preface to "The Real Manuscript of Yi Gin Ching"
By Herbalist Li Jing, Tarng Jen Guan 2nd Year (629 A.D.)

真本秘笈易筋經原序
唐貞觀二載李靖藥師

(In the time of) the late Emperor Wey Shiaw Ming in the Tay Her period, the great teacher Da Mo came to Wey from Liang, and faced the wall in the Shaolin temple. One day, he asked his disciples and said: "Why don't you describe what you know and (I) will tell you the achievement you have accomplished." (Therefore) each disciple described what he had cultivated. Teacher said: "You have acquired my skin, you have acquired my meat, and you have obtained my bone." Solely to Huoy Kee: "You have obtained my marrow." Later, people explained wrongly and thought (he meant) the depth of entering the Tao. (They) don't know (he) really meant something (specific). It was not a casual comment.

後魏孝明帝太和間，達磨大師自梁適魏，面壁於少
林寺。一日，謂其徒眾曰："盍各言所知，將以占造
詣。"眾因各陳其進修。師曰："某得吾皮，某得吾肉
，某得吾骨。"惟於慧可曰："爾得吾髓"云云。後人
漫解之，以為入道之淺深耳，蓋不知其實有所指，
非漫語也。

Between 420 A.D. and 589 A.D. (a total of 169 years), there were several emperors who divided China into separate countries. It was called "Epoch of the Division Between North and South." According to the available records, Da Mo was invited to China by the Liang emperor in 527 A.D. and later entered the Wey territory, staying at the Shaolin temple. This document errs about the timing. Wey Shiaw Ming was emperor from 516 A.D. to 528 A.D., and also, the Tay Her period was from 477 A.D. to 500 A.D. during the reign of emperor Wey Shiaw Wen. Because of this conflict within the document, the dates cannot be trusted.

Huoy Kee was a disciple of Da Mo who was said to have obtained the secret of Shii Soei Ching Chi Kung, which teaches a monk how to reach the final goal of Buddhahood. "Marrow" refers to the training techniques which he had learned, and not to the depth of his Taoist achievement.

After 9 years, the achievement was accomplished and (he) died, buried at the root of Bear's Ear Mountain. Then he left his shoes and went. Later, the wall he was facing was damaged by wind and rain, Shaolin monks repaired it and found a metal box. The box was closed with no seal or lock, (but) hundreds of methods could not open it. One monk comprehended and said: "This must be caused from the strength of glue. We should use fire." The box then opened. It was found the box was filled with wax which kept the box closed. (They) acquired two classics: one named "Shii Soei Ching," one named "Yi Gin Ching."

迨九年功畢示化，葬熊耳山脚，乃遺隻履而去．後面壁處碑砌，壞於風雨，少林僧修葺之，得一鐵函，無封鎖，有際會，百計不能開，一僧悟曰："此必膠之固也，宜以火"函遂開．乃鎔蠟滿注而四著故也。得所藏經二帙：一曰└洗髓經┘，一曰└易筋經┘。

This is the only document which tells where Da Mo was buried, though the exact location is still unknown. In China, when someone has achieved Buddhahood he is said to have left his shoes and gone. This implies that although he is gone, some of his accomplishments were left behind for those following him. In ancient times, wax was commonly used to glue things together. Again, it is not known whether the classics were really found where Da Mo had been meditating. It is most probable that this story was made up.

The Shii Soei Ching says a man's body (is) touched by love and desire, and formed with shape, contaminated by sediment and dirtiness. If you wish to cultivate the real meaning of Buddhism, (spirit) moving and stopping at will, (then) the five viscera and six bowels, four limbs and hundreds of bones must be completely washed clean individually. (When they are) pure and (you) are able to see the calmness and peace, then (you) can be cultivated and enter the domain of Buddhahood. (If you) do not cultivate this (way), (obtaining the Tao) will not have foundation and origin. Read till here, then know that the believers thought that "acquiring the marrow" was not a comparison.

洗髓經者，謂人之生，感於愛欲，一落有形，悉皆淳穢；欲修佛諦，動障真如，五臟六腑，四肢百骸，必先一一洗滌淨盡，純見清虛，方可進修，入佛智地，不由此經進修，無基無有是處；讀至此，然後知何者所謂得髓者，非譬喻也．

Shii Soei Ching teaches you how to clean yourself internally, including the internal organs, which are related to your thoughts. Only when you have regulated your thoughts and led your mind into a stage of peacefulness can your physical body be cleaned. Then you have laid the foundation for entering the Tao. This paragraph again points out that "acquiring the marrow" refers to Marrow/Brain training, and not to the depth of Tao cultivation.

The Yi Gin Ching says that outside of the bone and marrow, under the skin and meat (i.e., muscles), (there is) nothing but the tendons and vessels which connect the entire body and transport the blood and Chi. All of these are post-birth body, (and) must be promoted (i.e., trained); borrow them to cultivate the real (Tao). If you do not assist and promote them, (you will) see weakening and withering immediately. (If you) see (this training) as ordinary (training), how could you reach the final goal? (If you) give up and do not train them, then there is no strength for cultivation, and nothing can be achieved. (When I) read till here, then I know that what were called skin, meat, and bones are also not a comparison and not a casual comment.

易筋者，謂髓骨之外，皮肉之內，莫非筋聯絡周身，通行血氣，凡屬後天，皆其提挈，借假修真，非所贊勷，立見頹靡，視作泛常，烏臻極至？舍是不為，進修不力，無有是處；讀至此，然後知所謂皮肉骨者，非譬喻，亦非漫語也。

This paragraph explains that the Yi Gin Ching is used to train the physical body including skin, muscles, vessels, and bones. This physical body must be used temporarily (borrowed) for your internal cultivation as you reach for the final goal. Therefore, you must train your physical body and keep it healthy. If you do not train it, then you will not have a strong, healthy body for your spiritual cultivation. Therefore, when the first paragraph referred to the "acquiring of skin, meat, and bones," they are again not commenting on the depth of Taoist cultivation, but rather they are referring to actual training.

The Shii Soei Ching belonged to Huoy Kee, together with the robe and the bowl passed down secretly. Later generations rarely saw it. Only the Yi Gin Ching was kept, and stayed at Shaolin in memory of the teacher's morality. The words in the classic were all in Indian, none of the Shaolin priests could translate it completely. Even when they were translated, it was only one or two among ten (i.e., 10 or 20%). Again, because nobody was able to pass the secrets, then everyone used his own explanations, training, and practices. (Their) training

tends to enter the side way and become the branches and leaves. Consequently the real techniques for entering Buddhism were lost. Till now, Shaolin priests were able to use (the training) only for martial arts, is an example of this classic.

洗髓經帙，歸於慧可，附衣缽共作祕傳，後世罕見，惟易筋經，留鎮少林。以永師德，第其經字，皆天竺文，少林諸僧，不能徧譯，間亦譯得具十之一二，復無至人口傳密祕。遂各逞己意，演而習之，意趨旁徑，落於枝葉，遂失作佛真正法門。至今少林僧眾，僅以舟藝擅場，是得此經之一班也。

Huoy Kee was the best disciple of Da Mo, and it is said that he was the one who obtained the Shii Soei Ching. When Chinese refer to a teacher's "morality," they are referring to his great achievement, and to the teachings that he passed on.

The original text by Da Mo was in an Indian language, and there were very few people who could really translate it. Although some priests were able to translate part of it, they were not able to get the complete meaning. The training drawn from these limited translations led the Shaolin priests away from the correct path. Because what they were studying was the branches and leaves of the art, and not the root and main trunk, they were only able to use it for the martial arts. The training for the real final goal of achieving Buddhahood was neglected.

Among them, there was a priest who had a unique, excellent idea. If great teacher Da Mo left the classic, how can it be limited only to the small techniques? If we cannot translate it today, there must be someone who can translate it. Therefore, (he) took the classic and traveled far away, reaching every mountain. One day (he) reached Shuu, ascended Ermei Mountain and was able to meet the holy Indian monk Ban Tsyh Mih Dih. He talked about this classic and explained the intention of his visit.

眾中一僧具超絕識念，惟達磨大師既留聖經，豈惟小技，今不能譯，當有譯者。乃懷經遠訪，遍歷山嶽。一日抵蜀，登峨嵋山，得晤西竺聖僧般剌密諦，言及此經，並陳來意。

Shuu was Szechuan province. Ermei mountain is another Taoist and Buddhist religious center located there. It is very possible that Indian priests had been invited to preach there.

The holy monk said: "(This is) the Buddha ancestor's secret inheritance, the foundation is here. However, the classic cannot be translated because the Buddha's language is profound and deep. (But if) the meaning of the classic can be translated and understood, it is also able to reach the holy place." Therefore, he discussed and explained the meaning in detail. Also, (he) stopped the priest from leaving the mountain, (helping him) to advance and cultivate. (In a) hundred days (his body was) strong, another hundred days (the Chi) was full in the entire body, another hundred days (the Chi) was circulating smoothly. He obtaining what is called "metal steel and strong ground (i.e., a strong physical body)." (The monk) understood that this priest had the wisdom of Buddha, and had built up the foundation of tendon strength.

聖僧曰："佛祖心傳，基先於此，然而經文不可譯，佛語淵奧也。經義可譯通，凡達聖也。"乃一一指陳，詳譯其義，且止僧於山，提挈進修，百日而凝固，再百日而充周，再百日而暢達，得所謂金剛堅固地，馴此人佛智地，洵(誠)為有基筋矣。

Because Buddhism was imported from India, many of the terms and references are impossible for a non-Indian to understand. A word by word translation of the text would be unintelligible. However, if you understand the meaning of the classic it would be possible to rewrite it in your own language and retain the original meaning. This means that the document which comes from Ban Tsyh Mih Dih was not a word by word translation of the original.

The (Shaolin) priest's will was strong and he did not want to re-enter the business of the world, so he followed the holy monk preaching and traveling on the sea and mountains. I do not know where he has gone. The guest Shyu Horng met him on the beach and obtained the secret meaning. He gave it to the guest Chyou Ran, and the guest Chyou Ran again gave it to me. (I) tried it and experienced the verification, then I believed that the sayings inside were true. Unfortunately I did not obtain the secret of the Shii Soei and so that I could travel to the domain of Buddha. Again it is unfortunate that (my) will is not strong and I cannot be like the priest, forgetting the business of the world. I am only able to use the small branches and flowers and use it to extend my life. I feel guilty inside.

僧志堅精，不落世務，乃隨聖僧化行海嶽，不知所之，徐鴻客遇之海外，得其秘諦，既授於虬髯客，虬髯客復授於予，嘗試之，輒奇驗，始信語真不虛，惜乎未得洗髓之秘，觀游佛境，又惜立志不堅，不能如僧不落世務，乃僅借六花小技，以勳伐終，中懷愧歉也。

Travelers in China are often called guests.

However, the marvelous meaning of this classic has never been heard in this world, I can only write this preface and explain where it comes from and let (you) know the beginning and the end. (I am) hoping that the reader who wishes to reach Buddhahood will not ceaselessly repeat the business of the world. If (you) are able to reach Buddhahood, then (you) will not feel regret for (not meeting) the intention of great teacher Da Mo. If (you) only talk about bravery and expect to be known in this world, then there are plenty of people who were known for the strength of their bravery. How could we record all of them?

然則此經妙義，世所未聞，謹序其由，俾知顛末，企望學者，務期作佛，切勿區區作人間事業也。若各能作佛，乃不負達磨大師留經之意，若曰勇足以名世，則古之以力聞者多矣，奚足錄哉。
　　　　　唐貞觀二載三月三日李靖藥師甫序

This last paragraph advises the reader not to use this classic only to increase the strength of his body. This training is the foundation of Buddhahood, and you should aim for the higher goal of self-cultivation and finally reach the "holy city."

B. Preface to 'The Real Manuscript of Yi Gin Ching" Internal and External Spiritual Bravery

By General Horng Yih, Song Shaw Shing 12th Year (1143 A.D.)

真本易筋經內外神勇序
宏毅將軍宗紹興十二年

I am a martial fighter, my eyes cannot read a single word. (I am) good at playing long spear and large sword, riding the horse and bending the bow are my happiness.

予武人也，目不識一字，好弄長搶大劍，帶馬彎弓以為樂。

The author of this work was General Horng Yih, who served under Marshal Yeuh Fei. Since he was illiterate, he must have dictated it to someone.

It was the time that the center plain (i.e., central China) was lost, and the Huei and Chin emperors were kept in the North. The muddy horse passed the (Yangtze) river, many events happened south of the river. Because I was in Marshal Yeuh's staff, assigned as an assistant officer, I often won victories, finally becoming a general.

值中原淪喪，徽欽北狩，泥馬渡河，江南多事；予因應我少保岳元帥之幕，署為偏裨，屢上戰功，遂為大將。

In the Song dynasty (1101-1127 A.D.), the Huei and Chin emperors were seized by the Gin race and kept captive in the North. In order to

-33-

continue the Song empire, the new emperor moved the kingdom south of the Yangtze river. The wars were continuous. The expression "muddy horse" is a way of describing very heavy fighting, because the horses and soldiers would get very dirty while fighting "tooth and nail."

I recall when I was assigned by Marshal (Yeuh) to a battle, later (when) the army returned to the Eh. On the way back, I suddenly saw a spiritual monk, whose look was different and strange; he looked like a Buddha. He hand carried a letter and entered the camp. (He) told me to give it to Shao Bao (Marshal Yeuh). I asked him the reason. He said: "Do you generals know Shao Bao has spiritual power?" I said: "Don't know. But I saw Shao Bao is able to bend a bow of hundreds of stones."

憶昔年奉少保將令出征，後旋師還鄂，歸途忽見一
神僧，狀貌奇古，類阿羅漢像，手持一函入營．囑
余致少保，叩其故，僧曰：「將軍知少保有神力乎？」
予曰：「不知也，但吾見少保能挽百石之弓耳。」

Eh was where the Song kingdom was located, in today's Hubei province. Shao Bao was a nickname for Marshal Yeuh Fei. In ancient times strength was measured by how many stones you could lift, and the strength of a bow was also measured this way.

The monk said: "Is the spiritual power given by heaven?" I replied: "Yes." The monk said: "It is not. I taught him so. When Shao Bao was young, he served me and trained until he was successful in spiritual power. I asked him to follow me and enter the Tao, he didn't and got involved in human affairs. Although he has achieved establishing his reputation, he will not be able to complete his will. It is heavenly destiny and his fate. What can we do? The date (of his death) is about to arrive. Please pass this letter and (he) might be able to avoid it."

僧曰：「少保神力天賦之歟。」予曰：「然。」僧曰：「非也
，予授之耳。少保少嘗從事於予，神力成功，予囑
具相隨入道，不之信，去而作人間勳業，事名雖成
，志難竟，天也，命也，余若何！今將及矣，煩致
此函，或能反省獲免。」

The monk is saying that Yeuh Fei chose not to become a hermit and stay away from everyday human affairs, such as seeking things like money and fame, and fulfilling his personal desires.

I heard the saying and could not help but feel terrified. I asked his name but he did not reply. I asked where he was going to go, he said "To the west to visit teacher Da Mo." I was terrified by his spiritual sternness and dared not detain him. He departed gracefully.

予聞言，不勝悚異，叩姓氏，不答；叩所之曰：「西

訪達師。"予懼其神感，不敢挽留，竟飄然去。

At that time Da Mo had been dead for six hundred years, so the monk meant a spiritual visit. It was believed that when Da Mo died, he became a Buddha and his spirit lived in the Western Holy City (India) where all of the Buddhas were thought to live.

Shao Bao received the letter, read it and before finishing, started to cry and said: "My teacher is a spiritual monk. I don't have to wait (to see), my life is ended." Therefore he took out a volume from his pocket and gave it to me. (He) said: "Keep this volume carefully. Select the person and teach him. Do not let the techniques of entering the door of Tao be terminated. (It would be) ungrateful to the spiritual monk." In no more than a few months, as expected, (Shao Bao) was murdered by the cunning minister. I am so sorry for Shao Bao, my depression and resentment cannot be dispersed, I look on this meritorious services as dung and earth. Therefore, (I have) no more desire for human life. I think about the instruction of Shao Bao and cannot go against his will. I hate that (I am) a martial fighter and have not giant eyes and do not know who would have a strong will for Buddhahood in this world and deserve this volume. To choose (the right) person is difficult and teaching without choosing is in vain. Today (I) hide this volume in the stone wall in Song mountain and let the person who has the pre-destiny of Tao acquire it and use it as the way of entering the door of Tao. I can avoid the guilt of the abuse of teaching anyone. Then I can face Shao Bao in heaven without feeling guilty. Song, Shaw Shing 12th year. The great general of Eh under Marshal Shao Bao (Yeuh Fei). Horng Yih General, Niou Gaw, Tang Yin, Heh Jeou Fuu.

少保得函，讀未竟，泣數行下曰："吾師神僧也，不吾待，吾其休矣。"因從襟袋中出册付余，囑曰："好掌此册，擇人而授，勿使進道法門，斬焉中絶，負神僧也。"不數月，果為奸相所構。予心傷少保，寃憤莫伸，視功勳若糞土，因無復人間之想矣。念少保之囑，不忍負。恨武人無巨眼，不知斯世誰具作佛之志，堪傳此册者。擇人既難，妄傳無益，今將此册藏於嵩山石壁之中，聽有道緣者自得之，以衍進道之法門，庶免妄傳之咎，可酬對少保於天上矣。

宗紹興十二年鄂鎮大元帥少保岳麾下宏毅將軍湯陰牛臯鵬九甫序

Marshal Yeuh Fei was poisoned in prison by the cunning minister, Chin Kua. When Marshal Yeuh died, he was only 39 years old. Yeuh was credited with the creation of the Chi Kung set Eight Pieces of Brocade and the internal martial style Hsing Yi. Eagle claw style also claims that Marshal Yeuh Fei was its creator. The last sentence in this paragraph is the general's name, followed by the province and county he was born in.

C. Preface to "The Real Manuscript of Yi Gin Ching"
A Narration of a Traveler on Mountain and Sea

真本易筋經
海岱遊人敍記

When I was young, I was delayed by poets and books; until I was older, I liked to make friends with the people outside of the square (i.e., monks). When I had leisure, I liked to travel among the oceans and the mountains. One day I was at Chang Bae mountain with my friends carrying boxes and pots, walking on the beach and lay down a mat to sit. Suddenly I saw a person of the western Chiang traveling from the west to the east, passing through and (stopping) for a short rest. Seeing he had an elegant and cultivated look, I stopped him and offered him a drink.

余少時為詩書誤矣，及暮年好與方外人友，暇輒遊行海岱之間。一日至長白山，偕友挈盒提壺，步於海濱，席草而坐，忽一西羌人自西而東，經此暫想，予見其修雅可觀，乃止之飲。

    To the Chinese, lay society is considered "in the square" because the people are always preoccupied with emotions and desires, and tend to be too rigid and inflexible. The expression "outside of the square" (Fan Wai) is commonly used in reference to monks because they are outside of the influence of lay society. Chang Bae mountain is a very famous mountain in Shandong province in China. "Boxes and pots" refers to containers for food and wine. The Chiang is a small ethnic minority living on the western border of China near India.

I asked: "Where (are you) going? He said: Jiau Lau (is going to) visit the teacher of my teacher. I asked again: "What can he do?" He said: "Spiritual bravery." I asked: "What is spiritual bravery?" He said: "Closed fingers can penetrate a cow's stomach, side of palm can cut a cow's head off, fist is able to chop the tiger's chest. (If you) do not believe, please test my stomach." Therefore, I let a stronger man use wood, stone, and metal pestles to strike (him). It seems nothing happened. Again I used a long rope to tie up his testicles and also the wheel of a cow cart. He dragged the wheel and walked like running. Again, I tied up his two lower feet, and ask five or six strong men to pull, they could not move (him). All the people were shocked and said: "Alas! Is this given by heaven or from human training?" He said: "From man and not from heaven."

問：″所之？″曰：″膠嶗訪師之師也。″又問：″何能？″曰：″神勇。″問：″何神勇？″曰：″並指可貫牛腹，側掌可斷牛項，擎拳可劈虎胸，不信請試吾腹。″乃以木石鐵椎，令壯漢擊之，若罔知焉；又以長繩繫睪丸，綴以牛車之輪，曳輪而走，若馳也；又繫其雙足跟，令五六壯者曳之，屹立不移。眾愕然曰：「有是哉！天賦之歟？抑人功歟？」曰：「人也，非天也。」

Jiau Lau may be the name of the traveler. Since bravery comes from the raising up of the spirit, it is also referred to as spiritual bravery (Shen Yeong). When the spirit is raised, the physical body can become very strong, and resistant to outside force. This can be tested by striking the body. The root can also be developed. Even the genitals can be strengthened so that they can support or pull a considerable weight.

I asked what were the uses of it (i.e., spiritual power). He said: "Repelling sickness is one. Never sick is two. Entire life as a strong man is three. Not be afraid of hunger and cold is four. More male property, smart and beautiful is five. A hundred wins in the bedroom war is six. To pick up the pearl from the muddy water is seven. To defend against an attack without fear is eight. After the training, the achievement will not decay is nine. These are still the small uses. Using this as a foundation for entering the Tao of Buddhahood is the final goal.

叩其用。曰：「却病一，永不生病二，終身壯漢三，飢寒不怕四，多男靈秀五，房戰百勝六，泥水採珠七，禦侮不懼八，功成不退九，此其小用者也。基之成佛了道，乃其至也。」

"Repelling sickness" means when you are coming down with an illness to be able to resist it. "Never sick" means that when your body is trained to a higher level, you will never get sick. The training is able to change you from weak to strong so you will look and behave like a handsome, strong man. The "bedroom war" refers to sexual activity. "Picking up the pearl from the muddy water" means to refine and purify your spirit in this impure society.

I asked who his teacher is. He said: "My teacher is a monk and his teacher is an immortal. They passed down (the training) with its rules. Thereupon he took out a volume and let us read it. Then we knew that spiritual bravery can be reached from changing the tendons, and the accumulation of Li originates from accumulation of Chi. After drinking, this Chiang person wished to leave. We could not keep him longer. He said: "I see your spirit and shape are different from others, I would like to give you this volume. This meeting is our destiny. I (will) visit the spiritual monk and expect to tour the Buddha domain, I do not have time to stay long." Therefore, he went and left this book. The book was prefaced by herbalist Li. Can this herbalist speak recklessly?

問其所傳？曰：「吾師僧，僧師神，遞有傳授。」因出

書一冊閱之，乃知神勇之由筋可易，而積力由於積
氣也。酒已，羌人欲出，挽之不可，曰：「觀爾神形
異於眾，願以此贈，迨緣會耳。吾訪神僧，期遊佛
境，不暇長留也。」遂別去，留此書；書為李藥師序
，藥師豈妄語哉？

The next-to-last sentence indicates that the document already had
the preface, given above, by the herbalist Li.

**It is said in the classic: Use this as the foundation for becoming
a Buddha. This is the transcendence of the ancient Indian Mr.
Day. It is not what the central plain people are able to see.
How can we face the (Yeuh) Wu Mu when we die and together
with him visit the spiritual monk beyond the heavens?**
**Ching dynasty, Shuenn Jyh (1644 A.D.). Traveler on Mountain
and Sea, Chang Yeuh-Feng.**

經云：基之成佛，比則古西竺戴先生之超越，實非
中原人之所可遽視也。噫！安得起韋公武穆於九泉
，與之共訪神僧於天外哉！
順治辛丑海岱遊人張月峯記

There is no further information about this Indian Mr. Day. I believe
that it refers to Da Mo. The central plain means China. In this paragraph, it is clear that the document which the writer received was the
same as the one for which Marshal Yeuh Fei's general wrote the
preface and foreword.

Chapter 3

Buddhist and Taoist
Chi Kung

Because it was kept so secret, religious Chi Kung did not become as popular as the other categories in China before the Ching dynasty. It was not until this last century, when the secrets were gradually released to the public, that religious Chi Kung has become popular in China. Religious Chi Kung is mostly Taoist and Buddhist, and its main purpose is to aid in the striving for enlightenment, or what the Buddhists refer to as Buddhahood. They are looking for a way to lift themselves above normal human suffering, and to escape from the cycle of continual reincarnation. They believe that all human suffering is caused by the seven emotions and six desires. If you are still bound to these emotions and desires, you will reincarnate after your death. To avoid reincarnation, you must train your spirit to reach a very high stage where it is strong enough to be independent after your death. This spirit will enter the heavenly kingdom and gain eternal peace. This is hard to do in the everyday world, so religious Chi Kung practitioners frequently flee society and move into the solitude of the mountains, where they can concentrate all of their energies on self-cultivation.

Religious Chi Kung practitioners train to strengthen their internal Chi to nourish their spirit (Shen) until this spirit is able to survive the death of the physical body. Many monks consider Yi Gin Ching Chi Kung a necessary step in their training because it enables them to build up abundant Chi. Shii Soei Ching is then used to lead the Chi to the forehead, where the spirit resides, and to raise the brain to a higher energy state. Shii Soei Ching used to be restricted to only a few priests who had reached an advanced level of Chi Kung training. Tibetan Buddhists were also involved heavily in similar training. Over the last two thousand years the Tibetan Buddhists, the Chinese Buddhists, and the Taoists have followed the same principles to become the three main religious schools of Chi Kung in China.

The striving toward enlightenment or Buddhahood is recognized as the highest and most difficult level of Chi Kung. Many Chi Kung practitioners reject the rigors of this religious striving, and practice Yi Gin Ching and Shii Soei Ching Chi Kung solely to increase their longevity. It was these people who eventually revealed the training secrets to the outside world. The Yi Gin Ching will be discussed in the second part of this book, while the Shii Soei Ching will be discussed in the third part.

As you examine this book, you will see that the major portion of the documents come from the Taoists. For this reason we would like to give a brief introduction to Buddhist and Taoist Chi Kung, followed by a comparison of their training. We will also list the differences between the Buddhist and Taoist Yi Gin Ching and Shii Soei Ching training. In order to help you understand Taoist Chi Kung better, we will then review two major styles or attitudes of Taoist Chi Kung practice. We would like to remind you here that Yi Gin Ching and Shii Soei Ching training is only part of the Taoist training; there are many other Taoist Chi Kung practices which we plan to discuss in a later volume: "Taoist Chi Kung (Dan Diing Tao Kung)."

3-1. Buddhist and Taoist Chi Kung

Buddhist Chi Kung:

Three main schools of Buddhist Chi Kung have developed in Asia during the last two thousand years: Indian, Chinese, and Tibetan. Because Buddhism was created in India by an Indian prince named Gautama between 558 B.C. and 478 B.C., Indian Buddhist Chi Kung has the longest history. Buddhism was imported into China during the Eastern Han dynasty (58 A.D.), and the Chinese Buddhists gradually learned its methods of spiritual cultivation. Their practice was influenced by the traditional Chinese scholar and medical Chi Kungs, which had been developing for about two thousand years. What resulted was a unique system of training which was different from its ancestors.

According to the pieces of documents that are available, it is believed that at least in the first few hundred years after Buddhism's importation, only the philosophy and doctrines had been passed down to the Chinese. The actual methods of cultivation and Chi Kung training were not known. There are several reasons for this:

1. Because of the difficulty of transportation and communication at that time, the transferral of Buddhist documents from India to China was limited. Although a few Indian priests were invited to China to preach, the problems remained.

2. Even if the documents had been transferred, because of the profound theory and philosophy of Buddhism, very few people were qualified and could really translate the documents accurately from Indian to Chinese. This problem was enhanced by the different cultural backgrounds. Even today, different cultural backgrounds are always the main problem in translating accurately from one language to another.

3. The main reason was probably that most of the actual training methods must be taught and guided personally by an experienced master. Only a limited amount can be learned from the documents. This problem was enhanced by the tradition of passing information secretly from master to disciples.

You can see that the transferral process was very slow and painful, especially with regard to the actual training methods. For several hundred years it was believed that as long as you were able to purify your mind and sincerely strive for Buddhahood, sooner or later you would succeed. As mentioned in the last chapter, this situation was not improved until Da Mo wrote the Yi Gin Ching and Shii Soei Ching; then finally there was a firm direction in the training to reach the goal of Buddhahood.

Before Da Mo, Chinese Buddhist Chi Kung training was very similar to Chinese scholar Chi Kung. The main difference was that while scholar Chi Kung aimed at maintaining health, Buddhist Chi Kung aimed at becoming a Buddha. Meditation is a necessary process in training a priest to stay emotionally neutral. Buddhism believes that all human suffering is caused by the seven passions and six desires (Chii Ching Liow Yuh). The seven passions are joy, anger, sorrow, fear, love, hate, and lust. The desires are generated from the six roots which are the eyes, ears, nose, tongue, body, and mind (Hsin). Buddhists also cultivate within themselves a neutral state separated from the four emptinesses of earth, water, fire, and wind (Syh Dah Jie Kong). They believe that this training enables them to keep their spirits independent so they can escape from the cycle of repeated reincarnation.

Tibetan Buddhism has always been kept secret and isolated from the outside world. Because of this, it is very difficult to decide when exactly Tibetan Buddhism was established. Because Tibet is near India, it is reasonable to assume that Tibetan Buddhism started earlier than that of China. Naturally, it is again reasonable to assume that Tibetan Chi Kung training has had more influence from India than Chinese Chi Kung has. However, over thousands of years of study and research, the Tibetans established their own unique style of Chi Kung meditation. The Tibetan priests are called Lamas (Laa Ma), and many of them also learned martial arts. Because of the different cultural background, not only are the Lamas' meditation techniques different from those of the Chinese or Indian Buddhists, but their martial techniques are also different. Tibetan Chi Kung meditation and martial arts were kept secret from the outside world, and were therefore called "Mih Tzong," which means "secret style." Because of this, and because of the different language, there are very limited documents available in Chinese. Generally speaking, Tibetan Chi Kung and martial arts did not spread into Chinese society until almost the Ching dynasty (1644-1911 A.D.). Since then, however, they have become more popular.

Even though Tibetan Chi Kung training techniques are sometimes different from those of the Chinese and Indian Buddhists, they still have the same goal of Buddhahood. According to the available documents, Tibetan Chi Kung training emphasizes spiritual cultivation through still meditation, although they also use many physical Chi Kung exercises which are similar to Indian Yoga.

Taoist Chi Kung:

Like the Buddhists, the Taoists believe that if they can build up their spirit (Shen) so that it is independent and strong, they will be able to escape from the cycle of repeated reincarnation. When a Taoist has reached this stage, he has reached the goal of enlightenment. It is said that he has attained eternal life. However, if he cannot build his spirit quite strong enough before he dies, his soul or spirit will not go to hell, and he will be able to control his own destiny, either remaining a spirit or being reborn as a human. They believe that it is only possible to develop the human spirit while in a body, so that the continual cycle of rebirth is necessary to attain enlightenment.

The Taoist monks found that in order to enhance their spirit, they had to cultivate the Chi which was converted from their Jieng (Essence). The normal Taoist Chi Kung training process is 1. To convert the Jieng (Essence) into Chi (Liann Jieng Huah Chi); 2. To nourish the Shen (spirit) with Chi (Liann Chi Huah Shen); 3. To refine the Shen into nothingness (Liann Shen Faan Shiu); and 4. To crush the nothingness (Feen Suory Shiu Kong).

The first step involves firming and strengthening the Jieng, then converting this Jieng into Chi through meditation or other methods. This Chi is then led to the top of the head to nourish the brain and raise up the Shen. When a Taoist has reached this stage, it is called "the three flowers meet on the top" (San Huea Jiuh Diing). This stage is necessary to gain health and longevity. Finally, the Taoist can start training to reach the goal of enlightenment. However, the biggest obstacle to achieving this goal is the emotions, which affect the thinking and upset the balance of the spirit. This is the reason why they hid themselves away in the mountains, away from other people and their distractions. Usually they also abstained from eating meat, feeling that it muddied thinking and increased the emotions, leading the spirit away from self-cultivation.

An important part of this training to prolong life is Yi Gin Ching and Shii Soei Ching Chi Kung. While the Yi Gin Ching Chi Kung is able to strengthen the physical body, the basic idea of Shii Soei Ching Chi Kung is to keep the Chi circulating in the marrow so that the marrow stays clean and healthy. Your bone marrow manufactures most of your blood cells. The blood cells bring nourishment to the organs and all the other cells of the body, and also take waste products away. When your blood is healthy and functions properly, your whole body is well-nourished and healthy, and can resist disease effectively. When the marrow is clean and fresh, it manufactures an enormous number of healthy blood cells which will do their job properly. Your whole body will stay healthy, and the degeneration of your internal organs will be significantly slowed. Your body is not unlike an expensive car. It will run a long time if you use a high quality fuel, but if you use a low quality fuel the car engine will deteriorate a lot faster than it needs to. In order to reach the goal of enlightenment, you must also learn how to lead the Chi to the brain to nourish it and also raise up the spirit.

For longevity, although the theory is simple, the training is very difficult. You must first learn how to build up your Chi and fill up your eight Chi vessels, and then you must know how to lead this Chi into the bone marrow to "wash" the marrow. Except for some Taoist monks, there are very few people who have lived more than 150 years. The reason for this is that the training process is long and hard. You must have a pure mind and a simple lifestyle so that you can concentrate entirely on the training. Without a peaceful life, your training will not be effective.

Do not be misled into thinking that the Buddhist Charn (Zen) meditation is inferior to the Taoist approach in achieving enlightenment or Buddhahood. In fact, the Buddhists often had much greater success in reaching enlightenment than the Taoists through their use of still meditation. Additionally, many of the Taoist Chi Kung practices originated with the Buddhists. The Taoists then modified them to suit their own circumstances and purposes, and some of the practices, like Shii Soei Ching, were practiced much more widely by the Taoists than the Buddhists.

Many Taoist Chi Kung styles are based on the theory of cultivating both the spirit and the physical body. In Taoism, there are generally three ways of training: Golden Elixir Large Way (Gin Dan Dah Tao), Double Cultivation (Shuang Shiou), and Herb Picking Outside of the Tao (Tao Wai Tsae Yaw).

Golden Elixir Large Way teaches the ways of Chi Kung training within yourself. This approach believes that you can find the elixir of longevity or even enlightenment within your own body.

In the second approach, Double Cultivation, a partner is used to balance one's Chi more quickly. Most people's Chi is not entirely balanced. Some people are a bit too positive, others too negative, and individual channels also are positive or negative. If you know how to exchange Chi with your partner, you can help each other out and speed your training. Your partner can be either the same sex or the opposite.

The third way, Herb Picking Outside of the Tao, uses herbs to speed and control the cultivation. Herbs can be plants such as ginseng, or animal products such as musk from the musk-deer. To many Taoists, herbs also means the Chi which can be obtained from the sexual practices.

According to the training methods used, Taoist Chi Kung can again be divided into two major schools: Peaceful Cultivation Division (Ching Shiou Pay) and Plant and Graft Division (Tzai Jie Pay). This division was especially clear after the Song and Yuan dynasties (960-1367 A.D.). The meditation and the training theory and methods of the Peaceful Cultivation Division are close to those of the Buddhists. They believe that the only way to reach enlightenment is Golden Elixir Large Way, according to which you build up the elixir within your body. Using a partner for the cultivation is immoral and will cause emotional problems which may significantly affect the cultivation.

However, the Plant and Graft Division claims that their approach of using Double Cultivation and Herb Picking Outside of the Tao in addition to Golden Elixir Large Way makes the cultivation faster and more practical. For this reason, Taoist Chi Kung training is also commonly called "Dan Diing Tao Kung," which means "the Tao Training in the Elixir Crucible." The Taoists originally believed that they would be able to find and purify the elixir from herbs. Later, they realized that the only real elixir was in your body.

According to my understanding, the major difference between the two Taoist schools is that the Peaceful Cultivation Division aims for enlightenment in a way similar to the Buddhists' striving for Buddhahood, while the Plant and Graft Division uses the training to achieve a normal, healthy, long life. We will discuss these two major Taoist schools more extensively in the third section of this chapter.

You can see that Taoism has already been a religion and a scholarly study of Chi Kung methods. As a modern and scientific Chi Kung practitioner, you should only adopt the Chi Kung training methods which can benefit you. Superstition should be filtered out. However, you need to know the historical background so that you will understand the root and the motivation of the training.

3-2. The Differences between Buddhist and Taoist Chi Kung

In order to help you understand more clearly about Buddhist and Taoist Chi Kung, we would like to list and briefly discuss the general differences between these two religious Chi Kung training methods. Then we will discuss their differences with regard to the training of Yi Gin Ching and Shii Soei Ching Chi Kung.

General Differences between Buddhist and Taoist Chi Kung:

1. From the point of view of training philosophy, Buddhism is conservative while Taoism is open minded. It was discussed in the last chapter that because religious Taoism was formed by absorbing the imported Buddhist culture into the traditional scholar Taoism, their doctrine, generally speaking, is open minded. Whenever the Taoists could find any training method or theory which could help their training and cultivation proceed faster and more effectively, they adopted it. This was almost impossible for the Buddhists, who believed that any philosophy other than Buddhism was not accurate. In Buddhist society, new ideas on cultivation would be considered a betrayal. For example, the sixth Charn ancestor Huoy Neng, who lived during the Tarng dynasty, changed some of the meditation methods and philosophy and was considered a traitor for a long period of time. Because of this, the Charn style divided into Northern and Southern styles. This is well known among Buddhists, and is called "Sixth Ancestor Disrupting the Passed Down Method" (Liow Tzuu Shwo Chwan Faa). Because of this attitude, the Taoists have had more opportunities to learn, to compare, and to experience. Naturally, in many aspects they have advanced faster than the Buddhists. For example, in health and longevity Chi Kung training, Taoist theory and training methods are more systematically organized and more effective than those of the Buddhists.

2. Though both Buddhists and Taoists kept their training secret for a long time, the Buddhists were stricter than the Taoists. This is especially true for the Tibetan Buddhists. Before the Ching dynasty, although both Buddhist and Taoist Chi Kung were kept from laypeople, at least the Taoist monks were able to learn from their masters more easily than the Buddhists were. In Buddhist society, only a few trusted disciples were selected to learn the deeper aspects of Chi Kung training.

3. Taoists and Buddhists have different training attitudes. Generally, the Buddhist practices are more conservative than those of the Taoists. For example, in Chi Kung practice the Buddhists emphasize "cultivating the body" (Shiou Shenn) and "cultivating the Chi" (Shiou Chi). Cultivation here implies to maintain and to keep. However, Taoists will focus on "training the body" (Liann Shenn) and "training the Chi" (Liann Chi). Training means to improve, to build up, and to strengthen. They are looking for ways to resist destiny, to avoid illness, and to extend the usual limits on the length of one's life.

4. Buddhist Chi Kung emphasizes mainly becoming a Buddha, while Taoist Chi Kung focuses on longevity and enlightenment. While striving for Buddhahood, most Buddhist monks concentrate all their attention on the cultivation of their spirit. The Taoists, however, feel that in order to reach the final goal you need to have a healthy physical body. This may be the reason why more Taoists than Buddhists have had very long lives. In their nineteen hundred years of research, they found many ways to strengthen the body and to slow down the degeneration of the

organs, which is the key to achieving a long life. There have been many Taoists who lived more than 150 years. In Taoist society it is said: "One hundred and twenty means dying young." This does not mean that the Buddhists did not do any physical training. They did, but unfortunately it was limited to those who were doing Buddhist martial arts, such as Shaolin priests. Therefore, generally speaking, today's Buddhists can be divided into two major groups. One is Buddhist martial artists and some Buddhist non-martial artists who train both the physical body and the spirit, while the other group consists of those who still ignore the physical training and emphasize only spiritual cultivation.

5. Because of their emphasis, the Buddhists' spiritual cultivation has generally reached a higher level than that of the Taoists. For example, even though Charn meditation is only a branch of Buddhist spiritual cultivation, it has reached the stage where the Taoists can still learn from it.

6. Almost all of the Buddhist monks are against such training methods as "double cultivation" or "picking herbs from outside of the Tao" through sexual practices. They believe that using someone else's Chi to nourish your cultivation can lead to emotional involvement and may disturb your cultivation. The mind will not be pure, calm, and peaceful, which is necessary for spiritual cultivation. However, because many Taoists are training mainly for health and longevity instead of enlightenment, they consider these methods to be beneficial.

Now that you have a general idea of the attitudes and philosophy that the Buddhists and Taoists follow in their training, let us discuss what they think about Yi Gin Ching and Shii Soei Ching Chi Kung.

The Differences between Buddhist and Taoist Yi Gin Ching and Shii Soei Ching Training:

1. Although the Buddhists originated these two types of training, they kept them strictly secret, and so the training has not had much opportunity to develop and evolve. However, once the Taoists learned these two classics, they continued to research and develop them. Consequently, it seems that the Taoist training methods and theory are more complete and more systematically organized than those of the Buddhists.

2. The Taoists have revealed more of their training to the public than the Buddhists have. Because the Taoist training can be used to gain health and longevity faster and more effectively than the Buddhist training can, its techniques can be practiced by laymen who do not wish to give up their normal existence and become renunciates. For this reason, more Taoist training documents have been found than Buddhist. However, the very original theory, principles, and training methods are recorded in the Buddhist bibles.

3. Due to the above reason, many of the training techniques developed by the Taoists are more effective, and the training goals can be reached more quickly than with the Buddhist methods. This is especially true for those practices from the two classics which are used to improve health and increase longevity. However, when the training has reached a high level of spiritual cultivation in the Shii Soei Ching, it seems the Buddhist ways are more effective. The Buddhists focus on training for the future instead of the present, while the Taoists pay more attention to the present.

4. Taoists have developed many techniques such as "double cultivation" or "Picking the Herb from Outside of the Tao" to assist the Shii Soei Ching training. These are forbidden to the Buddhists. The Taoists of some sects allow or even encourage the practitioner to gain his/her Chi balance through two-person meditation or even sexual practices. Sexual Chi Kung training has always been forbidden in the Buddhist monasteries. This is probably the most significant difference in their training.

5. Taoist Shii Soei Ching training is both physical and spiritual, while the Buddhist approach is mainly spiritual. Taoist training begins with many physical exercises, such as massaging the testicles. The physical stimulation generates semen, which is then converted into Chi either physically or mentally. The Taoist documents discuss many physical training techniques, while the Buddhist training emphasizes meditation.

6. Taoists have been researching the use of herbs to help them in their Chi Kung training, while the Buddhists have never given much attention to this field. The Taoist documents have more herbal prescriptions than the Buddhist documents.

3-3. The Two Major Styles of Taoist Chi Kung

In this section, let us look more fully over the background of Taoist Chi Kung training. As with Buddhism, over thousands of years of study there developed many styles or divisions of Taoist Chi Kung. Every style or division, though the basic training theory and the final goal are the same, has its own theory and training methods to reach the goal of Tao.

As mentioned earlier, since the Song and Yuan dynasties (960-1368 A.D.), among all of these different divisions, two major ones have predominated: the Peaceful Cultivation Division (Ching Shiou Pay) and the Plant and Graft Division (Tzai Jie Pay).

It was also mentioned earlier that there are three general ways of training or cultivation which have been developed by the Taoists: Golden Elixir Large Way (Gin Dan Dah Tao), Double Cultivation (Shuang Shiou), and Picking the Herb from Outside of the Tao (Tao Wai Tsae Yaw). The meditation methods and training theory of the Peaceful Cultivation Division are closer to those of the Buddhists, and they prefer the Golden Elixir Large Way techniques. The Plant and Graft Division claims their methods are faster and more practical, and may utilize all three techniques. The major difference between the two Taoist schools is that the Peaceful Cultivation Division is aiming for enlightenment in a way similar to the Buddhists' striving for Buddhahood, while the Plant and Graft Division trains in order to achieve a long and healthy life. We will briefly discuss the differences between these two divisions.

Peaceful Cultivation Division (Ching Shiou Pay):

Ching means clear, clean, peaceful; Shiou means cultivation, study, training; and Pay means style or division. The basic rules of Peaceful Cultivation Division Taoists are to follow the traditions from the Taoist bibles. All of the training and study are based on the fundamental principles which Lao Tzu stated: "Objects are many, each returns back to its root. When it returns to its root, (it) means calmness. It (also) means repeating life."(*1) This means that all things have their

---

(*1). 老子云："夫物芸芸，各復歸其根，歸根曰靜，是謂復命。"

origins, and ultimately return to these origins. When things return to their origin, they are calm and peaceful. Then, from this state, life again originates. He also stated: "Concentrate the Chi to reach softness, you are able to be like a baby"(*2). You can see from these two sayings of Lao Tzu the emphasis on cultivating **CALMNESS, PEACE, HARMONY, AND SOFTNESS**. These are the basic rules of traditional Chinese Taoism, which originated from the observation of natural growth and cycles. It is believed that all life originated from and grows out of the roots of calmness and peace.

All of the Peaceful Cultivation Taoists emphasize "the method of Yin and Yang, harmony of the numbers (according to the I Ching), and the shape will follow the spirit and combine."(*3) This means that Yin and Yang must be harmonious and balance each other naturally, and the appearance of the physical body will ultimately follow the lead of the spirit. This division believes that purely spiritual cultivation is able to lead them to the final goal of enlightenment. Therefore, a strong physical body is not the main target of the training. The body is only temporarily used as a ladder to reach the final goal of spiritual enlightenment. Consequently, they emphasize sitting meditation, from which they learn to "regulate the body" (Tyau Shenn), "regulate the emotional mind" (Tyau Hsin), "regulate the breathing" (Tyau Shyi), "condense the spirit" (Ning Shen), "tame the Chi" (Fwu Chi), "absorb the Essence" (Sheh Jieng), and "open the crux" (Kai Chiaw). These are known as the seven steps of "internal Kung Fu" (Nei Kung), by which they cultivate, study, train, trace back to their root and origin (find the point of calmness and peace within themselves), and finally cultivate an eternal spiritual life. Through this cultivation they endeavor to reach the level of immortality and enlightenment.

We can see that the principles and training methods of the Peaceful Cultivation Division are similar to those of Charn (Zen) meditation in Buddhism. Their training and cultivation are based on calmness and peace. Once their mind is calm and peaceful, they look for the root and the real meaning of life, and finally learn to be emotionally neutral and reach the final goal of enlightenment.

Plant and Graft Division (Tzai Jie Pay):
Tzai means to plant, to grow, or to raise. Jie means to join, to connect, to graft. Pay means style or division. In training, Plant and Graft Division Taoists walk in the opposite direction of the Peaceful Cultivation Division Taoists. They maintain that the methods which are used by the Peaceful Cultivation Division, such as still meditation alone, breathing and swallowing saliva, using the Yi to lead the Chi to pass through the gates (Chi cavities) and open the vessels, are less effective and impractical. This viewpoint was expressed in the document Wuh Jen Pian (Book on Awakening to the Truth): "Within Yang, the quality of Yin essence is not tough (strong); to cultivate one thing alone is wasteful; working on the shape (body) or leading (the Chi)(only) is not the Tao; to tame the Chi (through breathing) and

---

(*2). 專氣致柔，能嬰兒乎．

(*3). 法於陰陽、和於術數、形與神俱。

dining on the rosy clouds are emptiness after all."(*4) The first sentence implies that still meditation is the Yin side of cultivation. The Yin essence that is found in the Yang world is not pure. You must also have Yang training methods which are different from purely still meditation. This criticizes the Peaceful Cultivation Division Taoists for seeking longevity and enlightenment only through meditation. It again says that trying to lead the Chi by controlling the breathing in meditation is like trying to make a meal of rosy clouds - it is empty and in vain.

The Taoist document Baw Poh Tzyy (Embracing Simplicity, which is also the Taoist name of the author Ger Horng) also said: "The Top Ultimate (i.e., the emperor) knows Taoist layman techniques, (which he) carefully keeps up and respects, of thoroughly studying the ultimate emptiness, enlivening all things, then viewing its repetition, finally obtaining the Tao and entering heaven."(*5) Layman techniques are those which were used by the Plant and Graft Taoists. When the ultimate emptiness is reached, all things start again from the beginning and are enlivened. When you understand that this cycle occurs continually throughout nature, you will comprehend the real Tao. This sentence emphasize that even the emperor, who practiced Taoist layman techniques, was able to reach the final enlightenment.

What then are the layman techniques of the Plant and Graft Division? They said: "(If) the tree is not rooted, the flowers are few; (if) the tree is old and you join it to a fresh tree, peach is grafted onto willow, mulberry is connected to plum; to pass down examples to people who are looking for the real (Tao), (these are) the ancient immortal's plant-grafting method; (then you will find that) the man who is getting old has the medicine to cure after all. Visit the famous teacher, ask for the prescriptions, start to study and immediately cultivate, do not delay."(*6) This says that when you are getting old, you can gain new life from a training partner. Mutual Chi transportation can be done through particular sexual practices or through special types of meditation.

They also say: "(When) clothes are torn, use cloth to patch; (when the) tree (is) senile, use (good) soil to cultivate; when man is weakening, what (should be used) to patch? (Use) Heaven and Earth to create the opportunity of variations."(*7) This sentence asks, how can a weakened person regain his energy if not from another person? You can see that the purpose of the Plant and Graft training is "similar types working together, spiritual communication between separate

(*4). 悟真篇云："陽裡陰精質不剛，獨修一物轉羸，夢形導引皆非道，服氣餐霞總是空。"

(*5). 抱朴子云："太上知玄素之術，守敬篤，致虛極，萬物並作，以觀其復而得道飛昇。"

(*6). 無根樹，花正微，樹老將新接嫩枝，挑寄柳、桑接梅，傳於修真作樣兒，自古神仙栽接法，人老原來有藥醫。訪名師，問方兒，下手速修莫太遲。

(*7). 衣破用布補，樹衰以土培，人損將何補，乾坤造化機。

bodies."(*8) Similar types of people who are working on the same training can help each other. Spiritual communication (Shen Jiau) means using your feelings and your partner's to guide your spirits to stimulate the production of hormones or Essence. This is the original source of the Chi which can be exchanged with and used to communicate with your partner. In the sexual practices, sexual feelings are used to stimulate hormone production, and particular sexual activities are used to protect and store the Chi, which can be used as the herb to cure aging. When the sexual practices are done correctly, neither side will lose Chi, and both will obtain the benefit of longevity.

You can see that this style of Taoism encourages a proper sex life. If the correct methods are practiced, both sides are able to benefit. However, with this approach it is difficult to achieve emotional neutrality, and so it is very difficult to reach the goal of enlightenment. As a result, this style mainly emphasizes a long and happy life. Han Shu Yih Wen Jyh (Han's Book of Art and Literature) says: "The activity in the (bed)room is the ultimate of the personality and emotions, is the ultimate of reaching the Tao. To restrain the external joy, to forbid the internal emotion. Harmony between husband and wife is the scholarship of longevity."(*9) This clearly implies that a correct sexual life is the way to longevity, because it enables you to balance your Chi and spirit.

In addition to sexual double cultivation, they also emphasize non-sexual double cultivation (Shuang Shiou). According to this theory, every person has a different level of Chi, and no one's Chi is completely balanced. For example, in the teenage years your Chi is stronger and more sufficient than at any other age. Once you pass forty, your Chi supply tends to weaken and become deficient. To be healthy, your Chi must be neither excessive nor deficient. Therefore, if you and your partner learn Double Cultivation meditation or other techniques, you will be able to help each other balance your Chi. The Chi balancing can be done by two males, two females, or male and female. It is said: "Yin and Yang are not necessarily male and female, the strength and the weakness of Chi in the body are Yin and Yang."(*10) It is again said: "Two men can plant and graft and a pair of women can absorb and nourish."(*11).

The Plant and Graft Taoists claim that there are four requirements for reaching the Tao: "money, partner, techniques, and place." Without money you have to spend time earning a living, and you will not have time to study and cultivate. Without a partner, you will not be able to find the "herb" and balance your Chi. Without the right techniques you will be wasting your time. Finally, without the right place to train, you will not be able to meditate and digest the herb you have taken.

As a Plant and Graft Taoist, after you have balanced your Chi with your partner, you must also know the techniques of retaining semen, converting this semen into Chi, and using the Chi to nourish your

---

(*8). 同類施工，隔體神交。

(*9). 漢書藝文志云：″房中者，性情之極，至道之極，制外樂，禁內情，和夫婦，及壽考之學也。″

(*10). 陰陽不必分男女，體氣強弱即陰陽。

(*11). 兩個男人可栽接，一對女人能採補。

Shen. If you are able to reach this level, you will be able to use your energized Shen to direct the Chi into your five Yin organs (heart, lung, liver, kidney, and spleen) so that they can function more efficiently. The Chi with which the organs carry out their functions is called Managing Chi (Ying Chi). Your Shen can also direct the Chi to the skin, where it can reinforce the energy field which protects you against negative outside influences. This Chi is called Guardian Chi (Wey Chi). Your Shen can also lead Chi into your bone marrow. This keeps the marrow fresh and clean so that the blood cells which are manufactured there will be fresh and healthy. When your blood is healthy, you are healthy, and the aging process will slow down. Taoists who reach this level have long and healthy lives. However, a Taoist who desires to reach even higher and attain enlightenment needs more than just this.

If a Taoist intends to reach the goal of enlightenment, he must use his Chi to build a "baby Shen" (Shen Tai or Shen Ing) or "spiritual baby" (Ling Tai) in his Upper Dan Tien. He must feed this baby and teach it how to be independent. Only when this baby is grown up and independent will he reach the goal of enlightenment. In order to reach this higher level, he must get rid of his emotions. It is usually necessary to leave normal society and become a hermit in order to find a quiet and peaceful place to cultivate the mind.

Even though the Plant and Graft techniques bring quick results, many Taoists and Buddhists are against them, and even despise them. There are two major reasons for this. First, since you are a human being, it is very easy for you to drop back into the normal state of emotional bondage during training. This will stop you from clearing your mind and concentrating. Second, they fear that many people who practice these techniques will not use them to balance the Chi for the mutual benefit of both partners, but instead will simply take the Chi that the partner offers, and not give anything in return. This is especially easy with a partner who does not know Chi Kung. This kind of selfishness is considered very immoral.

The Plant and Graft Taoists also use herbs to help in their Chi cultivation, believing that they offer significant help. The Peaceful Cultivation Taoists and the Buddhists also use herbs, but usually only for healing purposes.

Chapter 4

Kan and Lii

4-1. What are Kan and Lii?

The terms Kan and Lii occur frequently in Chi Kung documents. In the Eight Trigrams Kan represents "Water" while Lii represents "Fire." However, the everyday terms for water and fire are also often used. Kan and Lii training has long been of major importance to Chi Kung practitioners. In order to understand why, you must understand these two words, and the theory behind them.

First you should understand that though Kan-Lii and Yin-Yang are related, Kan and Lii are not Yin and Yang. Kan is Water, which is able to cool your body down and make it more Yin, while Lii is Fire, which warms your body and makes it more Yang. Kan and Lii are the methods or causes, while Yin and Yang are the results. When Kan and Lii are adjusted or regulated correctly, Yin and Yang will be balanced and interact harmoniously.

Chi Kung practitioners believe that your body is always too Yang, unless you are sick or have not eaten for a long time, in which case your body may be more Yin. When your body is always Yang, it is degenerating and burning out. It is believed that this is the cause of aging. If you are able to use Water to cool down your body, you will be able to slow down the degeneration process and thereby lengthen your life. This is the main reason why Chinese Chi Kung practitioners have been studying ways of improving the quality of the Water in their bodies, and of reducing the quantity of the Fire. I believe that as a Chi Kung practitioner, you should always keep this subject at the top of your list for study and research. If you earnestly ponder and experiment, you will be able to grasp the trick of adjusting them.

If you want to learn how to adjust them, you must understand that Water and Fire mean many things in your body. The first concerns your Chi. Chi is classified as Fire or Water. When your Chi is not pure and causes your physical body to heat up and your mental/spiritual body to become unstable (Yang), it is classified as Fire Chi. The Chi which is pure and is able to cool both your physical and spiritual bodies (make them more Yin) is considered Water Chi. However, your body can never be purely Water. Water can cool down the Fire, but it must never totally quench it, because then you would be dead. It is also said that Fire Chi is able to agitate and stimulate the emotions, and from these emotions generate a "mind." This mind is called Hsin, and is considered the Fire mind, Yang mind, or emotional mind. On the other hand, the mind that Water Chi generates is calm, steady, and wise. This mind is called Yi, and is considered to be the Water mind or wisdom mind. If your spirit is nourished by Fire Chi, although your spirit may be high, it will be scattered and confused (a Yang spirit). Naturally, if the spirit is nourished and raised up by Water Chi, it will be firm and steady (a Yin mind). When your Yi is able to govern your emotional Hsin effectively, your will (strong emotional intention) can be firm.

You can see from this discussion that your Chi is the main cause of the Yin and Yang of your physical body, your mind, and your spirit. To regulate your body's Yin and Yang, you must learn how to regulate your body's Water and Fire Chi, but in order to do this efficiently you must know their sources.

The first book in this series "The Root of Chinese Chi Kung" discussed adjusting your body's Water and Fire in general Chi Kung practice. Here we would like to discuss the Water and Fire training in Yi Gin Ching and Shii Soei Ching. Later you will realize that this discussion is more profound than those in the other book. This is because, in order to feel the Water and Fire adjustment, you usually need to have some level of understanding and experience in Chi Kung. Though the subject is profound and the training more difficult, once you understand and experience the keys, you will be able to advance your training rapidly.

4-2. Kan and Lii in Modern Science

In order to understand Kan and Lii clearly and to adjust them efficiently, you are urged to use the modern scientific, medical point of view to analyze the concepts. This will allow you to marry the past and present, and give birth to the future.

Before we continue our discussion, I would like to point out a few things. First, you should understand that relying on drugs is the worst way to cure an illness or gain a healthy body. The best way is to solve the problem at its root. Ancient China did not have our modern medical chemistry, and so they had to develop other ways of adjusting the body's Water and Fire. We could learn much from them. For example, many arthritis patients today commonly rely on medicine to reduce pain. While this may offer temporary relief from pain, it does not cure the problem. When the medicine is gone, the pain resumes. However, Chinese medicine and Chi Kung believe that the way to cure arthritis is to rebuild the strength of the joints. They therefore teach the patients how to increase the Chi circulation with slow, easy exercises, and how to massage the joints to strengthen them. These practices readjust the Yin and Yang balance, which allows the body to repair the damage and increase the strength of the joints. This approach cures the root of the problem.

Next, if we look carefully, we will discover that many modern medical practices are in conformity with Kan and Lii theory. For example, when the body temperature is very high, medicine and ice cubes are used to reduce the temperature. Again, when an injury is swollen, ice cubes are used to reduce the swelling. Whether you follow ancient medicine or modern medicine, the basic theory of healing remains the same: Kan and Lii adjustment. Naturally, we cannot deny that modern chemistry has brought us much that is marvellous. However, we cannot deny that chemical medicine has also brought many problems. The best approach is probably to borrow from both approaches and generate a whole new modern medicine.

The key to this new medical science is understanding Chi, or the bio-electric circulation in the human body. Controlling this will lead to strengthening both the physical and mental bodies and maintaining health, and will also allow doctors to correct irregular Chi even before the appearance of physical symptoms. It is even likely that the length of a person's life may be considerably extended.

From the point of view of modern bioscience, Yin and Yang are the results of bioelectric imbalance or abnormal circulation in the body. Scientifically, in order to have electric circulation, there must be an electromagnetic force (EMF). Without the EMF, the electric potential in the circuit will be the same throughout, and an electric current will not occur. The same principle applies to your body's electrical circuit. Therefore, the major causes of imbalance come from the EMF (electro-magnetic force) generated in the body. When the EMF is too strong, the current circulating in the body will be too strong and will therefore cause the body to be too Yang. When the EMF is too weak, the current will be weak and cause the body to be Yin.

You can see that in order to adjust Kan and Lii, you must first find the root or the origin of the problems. That means you must first understand how EMF is generated and how it affects the body's bio-electric circulation. Generally, there are four possible causes for the generation of EMF in the human circuit:

1. Through the influence of natural energy. That means the EMF generated in the human body circuit can be affected by external energy interference, for example from the sun and the moon. Alternatively, you may expose your body to a radioactive area or even an electromagnetic field which can influence the electrical circulation in your body.
2. From the conversion of food and air Essence. Whenever food and air are taken in, they are converted into bioelectric energy through biochemical reaction. This generates an EMF which causes the Chi to circulate.
3. From exercise. Whenever you move your muscles, part of the stored Essence in your body is converted into bioelectricity and generates an EMF in the exercised area.
4. From the mind and Shen (spirit). Your mind plays an important role in the generation of EMF. According to traditional Chi Kung theory, when you wish to move your arm your Yi generates an idea, which causes the Chi to flow and move your arm. If Chi is bioenergy, then when your mind generates an idea, the idea generates an EMF which moves the bioenergy. Exactly how this happens is a question still waiting for a complete answer.

In Chi Kung training for adjusting Kan and Lii, you are training to adjust your EMF through proper intake of food and air, Chi Kung exercises, and focused thought. In this chapter we will discuss how to use the mind and strategy to adjust Kan and Lii, which is the key to successful Yi Gin Ching and Shii Soei Ching Chi Kung training.

4-3. The Keys to Kan and Lii Adjustment

In this section we will discuss some of the main keys to regulating Kan and Lii in Chi Kung practice. These keys will help you build up a foundation of knowledge for the discussion of Yi Gin Ching and Shii Soei Ching Chi Kung in the second and the third parts of this book. Before we discuss these keys, we would first like to introduce the general concepts of how Kan and Lii relate to your breathing, mind, and spirit. Then, we will combine them together and construct a secret key which will lead you to the Chi Kung treasure.

Breathing's Kan and Lii

In Chi Kung, breathing is considered a "strategy" which enables you to lead the Chi effectively. For examples, you can use your breath to lead the Chi to your skin or marrow. Breathing slow or fast can make the Chi flow calm or vigorous. When you are excited your body is Yang, and you exhale more than you inhale to lead the Chi to the skin so that the excess will dissipate in the surrounding air. When you are sad your body is Yin, and you inhale more than you exhale to lead the Chi inward to conserve it. You can see that breathing can be the main cause of changing the body's Yin and Yang. Therefore, breathing has Kan and Lii.

Generally speaking, in the normal state of your body, inhaling is considered to be a Water activity because you lead the Chi inward to the bone marrow where it is stored. This reduces the Chi in the muscles and tendons, which calms down the body's Yang. Exhaling is considered a Fire activity because it brings Chi outward to the muscles, tendons, and skin to energize them, making the body more Yang. When the body is more Yang than its surroundings, the Chi in the body is automatically dissipated outward.

Normally, Yin and Yang should be balanced so that your body will function harmoniously. The trick to maintaining this balance is using breathing strategy. Usually your inhalations and exhalations should be equal. However, when you are excited your body is too Yang, so you may inhale longer and deeper to calm down your mind and lead the Chi inside your body to make it more Yin.

In Chi Kung practice, it is very important to grasp the trick of correct breathing. It is the exhalation which leads Chi to the five centers (face, two Laogong cavities, and two Yongquan cavities) and the skin to exchange Chi with the surroundings. Inhalation leads Chi deep inside your body to reach the internal organs and marrow. Table 4-1 summarizes how different breathing strategies affect the body's Yin and Yang in their various manifestations.

The Mind's Kan and Lii

In Chi Kung training, the mind is considered the "general" who directs the entire battle. It is the general who decides the fighting strategy (breathing) and control the movement of the soldiers (Chi). Therefore, as a general, you must control your Hsin (emotional mind) and use your Yi (wisdom mind) to judge and understand the situation, and then finally decide on the proper strategy.

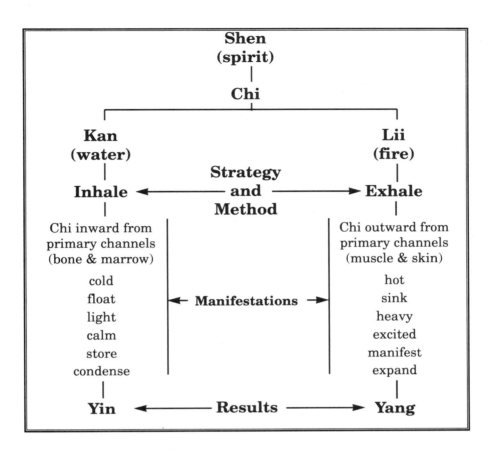

Table 4-1. The Effects of Breathing Strategies on the Body's Yin and
Yang in their Various Manifestations.

In Chi Kung, your wisdom mind must first dominate the situation
and generate an idea. This idea is the EMF which generates and exe-
cutes the strategy (breathing) and also is the force which moves the
Chi. Generally speaking, when your mind is excited, aggressive, and
energized, the strategy (breathing) is more offensive (emphasizing
exhalation) and the Chi circulation is more vigorous and expansive.
This aggressive mind is then considered a Fire mind, since it is able to
make your body more Yang. However, when the strategy is more
defensive (emphasizing inhalation), the Chi circulation will be more
calm and condensing. Therefore, a calm or depressed mind is considered a Water mind, since it can make your body more Yin.

You can see that the mind's Kan and Lii are more important than
breathing. After all, it is the mind which makes the strategy. Because
of this, regulating the mind and the breathing are two of the basic techniques for controlling your body's Yin and Yang. Regulating the mind
and the breathing cannot be separated. When the mind is regulated,
the breathing can be regulated. When the breathing is regulated, the
mind is able to enter a deeper level of calmness.

The Shen's Kan and Lii

Now it is time to consider the final and most decisive element in
winning a battle - the Shen (spirit). Shen is compared to the morale of

the general's officers and soldiers. There are many cases throughout history of armies winning battles against great odds because the morale of its soldiers was high. If a soldier's morale is high enough, he can defeat 10 enemies.

It is the same in Chi Kung training. It is the Shen which determines how successful your Chi Kung practice will be. Your Yi, which is the general who makes the strategy, must also be concerned with raising up the fighting morale (Shen) of the soldiers (Chi). When their morale is raised, the soldiers can be led more efficiently and, consequently, the strategy can be executed more effectively.

You can see that knowing how to use the Yi to raise the Shen is the major key to successful Chi Kung training. In Chi Kung, Shen is considered the headquarters which governs the Chi. As a matter of fact, it is the Yi and the Shen both which govern the Chi. They are closely related and cannot be separated.

Generally speaking, when the wisdom mind (Yi) is energized, the Shen is also raised. You should understand that in Chi Kung training, you want to raise up your Shen but not get it excited. When the Shen is raised, the strategy can be carried out effectively. However, if the Shen is excited, the body will become too Yang, and that is not desirable in Chi Kung practice. When you are practicing Chi Kung, you want to keep your Shen high all the time and use it to govern the strategy and the Chi. This will enable you to adjust or regulate your Kan and Lii efficiently.

Shen is the control tower which is able to adjust the Kan and Lii, but it does not have Kan and Lii itself. However, some Chi Kung practitioners consider the raised Shen to be Lii (Fire) and the calm Shen to be Kan (Water).

The Secret of Adjusting Kan and Lii

You may already have figured out the secret of Kan and Lii adjustment by yourself. Before we discuss this secret, let us first draw a few important conclusions from the above discussion:

A. Kan (Water) and Lii (Fire) are not Yin and Yang. Kan and Lii are methods which can cause Yin or Yang.
B. Chi itself is only a form of energy and does not have Kan and Lii. When Chi is too excessive or too deficient, it can cause the body to be too Yang or too Yin.
C. When you adjust Kan and Lii in the body, the mind is the first concern. The mind can be Kan or Lii. It determines the strategy (breathing) for withdrawing the Chi (Kan) or expanding it (Lii).
D. Breathing has Kan and Lii. Usually inhaling, which makes the body more Yin, is Kan while exhaling, which makes the body more Yang, is Lii.
E. The Shen (spirit) does not have Kan and Lii. Shen is the key to making the Kan and Lii adjustment effective and efficient.

Now that you understand the above conclusions, let us talk about the secret of Kan and Lii adjustment. These secrets are repeatedly mentioned in the ancient documents. The first key is that Shen and Breathing (Shyi) mutually rely on each other. The second key is that Shen and Chi mutually combine. We will discuss these secrets or keys of training by dividing them into two parts: theory and training.

1. Theory:

A. Shen and Breathing Mutually Dependent (Shen Shyi Shiang Yi) - Methods

We know that breathing is the strategy which directs the Chi in various ways and therefore controls and adjusts the Kan and Lii, which in turn control the body's Yin and Yang. We also know that the Shen is the control tower which is able to make the strategy work in the most efficient way. Therefore, Shen governs the strategy directly, and controls Kan and Lii and the body's Yin and Yang indirectly. You can see that the success of your Kan and Lii adjustment depends upon your Shen.

When the Shen matches your inhaling and exhaling, it can lead the Chi to condense and expand directly in the most efficient way. Your Shen must match with the breathing to be raised up or calmed down, and the breathing must rely on the Shen to make the strategy work efficiently. In this case, it seems that the Shen and breathing are depending on each other and cannot be separated. In Chi Kung practice, this training is called "Shen Shyi Shiang Yi," which means "Shen and breathing depend on each other." When your Shen and breathing are matching each other, it is called "Shen Shyi," or "spirit breathing," because it seems that your Shen is actually doing the breathing.

You can see that "Shen Shyi Shiang Yi" is a technique or method in which, when the Shen and breathing are united together, the Shen is able to control the Chi more directly.

B. Shen and Chi Mutually Combined (Shen Chi Shiang Her) - Result

When your Shen and breathing are able to match with each other as one, then the Chi can be led directly and therefore, Shen and Chi will become one. In Chi Kung practice, it is called "Shen Chi Shiang Her," which means "Shen and Chi mutually combined." When this happens, the Shen will be able to govern the Chi directly and more efficiently. You can see from this that the Shen and Chi combining is the result of the Shen and breathing being mutually dependent.

2. Training:

To discuss the training, we will start with a number of subjects which are related to Kan and Lii, and then get into the keys to the actual training.

A. Breathing and Chi Circulation:

First let us analyze how the Chi circulation relates to your breathing. As explained in the first volume "The Root of Chinese Chi Kung," there are eight Chi vessels (which function like reservoirs) and twelve primary Chi channels (which function like rivers) in your body. The Chi flow in the Conception and Governing Vessels and the twelve primary channels is related to the time of day. In the Conception and Governing vessels, the major Chi flow force moves up the back and down the front of the body according to the time of day, completing one cycle each 24 hours. In the twelve primary Chi channels, the major Chi flow force switches from one channel to another every 2 hours. This cycle is also completed every 24 hours.

In addition to the eight vessels and the twelve primary channels, there are millions of tiny channels branching out from the twelve channels to the surface of the skin to generate a shield of Guardian Chi

(Wey Chi). This Chi is responsible for hair growth and for defending against negative outside influences. These tiny channels also enter into the bone marrow to keep it healthy and producing blood cells.

Generally speaking, this circulation happens naturally and automatically in people who do not have Chi Kung training. However, an experienced Chi Kung master will be able to use his mind to generate an EMF to control the Chi circulation. When the average person exhales, he normally expands the Chi and leads it from the primary channels to the skin, and the body becomes more Yang. When he inhales, he draws in the Chi and leads it from the primary channels to the bone marrow, and the body become more Yin (Figure 4-1). When inhalation and exhalation are balanced, the Yin and Yang will be balanced.

As you get older, the length of your breath becomes shorter and shorter, and less Chi is led to the skin and the bone marrow. The Chi starts to stagnate in the skin and the bone marrow, and the skin starts to wrinkle, the hair turns gray or drops out. In addition, fewer blood cells are produced, and those that are are not as healthy as those produced when you were young. Since the blood cells carry nutrition and oxygen to the entire body, problems start to occur. In other words, you get sick more often, and start to age faster.

You can see that the first key or secret to maintaining your youth is learning how to regulate your breathing. This enables you to control Kan and Lii, and consequently the Yin and Yang of your body.

B. Fire Path, Water Path, Wind Path:

The most effective method of Kan and Lii adjustment in advanced Chi Kung practice is to use the various paths of Chi circulation. It was

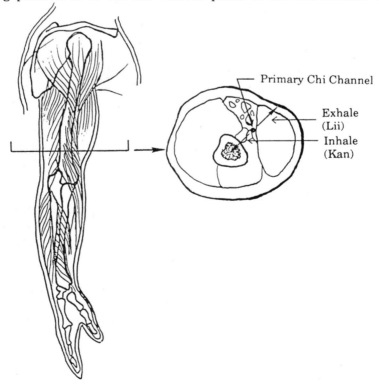

Figure 4-1. The Expansion and Condensing of Chi during Breathing

explained in the first volume, "The Root of Chinese Chi Kung," that there are three major paths which an advanced Chi Kung practitioner can use to govern the Chi flow rate: the Fire Path, the Wind Path, and the Water path.

In Fire path circulation, once you build up an abundance of Chi in your Lower Dan Tien, you circulate the Chi up the Governing Vessel and down the Conception Vessel. This fills up the Chi in these two vessels, which are the most important of the eight, and enables you to regulate the Chi circulation in the twelve primary channels, which are linked to the twelve internal organs. This strengthens your body. However, although your body is now strong and healthy because of the abundant Chi circulation, it will now also deteriorate more quickly because it is too Yang. In order to balance the Lii (Fire) training of the Fire path, you also need to practice Kan (Water) methods: the Wind path and the Water path. Fire path training will be discussed in the second part of this book.

In the Wind path, the Water Chi accumulated in the Lower Dan Tien is led upward to the Middle Dan Tien (solar plexus) to cool down the Fire Chi accumulated there. Fire Chi comes from the converted Essence of the food and air you have taken in, while Water Chi is converted from your Original Essence. Mixing Water Chi with the Fire Chi will cool down your body, even when you are circulating a great amount of Chi. You can see that in order to balance the Kan and Lii in your body you must learn the Fire path and the Wind path. This will also cause your body's Yin and Yang to be balanced and harmonious.

The Water path is the hardest but most effective method of balancing Kan and Lii. This method is found mainly in Shii Soei Ching Chi Kung. In Water Path training, the flow of Chi from the Lower Dan Tien is divided at the Huiyin cavity (Figure 4-2). One flow enters the Fire Path and circulates through the Conception and Governing Vessels, and the other flow is led upward through the marrow of the spine to nourish the brain. The Kan (Water) circulation through the marrow of the spine is used to balance the Lii (Fire) circulation in the Governing and Conception Vessels. In Shii Soei Ching Chi Kung, in order to increase the quantity of Chi going to the marrow and the brain, special techniques are used to increase the semen Essence production and improve the efficiency of the conversion of Essence into Chi. This will be discussed in the third part of this book.

When you practice adjusting Kan and Lii, regardless of which of the three paths you use, the most important key involves your Huiyin cavity and anus. In Fire path training, when the Huiyin cavity and anus are coordinating with the inhaling and exhaling, the Chi can be led from the Lower Dan Tien to the tailbone, and then upward to the head and around. If you do not know the trick of Huiyin and anus coordination, the built up Chi will be held at the Huiyin and the circulation will stagnate.

In the Wind path, coordinating the Huiyin and anus can slow down the Chi circulation in the Fire path so that your mind can lead the Chi up the front of the body to the Middle Dan Tien.

In the Water path, Huiyin and anus coordination allows you to regulate the Chi flow rate in the Fire and Water paths. In the Water path, the Chi flow enters the sacrum (Figure 4-2), and moves through the marrow of the spine to the brain. The Chinese call the sacrum the "immortal bone" (Shian Guu) because it is the key to success in Shii Soei Chi Kung and in reaching the goal of enlightenment and immortality.

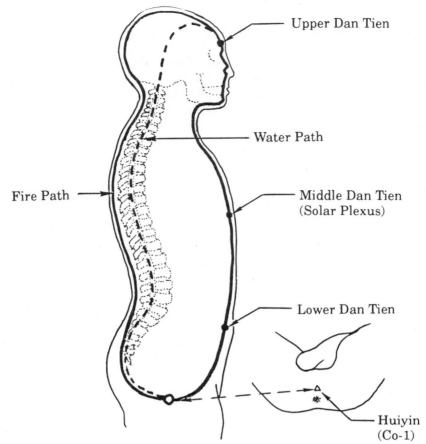

Figure 4-2. The Water and Fire Paths of Chi Circulation

Naturally, the methods of Huiyin and anus coordination are different in all three cases. The key point is the mind. After all, it is the mind which generates an EMF to cause the Chi to move. Next, we will introduce some simple Kan and Lii practices. Hopefully they will give you the experience you need for advanced Kan and Lii practice. However, even though they are simpler, they may still be difficult for those who have only limited experience with Nei Dan Chi Kung.

C. Training Methods:

Before you practice the following training, you should already understand the five main keys of general Chi Kung practice discussed in the first volume "The Root of Chinese Chi Kung." These five keys are: regulating the body, regulating the breathing, regulating the mind, regulate the Chi, and regulating the Shen. Among these five keys, regulating the mind is the most important. After all, it is the mind which controls the entire situation.

In addition, you must learn how to coordinate the Shen, breathing, and Chi, which we have discussed in the previous section. That is, Shen and breathing are mutually dependent, and Shen and Chi must mutually combine.

Breathing is the strategy for adjusting the body's Kan and Lii and determining the body's Yin and Yang. This is why breathing methods have become one of the most important subjects in Chi Kung research and practice. We would like to discuss a few of the well known ways of regulating the breath. This will help you to better understand Nei Dan Yi Gin Ching and Shii Soei Ching.

The following breathing and mind practices are listed from relatively easy to more difficult. If you are able to catch the knack of each one, you may be able to experience all of them is about three years. Be patient and learn each one before going on to the next one in the list. Only then will you be able to profoundly comprehend the theory.

a. Chest Breathing (Normal Breathing)

First you should learn how to regulate your normal chest breathing, inhaling and exhaling smoothly with the lungs relaxed. The mind must concentrate on the practice until it is neutral, calm, and peaceful. Then you will find that the breathing can be long and deep and the body can remain relaxed. When you have done this, the heart beat will slow down. You may practice in any comfortable position. Practice ten minutes each morning and evening until one day you notice that your mind does not have to pay attention to the chest. Then you may concentrate your mind on feeling the result of the training. The result can be that when you exhale you feel the pores on the skin open, and when you inhale the pores close. It seems that all of the pores are breathing with you. This is a low level of skin or body breathing. The feeling is very comfortable, even sensational. When you can do this comfortably and automatically, you have achieved the goal of regulating your Chest Breathing.

b. Buddhist Breathing

After you have completed the above training, you then learn how to control your abdominal muscles and coordinate them with the breathing. When you inhale, it expands, and when you exhale it withdraws. You should practice until the entire process becomes smooth and the entire body remains relaxed. Naturally, your mind must first concentrate on your abdomen in order to control the abdominal muscles. After practicing for some time, you will find the entire breathing process becoming natural and smooth. This means that you are now ready to build up Chi at the Lower Dan Tien.

Once you have reached this level, you should then coordinate your breathing with the movements of your Huiyin and anus. When you inhale, relax the Huiyin and anus, and when you exhale hold them up. Remember, you are gently holding up the Huiyin and anus, not tightening them. When you hold them up they can remain relaxed, but if you tighten them you will impede the Chi circulation. When you tense them you also cause tension in the abdomen and stomach, which can generate other problems. In the beginning, you will seem to need to use your muscles to do this, but after you have practiced for a time, you will find that the mind is more important than the movement of the muscles. When you have reached this stage, you will feel a wonderful and comfortable feeling in the area of the Huiyin and anus. You will also feel that the Chi is led more strongly to the skin then when you did Chest Breathing. It will feel like your entire body is breathing with you.

c. Taoist Breathing

After you have mastered Buddhist Breathing, you should then start Taoist breathing, which is also called Reverse Breathing. It is called this because the movement of the abdomen is the reverse of Buddhist Breathing, in other words, the abdomen withdraws when you inhale and expands when you exhale.

When you are learning Taoist Breathing, you should first stop your Huiyin and anus coordination until you can do the Reverse Breathing smoothly and naturally. Then resume the Huiyin and anus coordination, only now when you inhale you hold up your Huiyin cavity and anus, and when you exhale, you relax them.

After you have practiced for a while, you may discover that you can now lead the Chi to the skin more efficiently when you exhale than with the Buddhist method.

d. Shen Breathing

When you have accomplished Taoist Breathing, you must then train to combine your Shen and breathing. When you inhale, pay attention to your Upper Dan Tien and when you exhale, relax your concentration. Remember, you should not use force to achieve the concentration. Simply pay attention while your physical body and mind stay relaxed. One day you will realize that your Shen and Breathing have become one. This is the stage of Shen Breathing.

When you are able to do Shen breathing, your Shen can be raised so that it will be able to govern the Chi very efficiently. When you have reached this level, you have already built up a firm foundation for Yi Gin Ching and Shii Soei Ching Chi Kung.

e. Five Gates Breathing

After you have reached the level of Shen Breathing, you then learn how to regulate the Chi circulating to the five gates, or centers: the head (including the Upper Dan Tien and Baihui), the two Laogong cavities on the palms, and the two Yongquan cavities on the bottoms of the feet. Beginners use the Baihui gate on the head because it is easier for them to communicate with the surrounding Chi. Later, once it is opened, the Upper Dan Tien will be used instead.

In this training, when you inhale the Chi is led from the five gates to the Lower Dan Tien, and when you exhale the Chi is led to the gates, where it exchanges with the surrounding Chi (Figure 4-3).

f. Body Breathing

Body breathing is sometimes called "skin breathing." Actually, body breathing involves breathing with the entire body, not just the skin. When you exhale you lead the Chi to the muscles and the skin, and when you inhale you lead the Chi to the marrow and the internal organs. It should feel that your entire body is transparent to the Chi.

When you train this, the mind and the Shen are most important. When you inhale you draw Chi into your body from outside, and lead it to the Lower Dan Tien. When you are doing this, you should also feel that the Chi is being led inward to the internal organs and marrow. When you exhale, you lead this Chi from the Lower Dan Tien outward to your muscles, tendons, skin, and even beyond the skin. Again, the coordination of your Huiyin and anus remains the main key to successful training. When you breathe this way you will feel inflated like a beach ball. When you inhale

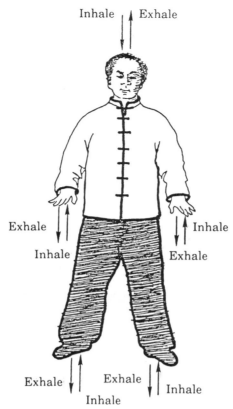

Inhale   Exhale

Exhale   Inhale

Inhale   Exhale

Exhale   Exhale   Inhale

Inhale

Figure 4-3. Five Gates Chi Breathing

the ball gets smaller, and when you exhale it gets larger (Figure 4-4). Inside the ball, the Chi flow is smooth, abundant, and natural. It seems that your entire body is transparent to the Chi. When you inhale you will feel light, and when you exhale you will feel heavier.

After you have completed the above training, you will not have any problems with the final stage of breathing: marrow and brain breathing, which we will discuss in the third part of this book.

4-4. Kan and Lii in Yi Gin Ching and Shii Soei Ching

By now you should have a good grasp of the important idea that when you train any style of Chi Kung, you must balance Yin and Yang by controlling Kan and Lii. For example, when you practice Tai Chi Chuan, you learn the slow meditative movements that are Lii, and may cause your body to become too Yang. You must also learn still meditation, which is Kan, and neutralizes the excessive Yang. Again, in the moving Tai Chi forms, there is also Kan and Lii adjustment. While the moving is Lii which causes Yang, the calm mind is Kan, and it may neutralize the Yang. In still meditation, while the stillness is Kan and causes Yin, the Chi must be led to circulate, which is Lii and balances the Yin. This means that in all of the Chi Kung practices, if there is Yin, there must be Yang to balance it, and vice versa.

It is the same with the Yi Gin Ching and Shii Soei Ching training. They are based on this Yin and Yang concept. The Yi Gin Ching is Lii because it generates Chi and causes Yang, while the Shii Soei Ching is Kan, because it utilizes and stores the Chi and causes Yin. The Yi Gin

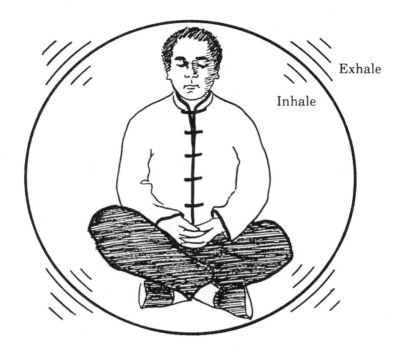

Figure 4-4. Body Breathing or Skin Breathing

Ching deals with the muscles and skin, which are visible externally, while the Shii Soei Ching deals with the marrow and brain, which must be felt internally. While the Yi Gin Ching training emphasizes the physical body, the Shii Soei Ching training focuses on the spiritual body. Therefore, Yin and Yang are balanced and coexist harmoniously.

In the Yi Gin Ching, the physical stimulation and exercises are considered Lii, and cause the body to become Yang, while the still meditation for the Small Circulation is Kan, which calms down the Lii and makes the body more Yin. Again, in the physical stimulation Lii training, external strength is Lii while internal strength is Kan. We will discuss external and internal strength in the second part of this book. In still meditation, the physical body is still and is Kan, while the Chi moving inside is Lii.

The same theory prevails in Shii Soei Ching training. The physical stimulation to increase the Original Essence production is Lii, while the techniques of internal cultivation which are used to lead the Chi to the marrow and brain are Kan.

You can see from this discussion that the basic key to successful Chi Kung training is Yin and Yang balance, and the trick to reaching this goal is Kan and Lii adjustment. Once you understand this fundamental theory, you will not have too much difficulty understanding the rest of this book.

PART TWO

MUSCLE/TENDON
CHANGING CHI KUNG
(Yi Gin Ching)

Chapter 5

Theories and Principles

5-1. Introduction

Theories and principles are always the guidelines for correct and smooth training. They give you the Why, How, and What, which are the keys to successful practice. You should read this chapter carefully, ponder it, and understand it.

Before we discuss this subject, you should know that even though there are many documents about the Yi Gin Ching available, very few of them actually discuss the training theory and principles clearly and in depth. It is believed that traditionally, most of the theory and principles, which are the keys to the training, were passed down orally from master to disciple. While many documents offer some theory and training methods, many others, although they also include some simple forms of training, emphasize mainly the history and talk about the great achievements that this Chi Kung training can provide. There are some others in which the text of the Yi Gin Ching training is mixed with Buddhist theory. If you have only a few of these faulty documents, it is very difficult to grasp the complete concept of the training.

However, in all these documents, no matter how deeply or superficially the subject is discussed, the basic theory remains the same. If you gather enough of them, and go over them again and again, you will be able to grasp the general concepts and the roots of the training. Suddenly, all of these documents become pieces of a puzzle. Once you throw away the extraneous parts and put the useful ones together, you can see the picture.

I am only a Chi Kung puzzle player who has collected a large number of the pieces. Although I have some in-depth understanding and experience in Chi Kung, many parts of the puzzle are new to me, and I still do not know where to place some of the pieces. Since this Chi Kung puzzle is so deep and wide, I may have missed some scenes or important points. However, I hope with this book to offer you an overview of the whole picture. There are still many details which others must follow up on. With your different background and experience, you may very well organize the puzzle somewhat differently than I have. However, as long as the main picture is correct, sooner or later hundreds of other small parts on your puzzle will become clearer and mesh together with the growth of your experience.

In this chapter we will discuss the theory and principles of Yi Gin Ching. In order to lead you into the traditional feeling of Yi Gin Ching, some selected documents will be translated and commented on in the second section. After you have tasted these traditional treasures, we will discuss the purposes, advantages, and disadvantages of Yi Gin Ching training in Section 3. In the fourth section we will review the general concepts of the two major cores of Yi Gin Ching training - Wai Dan and Nei Dan. This will prepare you for the discussion of Wai Juang (external strength) and Nei Juang (internal strength) in Section 5. Since many readers will have some understanding of Iron Shirt training, Section 6 will discuss the differences between it and Yi Gin Ching. Finally, the actual Yi Gin Ching training keys and theories will be discussed in Sections 7 and 8.

In the second chapter of Part Two we will study different traditional methods of Yi Gin Ching training. Since Yi Gin Ching has been studied and researched for more than fourteen hundred years, it is impossible to discuss all of the methods. Instead, we will only cover a number of typical and popular methods for each training category.

5-2. General Concepts from Old Documents

In this section we will translate parts of selected documents and make some comments. This will give you an overview of the Yi Gin Ching and a taste of the ancient documents. The excerpts selected emphasize the theory of the art.

1. The Purpose of Yi Gin Ching and Shii Soei Ching
易筋經與洗髓經之目的

Yi Gin Kung Fu is able to change the tendons and shape, Shii Soei Kung Fu is able to change the marrow and Shen. (They are) especially capable of increasing spiritual bravery, spiritual power, spiritual wisdom, and spiritual intelligence. Its training methods, compared with the Taoist family's Liann Jieng (train Essence), Liann Chi (train Chi), and Liann Shen (train spirit), are repeatedly mutually related in many ways, and its Yi of practice (i.e., goal) is completely the same.

易筋功夫，可換筋換形；洗髓功夫，可換髓換神；
尤可增加神勇、神力、神智、神慧。其功法與道家
之練精、練氣、練神，亦復脈脈相通，而用意則全
同。

Yi Gin (Muscle/Tendon Changing) and Shii Soei (Marrow/Brain Washing) Chi Kung training require a lot of time and great patience. This is why they are called Kung Fu (which literally means "energy-time"). Yi Gin Chi Kung is able to change the strength and the "shape" of the physical body. "Shape" includes the appearance of both the physical body, because it builds up the muscles, and the spiritual body, because you will look healthy and your spirit of vitality will be visibly high. Shii Soei Chi Kung is able to change the condition of the marrow, which, in Chinese medicine, includes the brain. If you accomplish these two exercises, you will be able to increase your bravery, power, wisdom, and intelligence. These qualities are related closely to the development of your spirit (Shen), which is the ultimate goal of these two exercises, and this is why they refer to "spiritual bravery" etc. The Buddhist method of training is similar in many ways to the Taoist: you must train your Essence and convert it into Chi effectively, and train how to lead the Chi to the brain to nourish the brain and spirit. Though the training methods are not completely the same, the final goal is the same for both Buddhists and Taoists.

However, (the Buddhist approach is) trained from external, while elixir family (i.e., Taoist approach) is trained from internal. Cultivating life (i.e., the physical body) is the major support of cultivating the Tao, it is the ladder and the voyage to Buddhahood. It serves the same purpose as "methods" (of cultivation). Once (you have) achieved the goal, the life and the methods should all be given up; not hesitating is the important point.

惟此乃由外練，而丹家則由內練也。修命乃修道之
拄杖，作佛之梯航，與法同其功用；及其成也，命
與法，俱應齊捨，不可執滯，是為要著。

The major difference between the training methods of the Buddhists and the Taoists is that the former emphasize training from the external, while the latter start from the internal. External means starting with Wai Dan training, while internal means Nei Dan training. As a matter of fact, according to other documents, both religions train both external and internal. Both believe that in order to reach the final goal of enlightenment or Buddhahood, you must first have a strong physical body (life). To them, the body is only a temporary residence for the spirit. Life is used as a ladder, a voyage, a tool for reaching the final goal of Buddhahood. Once you have reached the final goal, you will not need your physical body or the training methods, and you should give them up. If you persist, however, your spirit will stay in the physical body and keep you from becoming a Buddha.

This document does not discuss much of the "how" or "what" of the training theory. However, it clearly points out that the purpose of Yi Gin Ching and Shii Soei Ching is to change your body both physically and spiritually, leading you to a higher level of physical and spiritual life. In order to acquire the "how" and "what," you must first understand the general keys to Chi Kung training. These keys are learning how to regulate the body, the breathing, the emotional mind, the Chi, and the Shen. At this point, you are encouraged to study the first volume of the YMAA in-depth Chi Kung book series: "The Root of Chinese Chi Kung - The Secrets of Chi Kung Training."

2. Yi Gin Ching Training Secret
From Harn Fen Lou (Tower of Fragrance)

易筋經行功要訣

Man lives between heaven and earth, fearing cold and fearing heat, consequently he cannot (live) long in this world. (This) is not the original nature of created things (i.e., man). It is only (because) man forces himself.

人生天地間，畏寒惡熱，而不能久於世者，非造物
之本然，惟人自迫之耳。

In ancient China, it was believed that the earth was flat, and mankind lived between heaven (sky) and the earth (ground). After a person is born, he is afraid of extreme cold and heat, and therefore finds ways to protect himself. Gradually he loses contact with his original nature, as well as his inborn ability to adapt to the environment and protect himself from disease and the elements. Because of this, his body becomes weak and cannot live long. This is not the way it was meant to be, it is not the "original nature" of man. The original nature of the created being called man is to be strong of body and mind, able to face nature and adapt to it. Once we learned how to protect ourselves from the weather by wearing clothes and living in houses, we gradually lost our natural ability to protect ourselves. Our bodies became weak and, therefore, people die easily whenever they are sick. All of these things we have done to ourselves.

Therefore, person who is looking for the Tao, before anything else protect Jieng Shen (spirit of vitality), nourish Chi and blood, conduct (i.e., train correctly) the tendons and bones. When Jieng and Shen are full, then Chi and blood are abundant; when Chi and blood are abundant, then Li (muscular strength) is also sufficient. When tendons and bones are conducted, then Chi and blood transport smoothly, hundreds of sicknesses will not be generated.

故求道者，莫先於保精神、養氣血、導筋骨。蓋精
神足，則氣血足，氣血足，則力亦足。筋骨導，則
氣血通暢，百病不生矣。

If you are looking for the Tao (the natural way), there is no other way than first learning how to protect your Jieng (Essence) and Shen (spirit), how to nourish your Chi and blood, and also how to properly train your tendons and bones to make them strong.

Jieng is the source of Chi, and Shen is the headquarters of Chi, so when Jieng is full and the Shen is raised, the Chi and blood will be abundant. Chi and blood cannot be separated. Chi keeps the blood cells alive, and blood is the major carrier of Chi. They are always relating to each other. Where there is blood, there is Chi. Only when your Chi and blood are abundant can they effectively energize and strengthen the muscles.

When you have plenty of Chi and blood, you must also train your muscles (tendons) and bones. Only when they are strong and healthy will Chi and blood circulate smoothly and will your health be maintained.

Men today only know that when the blood is flourishing, then the Li is also strong. (They) don't know that blood is born of Chi, (and when) Chi is sufficient then the Li can be strong. Therefore, when man's life has blood and Chi, (he) has Li. (When) they are used - they exist, (when) ignored - they die. The way is nothing other than training. To build the foundation, use lead equipment.

今人但知血盛則力亦壯，而不知血生於氣，氣足而
後力壯也。然則人生有血氣，即有其力，用之則存
，忽之則亡。其要法不外乎行功，築基運用鉛器。

Most people in the time when this document was written knew that as long as they had plenty of blood, their Li (strength) would be strong. However, the life and health of the blood depends on the Chi. Therefore, in order to make your physical body (which generates Li) strong, you need to put your attention on your Chi, rather than your blood. When you have plenty of Chi and blood, you will have Li and be healthy. Chi and blood must be used continuously. The more they are used, the more abundant they will be and the smoother they can circulate. If you ignore them, and do not train and use them, they will become weak and degenerate quickly, and the circulation will become stagnant. In this direction lies death. How do we keep our Chi and blood abundant and circulating smoothly? There is no other way than proper training. The foundation of this training involves the use of lead equipment.

This paragraph explains that Chi is the most important factor in the training to strengthen your physical body. In order to keep the Chi strong and the blood abundant, you must use certain equipment. Because this article was written in ancient times, when only a few metals were available, it recommends lead. There were several reasons for using lead. First, it was easy to obtain. Second, lead is considered a Yin material which is able to absorb the excess Chi (Yang Chi) during training. Third, lead is heavier than other metals, and the equipment can be smaller. Fourth, lead has a low melting point, so it is easier to work with than most other metals. We will discuss some of the training equipment later.

The Tao (way) to build the foundation, begin at Tzy (midnight), Wuu (noon), between Tzy-Wuu (sun rise); or begin at Wuu-Tzy (sunset) when the variations are many, the Yin and Yang are exchanging, mutually turning and cooperating. If (you) are able (to train) day and night ceaselessly, not even a second ignored, then Heaven and man can unite. When trained for seven-seven (forty-nine days), Chi and blood will be sufficient and abundant. When trained for ten-ten (100 days), immortality can be gradually achieved.

築基之道，或起於子、午、子午、或是起於午子變
化多端，顛倒陰陽，更轉互屬，茍能晝夜不息，時

刻無訛，則天人會一，功至之之，氣血充足。功之
十十，仙亦日成。

This paragraph discusses the times for training. When you train Yi Gin Ching you may start at midnight, noon, dawn, or sunset, because at these times Yin and Yang are exchanging (Figure 5-1). According to the I Ching (Book of Change), at midnight the Yin is the strongest and the Yang starts to grow; and at noon the Yang is at its maximum and the Yin starts to grow. In addition, at dawn, the weak Yang starts to grow into the stronger Yang, and Yin is vanishing. At this time, all of the plants are converting from absorbing oxygen into absorbing carbon dioxide. At sunset, the strong Yang becomes weak Yang and the Yin starts to grow strong, and plants change from taking in carbon dioxide to taking in oxygen. These four times are the best for training because you are able to take advantage of the variations and exchanges of Yin and Yang - the variations being the continual change in the degree of Yin and Yang in your body, and the exchanges being when your body shifts from extreme Yin to extreme Yang or vice versa.

After you have trained for a period of time, you will be able to train at any time and any place. The training will have become a natural habit, and you will not have to pay too much attention to it. It is just like when you start jogging, you need to force yourself. Once you have built up a

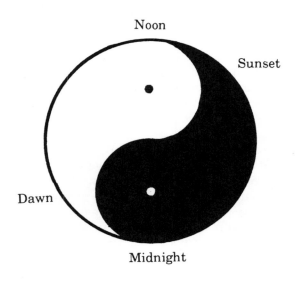

Figure 5-1. Yin and Yang and the Time of the Day

routine, it becomes much easier. When you have built up the routine of Yi Gin Ching practice, you can unite with heaven. This means your body will be able to adjust itself to nature automatically and reunite with it.

If you can train for forty-nine days, your Chi and blood will be sufficient and abundant. At this time, you will be able to see your body change from weak to strong. When you have trained for 100 days, you will have built up your training routine so that you can keep your body healthy, and you will have built a firm foundation for the Shii Soei Ching training. To Buddhists and Taoists, Shii Soei Ching training is necessary for reaching immortality.

Of most importance for training, (you) must seek movement within the calmness, look for the calmness within the movement. (Training should) be soft and continuous, gradually enter the sensational region. (When looking for) movement amidst the calmness, (because of the) calmness it is easy to fall asleep, it is best to shine peacefully. (When looking for) the calmness in the movement, (because of the) movement (it is) easy to disperse. (It is) best to condense (your Shen).

行功至要，務於靜中求動，動中求靜，綿密不間，漸入佳境。靜中動者，靜則易昏，最宜默照。動中靜者，動則易散，最宜收斂。

The most important thing during the training is to learn to find the movement when you are in a state of stillness. During the Nei Dan meditation which is part of the Yi Gin Ching training, when your body and mind are calm and peaceful, you must look for the Chi movement within your body. In this state of quietude, you can also easily lead the Chi smoothly. On the other hand, when you are doing the physically active part of the Yi Gin Ching training, you must take care that your mind does not become excited or agitated. When you train, your movements should be soft and continuous, and you will gradually begin to be able to sense what is going on inside your body.

When you are meditating, it is very common to fall asleep because you are so peaceful and calm. If you "shine peacefully" (raise your Shen) you will be able to clear your mind and still stay awake. When you are doing the active Wai Dan training it is hard to keep your mind from becoming scattered. If you condense your Shen and keep it in its residence you will be able to remain calm and keep your body from becoming over-excited.

The secret of shining peacefully is the secret of returning the Fire. The secret of condensing is the secret of adding Water. (If) the Fire does not return, then it flies away. (If) Water is not added, then you wither.

默照之訣，即返火之訣也。收斂之訣，即添水之訣也。火不返，則飛。水不添，則竭。

"Returning the Fire" means to return your body to a more fiery (Yang) state when it is becoming too Yin. During still meditation the heart beat slows down, the length of your breath increases, your mind is calm and peaceful, and the unnecessary activity of the body gradually slows down and stops. When this happens, it is very easy to fall asleep. The secret to staying awake is to raise your Shen (shine peacefully) so that the Fire in the body increases.

During Wai Dan training, condensing the Shen and firming your mind is the secret of adding Water to cool down your excited body and fiery mind (Hsin). During Nei Dan still meditation, if you fail to return the Fire and you fall asleep, your training will "fly away" and be in vain. However, when you are training your Wai Dan Yi Gin Ching, if you do not know how to add Water to cool down your excited mind and body, your physical body will degenerate and weaken.

You can see that during Yi Gin Ching training, you must learn how to adjust your Yin and Yang or Water and Fire (Kan and Lii). Only then will you be able to really achieve your purpose.

The method is to "keep the heavenly gate" and "stabilize the earth axis." Keeping the heavenly gate is the training of Wuu-Tzy (sunset), the secret of returning the Fire. Stabilizing the earth axis is the training of Tzy-Wuu, the secret of adding Water. The two of them mutually relate; train long and patiently. Thousands of variations and millions of derivations are within them (i.e., Water and Fire), there is nothing but what originates from these sources.

其法在守天關，定地軸而已。守天關者，即午子之功，返火之訣也。定地軸者，即子午之功，添水之訣也。二者相兼，久久行去，其間千變萬化，皆不外此根源。

What are the methods of returning the Fire and adding Water? The answer is learning to "keep the heavenly gate" and "stabilize the earth axis." Heavenly gate means the Baihui cavity (or called "Ni Wan Gong" by Taoists). It is believed that the top of your head is the gate which corresponds with the heaven energy. When you are able to lead the Chi to reach this cavity, you have led the Chi to the brain to nourish it, and this will also raise up the Shen. The best time to train raising your Shen is at sunset, when the Yin is getting stronger and the Yang is weakening. If you train at this time, you will be able to return the Fire to your body. Normally at sunset, after a whole day of thinking and working, your body is tired and your mind is scattered. If you meditate at this time, when your body is becoming more Yin, you can fall asleep easily. To prevent this you must return the Fire.

The earth axis means the Lower Dan Tien area, where the center of gravity is located, as well as the center of the body. The trick of cooling down the body's Fire is to add Water Chi to the Lower Dan Tien at dawn. At this time, Yang is getting stronger and Yin is weakening. Your body is well rested and energy is again abundant. Now you should learn how to accumulate Water Chi in the Lower Dan Tien. When you use this Chi to nourish your brain and Shen, you will be able to condense your Shen and calm down the excited body and mind.

Yin and Yang (or Kan and Lii) are mutually related. When you are able to grasp the tricks of controlling and adjusting your Yin and Yang (Kan and Lii) through long and patient training, you will be able, as the Chinese say, to generate thousands or even millions of variations of Yin and Yang, and accomplish anything you wish.

Again, use the lead equipment, gradually opening up the stagnation (of Chi and blood). On the left, smoothly move to the right. On the right, smoothly move to the left. (This will) enable the left and right to meet each other, Chi and blood will be abundant. (In this case), how (can a person) fear cold and die at a young age? The person who is looking for the Tao (should) keep these marvelous techniques, one thread connects them (sequentially); (train) sincerely and ceaselessly, then (you will) enter the door of the large Tao and acquire the secret of heaven. Practice diligently! Practice diligently!

而又運用鉛器，以漸漸疏通其凝滯。在左以順於右，在右以順於左，使左右逢源，氣血充足．焉有寒冷夭喪之患乎？求道者守此妙法，一線串成，至誠無息，則大道入門，天機自得矣，勉之勉之。

In addition to Yin and Yang training involving still meditation and Wai Dan Yi Gin exercises, you must also use the lead equipment to beat your physical body. This will gradually eliminate the stagnation of your Chi and blood circulation. You start on the sides of your body and move to the center. This will lead the Chi and blood to the center and make them abundant.

If you can train your body according to the above methods, how can you be afraid of cold and heat and die at a young age? You must train them continuously and patiently, and one day you will be able to enter the field of the large Tao.

This document makes several important points:
1. The key to maintaining health and strengthening the physical body is to protect your Jieng, raise your Shen, make your Chi and blood abundant, and train your physical body (muscles/tendons and bones).
2. The best training times are: midnight, sunrise, noon, and sunset.
3. You must look for the movement during calmness, and seek the calmness during movement. The trick is learning how to return the Fire and add Water.

3. The Total Thesis of Yi Gin Ching
真本易筋經總論

The translation says: The basic meaning of what the Buddha said was that whoever has advanced himself and verified the results (of Buddhist cultivation), his primary foundations are two: one is Clean and Empty, one is Drop Off and Change.

譯曰：＂佛祖大意，謂登證果者，其初基有二：一曰清虛、一曰脫換。

This document was originally translated by an Indian priest, and later was edited by a Chinese Taoist. Though I believe that some of the translation may be somewhat different from the original meaning, which is hard to avoid because of cultural differences, the general concept is most likely correct.

This first paragraph clearly points out that in order to become a Buddha, you must have two primary foundations. One of them is that your mind must be clean (pure and calm) and empty (of desires and emotional bonds). The other is that you must "drop off" your weak body and change it into a strong one. The cultivation of both the physical and the spiritual body is called "Shing Ming Shuang Shiou" (double cultivation of human body and nature). Therefore, in order to reach the goal of Buddhahood, you must have a strong and healthy body which provides a balanced physical foundation for your spiritual work.

(If) able to be pure and empty, then no barriers. (If) able to drop off and change, then no obstacles. (If) no barriers and obstacles, then able to enter the "steadiness" and exit the "steadiness." Knowing these, then there is a foundation for approaching the Tao. What was meant by clean and empty is Marrow/Brain Washing; by drop off and change is Muscle/Tendon Changing.

能清虛則無障，能脫換則無礙；無障無礙，始可入
定出定矣。知乎此，則進道有其基矣．所云：清虛
者，洗髓是也；脫換者，易筋是也．

If your mind is pure, calm, and free from emotional disturbance, then your spiritual cultivation will not be hindered. If your body can be changed from weak into strong, then you do not have to worry about weakness and sickness of your physical body. Therefore, there is no obstacle to your cultivation. Only when you are able to reach these two requirements will you be able to lead your spiritual mind in and out of the "steadiness." Steadiness means the state of still meditation which is necessary for cultivating the spirit. These are the foundation which you need before you can enter the Tao.

The text of Marrow/Brain Washing says: when a man is born, (he is) touched by emotional desire, resulting in a body with shape. In addition, the viscera, bowels, limbs, and bones are all contaminated by dirtiness, (they) must be washed and cleaned completely until not one tiny spot of defect (remains), then (he) is able to step in the door of transcending worldliness and attaining holiness. Apart from this then, there is no (other) foundation for entering the Tao.

其洗髓之說，謂人之生，感於情欲，一落有形之身
，而臟腑肢骸，悉為渾穢所染，必洗滌淨盡，無一
毫之瑕障，方可步超凡入聖之門．不由此，則進道
無基．

It is believed by the Buddhists that before birth the human spirit was originally pure, clean, and without shape. Once you are born, your mind is affected by emotional desires which shape your physical body. This physical body is contaminated by the dirtiness contained in food and air. In order to enter the domain of holiness, you must first clean your mind and physical body until there is not the slightest bit of contamination remaining.

In order to clean your spiritual body, you must "clean" your brain. Clean means to lead Chi to the brain to nourish it, wash it, and to keep it in a healthy condition. Only in this case will you be able to use your mind to build up an independent spirit and become a Buddha. In order to clean your physical body, you must first clean the blood. Since blood cells are produced in the bone marrow, you must also clean your bone marrow and keep it healthy.

It says: Washing the Marrow/Brain is cleaning internally; changing Muscle/Tendon is strengthening externally. If able to (be) clean and calm internally, strong and firm externally, (then) ascending into the holy city is as easy as turning your palms. Why worry (any more about) the Muscle/Tendon?

所言：洗髓者，欲清其內；易筋者，欲堅其外；如果能內清靜，外堅固，登聖城，在反掌之問耳，何患無筋？

In Shii Soei Ching, Chi is led deep inside your body. Yi Gin Ching is more external, and the results are visible. If you train both ways, you have prepared your whole body, and the further spiritual training for Buddhahood will be as easy as turning over your hand. Once you have reached Buddhahood, you will no longer have any need or interest in training the external part again.

It also says: what is Muscle/Tendon Changing? It is said that when man's body's muscles/tendons and bones (are) formed in the beginning in the embryo, some muscles/tendons are loose, some muscles/tendons are skinny, some muscles/tendons are withered, some muscles/tendons are weak, some muscles/-tendons are slack, some muscles/tendons are strong, some muscles/tendons are stretchable, some muscles/tendons are springy, some muscles/tendons are harmonious, all kinds and not (just) one. All of these are mainly (caused) by embryonic water. If muscles/tendons are loose, then sick; muscles/tendons are tiny, then skinny; muscles/tendons are withered, then weakening; muscles/tendons are weak, then inattentive; muscles/tendons are spasmodic, then dying; muscles/tendons are strong, then powerful; muscles/tendons are stretchable, then extendible; muscles/tendons are springy, then forceful; muscles/tendons are harmonious, then healthy. If one cannot be clean and empty internally and has barriers, as well as cannot be strong and tough externally and has obstacles, how can (he) enter the Tao? Therefore, to enter the Tao, (there is) nothing else but first changing the muscles/tendons to toughen the body, and strengthening

ening the internal to support the external. Otherwise, the Tao is again hard to reach. When talking about the Muscle/Tendon Changing, (the theory of) "change" is marvelous.

且云：易筋者，謂人身之筋骨，由胎稟而受之，有筋弛者、筋攣者、筋靡者、筋弱者、筋縮者、筋壯者、筋舒者、筋勁者，種種不一：大之由胎水，如筋弛則病，筋攣則瘦，筋靡則痿，筋弱則懈，筋縮則亡，筋壯則強，筋舒則長，筋勁則剛，筋和則康；若其人內無清虛而有障，外無堅固而有礙，豈許入道哉？故入道莫先於易筋，以堅其體，壯內以助其外；否則道亦難期；其所宜易筋者，易之為言大矣哉。

This paragraph explains that the many muscles and tendons in our bodies are in many different kinds of condition, and all of these conditions affect our health. The muscles/tendons can be loose, skinny, withered, weak, spasmodic, strong, extensive, springy, or harmonious. The Chinese people believe that all of these conditions originate while still in the womb. The purpose of Yi Gin Ching Chi Kung is to "change" all bad conditions into good ones. Only when you have changed your physical body from weak into strong, and cleaned yourself internally, will you have eliminated the obstacles to your internal cultivation. You can see that "change" is the first step of the real Tao.

"Change" is the Tao (or way) of Yin and Yang. Change is the change of variation. The variations of change exist between Yin and Yang; however, the variation of Yin and Yang, as a matter of fact, (also) exist in man. (Man) is able to handle the sun and moon in the pot, play Yin and Yang on the palms. Thus, when these two are coordinated in man, nothing cannot be changed.

易者，乃陰陽之道也，易即變化之易也：易之變化，雖存乎陰陽；而陰陽之變化，實有存乎人；弄壺中之日月，搏掌上之陰陽。故二豎係之，在人無不可易。

Yin and Yang are the names of the two extremes which everything falls between. It is the nature of everything to change, and so everything is continually moving and changing is the continuum between the two extremes. It is like the universe is a box, and Yin and Yang are the names of the two ends of the box. Everything in the universe is in the box, and is continually moving around, sometimes closer to one end, sometimes closer to the other end. To go deeper into this philosophy, since extreme Yin becomes extreme Yang, and vice versa, you can also say that the box is donut-shaped, like Einstein's concept of the universe, and you can move directly from one end to the other end.

It is the same with the human body. But while the state of the body is continually changing, it is possible for you to control the change. You can control the Yin and Yang (moon and sun) throughout your body, from deep inside your body in the cauldron (pot) where alchemical or spiritual transmutations are completed, to more externally (palm). Sometimes other terms are used for Yin and Yang, such as Kan and Lii, Water and Fire, and lead and mercury. The Taoists used the terms "lead and mercury" when they adjusted the Yin and Yang of the "elixir."

Therefore, (if it is) too void or too full, change it; too cold or too hot, change it; too hard or too soft, change it; too calm or too active, change it. High or low can be changed by rising or sinking; first or latter can be changed by slowing or speeding; smooth or stagnant can be changed by moving around. Danger changed into safety; disorder changed into order; disaster changed into luck; the dead changed into the living; the Chi being numbered (i.e., limited life) can be changed and saved. Heaven and earth can be reversed by change. Then as to man's muscles/tendons, how can't they also be changed?

所以，為虛為實者，易之；為寒為暑者，易之；為剛為柔者，易之；為靜為動者，易之；高下者易其升降，先後者易其緩急，順逆者易其往來，危者易之安，亂者易之治，禍者易之福，亡者易之存，氣數者可以易之挽回，天地者可以易之反覆，何莫非易之功也。至若人之筋骨，豈不可以易之哉。

Usually, the extremes balance each other in the body, so when there is an excess, there is also a deficiency. Therefore, change usually means to bring into balance. This paragraph emphasizes that conditions can be changed. When the Chi is numbered or limited, it is called "Chi Shuu." Generally, when a living thing is healthy and strong, the Chi is abundant and it can live for a long time. Chi production is unlimited, and the Chi cannot be numbered. However, if the living thing is weak or sick, the condition of the Chi is weakening, and the Chi can be numbered. That means that life is also limited. Heaven and earth represent the natural Yang and Yin powers.

However, the muscles/tendons are (related to) man's Ching and Lou. (These channels are located) outside of the bone joints and within the muscles. Four limbs and hundreds of bones, nowhere has no muscles/tendons, (if there is) no Ching, must have Lou. They connect and communicate the entire body, transport and move the blood, and are the external assistance of the Jieng-Shen (spirit of vitality). Just like a man's shoulder is able to carry, hands are able to grab, feet are able to walk, entire body is able to be agile and animated, all because of the functioning of the muscles/tendons. Then how can (we) allow them to degenerate and weaken; and those who are sick and weak, how can they enter the way of the Tao?

然筋人生之經絡也，骨節之外，肌肉之內，四肢百骸，無處非筋，無經非絡，聯絡周身，通行血脉，而為精神之外輔，如人肩之能員，手之能攝，足之能履，通身之活潑靈動者，皆筋之挺然者也，豈可容其弛攣靡弱哉。而病瘦痿懶者，又寧許其入道乎

Just as the muscles/tendons are distributed throughout the entire body, so are the Ching and Lou. The Ching are the twelve primary Chi channels, and the Lou are the millions of small Chi channels branching off from the primary channels out to the surface of the skin and inward into the bone marrow. The Ching and Lou are distributed throughout the body among the muscles and tendons. They are the Chi circuitry which connects the entire body and energizes the muscles and tendons. They are also responsible for transporting the blood and raising up the spirit of vitality. They are so absolutely necessary for life and movement; how could we possibly let them deteriorate?

Buddha used the method to turn around the situation, make the withered muscles able to extend, weak muscles able to change to strong, tensed muscles able to be harmonious, shrunken muscles able to be lengthened, and the degenerating muscles able to be strong. Then even the cotton soft body is able to be made (strong like) metal and stone. (All of these) are nothing but the result of the changing. (This is the source of the) body's benefit, and the foundation of holiness. This is one of the reasons.

佛祖以挽回斡旋之法，俾筋攣者易之以舒，筋弱者易之以強，筋弛者易之以和，筋縮者易之以長，筋靡者易之以壯，即綿弱之身，可以立成鐵石，何是非易之功也，身之利也，聖之基也。此其一端耳。

The Chinese Buddhists consider Da Mo to be a Buddha, and it is to him that the text refers. Da Mo taught people the methods and theory of the Yin and Yang so they could change their physical bodies. Even if your body is soft like cotton, you will be able to make it strong like metal or stone. You must have this strong foundation if you wish to advance in your spiritual studies.

Therefore, Yin and Yang can be held (i.e., controlled) by men. If Yin and Yang are not controlled and are themselves, (then) men will be men. Men (should) not be governed by Yin and Yang, (they should) use the body of blood and Chi and change it into a body of metal and stone. (If) no barriers internally, no obstacles externally, then able to enter steadiness and exit from steadiness. (You must study) the cause of this Kung Fu carefully. Its training has its order, (its) methods include internal and external, Chi must be transported and used, moving has beginning and stop. Even the herbs and the training equipment, the timing, the diet and lifestyle, all generate verification of the training. Those who enter this door, first must firm their confidence, then build their sincerity,

advance firmly and bravely; (while) training follow the method ceaselessly, no one will not be able to promote (himself) to the domain of holiness.

故陰陽為人握也，而陰陽不得自為陰陽，人各成其人也。而人勿為陰陽所羅，以血氣之軀，而易為金石之體。內無障，外無礙，始可入得定去，出得定來。此着功夫，亦非細故也，而功有漸次，法有內外，氣有運用，行有起止，至藥物器制，火候歲年，飲食起居，始終各有徵驗，其入斯門者，務宜先辦信心，次立虔心，奮勇堅往精進，如法行持而不懈，無不立躋於聖域者云。

If you do not know how to control your Yin and Yang, you will remain human forever and never become an immortal. You should use your Chi and blood to change your physical body from weak into strong. That means you must study and train both internally and externally. Only then will you be able to enter the stage of steadiness, which is the necessary path to raising your spirit into enlightenment. All of the training must follow the correct timing and the proper sequence of methods. You must learn how to transport your Chi, and how to use the herbs and training equipment. As you do all of this, the results you achieve will verify whether you have been training correctly. You must train diligently and patiently, otherwise you will never reach the final goal of holiness.

Ban Tsyh Mih Dih said: This thesis discusses the great teacher Da Mo's original meaning of the general concept of Yi Gin. (I) translated it into this article, not daring to add any slightest personal idea, or even create a word.

般刺密諦曰：「此篇就達磨大師本意，言易筋之大概，譯而成文，毫不敢加以臆見、或創造一語。

This document was translated by an Indian Priest Ban Tsyh Mih Dih and edited by the Southern Continent, a traveler of mountain and sea, White Clothes Chang Yeuh-Feng.

This article then goes on to discuss the training methods. We will discuss all of the training methods mentioned in this document in the next chapter. Though this document explains some of the general theory, many points remain vague and unclear. However, if you already have some understanding of Chinese Chi Kung, especially the theory and methods of "change" (Yin and Yang, Water and Fire, Kan and Lii), you will not have any problem understanding this document.

4. Meaning of the Yi Gin Ching
From Harn Fen Lou (Tower of Fragrance)

易筋經意篇

Between the heaven and the earth, only man is most precious. (Man has) five viscera internally, five (sensing) organs externally. If the five (sensing) organs are not governed, the five viscera will be injured. Looking long injures the liver, listening long injures the kidneys, looking too much injures the spleen, and worrying too much injures the heart. Few men know in this world, therefore this classic is offered. (It) is the real achievable training of "five Chis toward the origins."

天地間惟人為貴，內有五臟，外有五官。若五官不治，五臟即傷，久視傷肝，久聽傷腎，多視傷脾，多慮傷心，世人罕知，予得是經，真五氣朝元之功也。

　　Heaven, earth, and man were considered the three most powerful things in nature, and were called collectively "San Tsair," or the "three powers." Of these three, man is considered the most precious. Of the human organs, the five viscera (Yin organs) are considered the most important in Chinese medical and Chi Kung societies. They are the Heart, Liver, Kidneys, Lungs, and Spleen. The Chinese believe that these five organs are linked to the five sense organs: the tongue, eyes, ears, nose, and mouth. Chinese medicine considers the five sense organs the openings of the corresponding internal organs. For this reason, when the five sense organs are not regulated, the internal organs can be injured. However, some of the the examples given in this paragraph do not match the usual Chinese medical relationships. Aside from these anomalies, however, the key point of this paragraph is to emphasize the importance of the correspondence between the internal organs and the sense organs. One of the goals of Chi Kung exercises is to regulate the Chi of the five Yin organs until they have returned to their original healthy state. This training is called "Wuu Chi Chaur Yuan" (five Chis return to their origins). The first step of regulating the five Yin organs is to regulate your five sense organs.

When you start the training, first lie down with the face up to stabilize the Shen, restrain your vision and don't look (at anything), (then) liver Chi will not be wasted. Withdraw ear correspondence and do not listen, the kidney Chi will not be wasted. Breathe smoothly through the nose and don't pant, the lung Chi will not be wasted. Use the hand(s) to massage the stomach area and expand the Chi, (this will) conserve the spleen Chi.

行功之始，先仰臥以定神，含眼光而不視，肝氣莫耗也。收耳韻而莫聽，腎氣莫耗也。勻鼻息而勿喘，肺氣莫耗也。用手撐胃寬大，脾氣莫耗也。

Yi Gin Ching training begins with massage, which is followed with slapping, pounding, beating, and striking. Many of these trainings must be done lying on your back. The first thing you should do is to stabilize your Shen, which has been discussed in the first book of the YMAA Chi Kung series: "The Root of Chinese Chi Kung." Close or half close your eyes to restrain your vision. This will help bring your mind from the outside world into your body and lead your liver into a stage of peace and calmness. Do not pay attention to any noise you hear around you. Simply calm down and pay attention to your body and feel it internally. If you are not listening to anything outside of you, your emotions will not be disturbed and the kidney Chi can be regulated. These two trainings in Chinese meditation are called "Shou Shyh Faan Ting" (withdraw your view and listen internally). In addition to these two, you must also regulate your breathing. When your breathing is regulated, the lungs will be relaxed and the Chi which is converted from the air can be used efficiently. Finally, you should massage your stomach area including your liver, stomach, and spleen. This increases the Chi circulation there and protects these three organs.

This paragraph teaches you how to start Yi Gin Ching massage and beating training. During this training you must first regulate your body, breathing, and mind, and stabilize your Shen. Only then will your mind be able to concentrate on the training and lead the Chi to the area you are training. This is the key to building up internal strength (Nei Juang). Nei Juang training will be discussed later in this chapter.

Keeping the center is the most important, (it) is the way. After massage, then pound. After pounding, then beat. After beating, then strike. Like this for a hundred days of Kung Fu, five Chis all abundant, the Shen condenses and the Jieng is full, (you will be able) to repel sickness and extend the years (of life), never hungry never cold. After completing the training, again train the Conception Vessel in the front and the Governing Vessel in the back until they are full and abundant (of Chi). (This is) the foundation of cultivating into immortality and becoming a Buddha. (If) not cultivating and advancing from these, there is no root for learning the Tao.

守中至要，是為法。揉而後杵，杵而後槌，槌而後打。如是百日工夫，五氣皆足，神凝精滿，却病延年，不饑不寒。再行功完，前任後督，二脈充盈，修仙成佛之基地。不由此而進修，學道無根。

In the massage and beating training, the most important thing is to keep your mind centered at the stomach area. The stomach area is where the Yi Gin Ching training starts, and it is considered to be the "center" of the entire training. You must build up both the internal and external strength here first, and then gradually expand the area until the training covers the entire body. We will discuss the concept of "center" when we talk about massage in the next chapter. During the training, if your mind is not at this center and is placed somewhere else in order to avoid the feeling of pain, then your mind will not be able to build the Chi and strength internally.

In the first year of Yi Gin Ching training, there are four training steps: 1. massaging; 2. pounding or slapping; 3. beating; and 4. striking. Massage will loosen up the stomach area ("center") and allow the Chi to circulate smoothly. Massage can also help to accumulate Chi here. After massage, you slap or pound with the equipment. When slapping or pounding, the power will not penetrate into the deeper layers. The purpose of this step is to build up the Chi, to stimulate the muscles/-tendons, and to toughen the skin. After the skin and muscles/tendons have been stimulated to a high energy state, the pain will be reduced. Then you start to use the heavier equipment. Beating makes the power more penetrating and will build up the strength more internally. After beating, you strike. Striking involves using full power blows even to the vital areas. When you have reached this stage, you will have built the strength both internally and externally. This is the primary stage of "Iron Shirt." After you have strengthened the stomach area, you gradually expand your Chi to a wider area and extend your striking area to the chest to complete the Conception Vessel training, then to the back to complete the Governing Vessel training. Only when you have made the Conception and Governing Vessels full will you have built up the foundation for the Shii Soei Ching training. The abundant Chi accumulated in the Conception and Governing Vessels is considered the "root" of Buddhahood training. Finally, you incorporate the limbs to complete Grand Circulation training. The training procedures will be discussed in detail in the next chapter.

Da Mo traveled to the East to teach these two Yi Gin and Shii Soei classics, (it was) really our great luck. A bird like the crane is able to live long, an animal like the fox can be immortal, a human who cannot learn from these classics is worse than the birds and animals. Obtaining but not training (these two classics) may be caused by suspicion that it is a false creation, or fear the training is too long; (all of these) are generated from oneself. If (you are) able to believe it and train, after three years, (you will see your) bravery becomes like King Shiang's, and your strength though old will be able to conquer Wu Huoh. (Having) strength your entire life, never fearing hunger of cold, winning the bedchamber war, and finding the pearl in the muddy water, (these) are only the smaller uses. Cultivate to be an immortal and become a Buddha, nothing else but this. Those who have the predestined fate and train this will see the results later, then you will see that what I said is not ridiculous.

達磨東來，授此洗髓易經二帙，實吾人之大幸也。夫禽有鶴而能壽，獸有狐而亦仙，世之不得此經者，將禽獸之不若也。得之而不行，或疑其事為虛誕，或畏其功太長久，直自棄耳。若能信而行之，三年以後，將見勇若項王、力邁烏獲，終身堅壯，不畏饑寒，房戰取勝，泥水探珠，猶小用耳。修仙成

佛，要不外是。有緣者行之，自有應驗，彼時始知
予言之不謬也。

It is believed that Da Mo was the one who brought the Yi Gin Ching
and Shii Soei Ching knowledge from India to China. The Chinese
believe that cranes can live a long time because they know how to regulate and train their Chi internally. The Chinese also believe that if even
a fox learned how to train itself, it would be able to achieve immortality.
There are many ancient Chinese stories which tell of how a fox was able
to reach immortality and change into human form.

If the birds and animals are able to reach this goal of cultivation,
why can't people reach it too? The reasons are: lack of confidence and
loss of patience. In this case, men are worse than birds and animals.
If you can train diligently and patiently, after three years you will be
as brave as King Shiang. King Shiang, named Shiang Yu, was a
great warrior who contested the throne of the founding emperor of the
Han dynasty, Liou Ban. Wu Huoh was the chief of a tribe near Tibet
which invaded China often during the Three Kingdoms Period.
Pearls are found in oysters, which live in muddy water. This
metaphor means that you will be able to find valuable results even in
this muddy world. All of these are only small achievements. For the
great achievement, you may use these methods to cultivate yourself
and become an immortal or Buddha.

This article gives you an idea of how to start the training. It clearly
tells you that you will need 100 days of foundation training for
massage, pounding, beating, and striking. To complete the entire
training, you will need at least three years.

5-3. Purposes, Advantages, and Disadvantages

Before we go into the theory of the Yi Gin Ching, we would like to
discuss the purposes of Yi Gin Ching Chi Kung, as well as its advantages and disadvantages. Although we discussed this subject in Part
One, we will cover it now in greater depth. If you have a clear understanding of this art, you will be more confident in your training, and
better able to predict and expect results.

1. Purposes of Yi Gin Ching Chi Kung:

A. To strengthen the physical body and maintain health. This is the
most common goal for most practitioners. Many Chi Kung sets were
based upon the same principles to achieve this same goal, such as
"The Eight Pieces of Brocade" or "Da Mo's Strengthening Chi Kung"
(Da Mo Juang Chi Kung). Most of these sets are purely Wai Dan,
and emphasize building up Chi in the limbs, rather than in the body.
They provide a way for people to strengthen their bodies and maintain their health through simple, specifically designed movements.
They do not require any in-depth, detailed knowledge of how Chi
functions and circulates in the body.

B. To increase the Chi storage and circulation in the Governing and
Conception Vessels (Small Circulation). This is a higher purpose than
the last one. It is Nei Dan Chi Kung, and most practitioners who train
it tend to go on to Grand Circulation The Conception Vessel is responsible for the Yin Chi channels, while the Governing Vessel governs the

Yang channels. Opening and filling these two vessels are the first steps of Nei Dan Chi Kung training.

C. To eliminate stagnation in the twelve primary channels. Once you have filled the Conception and Governing Vessels with Chi, you learn how to lead the Chi to the twelve primary channels, which are related to the twelve organs. When you have reached this stage (called Grand Circulation), practicing will not only strengthen your limbs, it will also improve the condition of your internal organs.

D. To strengthen the Guardian Chi. After you are able to circulate the Chi smoothly in the twelve primary channels, you learn how to expand your Chi from these channels to the surface of your skin, eventually reaching the hair, nails, or even beyond your skin. This strengthens and enlarges your Guardian Chi shield and protects you from any negative influence from the surrounding Chi.

E. To increase martial abilities. Soon after the Yi Gin Ching was taught to the priests, it was applied to the martial arts. Its principles and exercises were used to develop Iron Shirt training, and to train martial artists to use their Chi effectively to energize their muscles to a higher level.

F. To build a firm foundation for Shii Soei Chi Kung practice. In Da Mo's Chi Kung training, Yi Gin Ching is considered the Yang training which emphasizes the physical body and builds up abundant Chi, while Shii Soei Ching is considered the Yin training which uses this Chi to nourish the marrow and brain. These two Chi Kung practices must be balanced. One generates the Chi and the other uses the Chi. One makes the body Yang, the other makes the body Yin. Therefore, in order to train the Shii Soei Ching and reach the final goal of enlightenment, you must first have plenty of Chi, which is obtained through Yi Gin Ching training.

Now that you have a better idea of the general purposes of Yi Gin Ching, you should have some idea as to what you want from your training. Next, we will list some of the advantages and disadvantages of Yi Gin Ching training.

2. Advantages of the Yi Gin Ching:

A. The Yi Gin Ching is easier than the Shii Soei Ching to understand and practice. The theory is simpler and the training is easier, and it is therefore more accessible to the average person.

B. With the Yi Gin Ching, you are able to see results in a short time. Because of this, more people are willing to accept the training.

C. More documents are available and, since the training is more popular, it is relatively easy to find a master. Because the Yi Gin Ching is easier than the Shii Soei Ching to understand and learn, more people have practiced it, more documents have been written about it, and therefore, more people are teaching it.

D. Compared to Shii Soei Ching, Yi Gin Ching training is safer. Because there are more documents available, more people have trained it, and more experiences have been shared with the public. In addition, Yi Gin Ching emphasizes the external physical body and does not directly involve the vital organs, as does the Shii Soei Ching.

3. Disadvantages of the Yi Gin Ching:

A. It is a Yang training. Though health can be gained, increase of longevity is limited. We mentioned earlier that the Yi Gin Ching teaches you how to strengthen your body and build up the Chi internally. All of this effort will lead your body into a Yang state. Although this strengthens your physical body and Guardian Chi, it also causes the body to degenerate faster. To increase the length of your life significantly, you must learn how to use the Shii Soei Ching training to utilize the Chi.

B. It may over-stress the physical body and cause Sann Kung. This is commonplace among martial practitioners of Yi Gin Ching training, because they are trained to lead their Chi to the limbs with heavy breathing. This will energize the muscles effectively, but it also builds up the muscles and over-stresses the lungs. Frequently, the muscles will be over-developed. Unfortunately, when these people get older, their muscles lose their flexibility and elasticity, and degenerate faster than the average person's muscles. This phenomena is called "Sann Kung" (energy dispersion) in martial arts society. In Yi Gin Ching training for health, however, you usually do not place as much emphasis on training your muscles, and this problem is not usually encountered.

You can see that there are more advantages than disadvantages. Furthermore, most of the disadvantages can be controlled easily if you know the theory of the training. It has been proven that Yi Gin Ching training is one of the most effective ways to change the quality of the physical body.

5-4. Wai Dan and Nei Dan Yi Gin Ching

Wai Dan means "external elixir" and Nei Dan means "internal elixir." Wai Dan Chi Kung (often called Wai Dan Kung) and Nei Dan Chi Kung (often called Nei Dan Kung) are the two major categories in Chi Kung practice. Since these two terms have been discussed in the earlier books: "Chi Kung - Health and Martial Arts" and "The Root of Chinese Chi Kung." We will only review their definitions here.

In Wai Dan Chi Kung training, you learn to build up the Chi in the limbs through special exercises, trainings, or treatments, and later you learn to allow the built-up Chi to flow back to your body and organs, thereby nourishing the organs and maintaining smooth Chi circulation. This means that Chi is built up on the surface of the body or in the limbs, and then flows "inward" to the body. Common Wai Dan Chi Kung practices are limb exercises, massage, and acupuncture. Because in Wai Dan you build up the Chi (or elixir) externally, it is called "external elixir."

In Nei Dan Chi Kung, the Chi (elixir) is built up in the body, and then led outward to the extremities. For this reason it is called Nei Dan (internal elixir). Nei Dan practice includes ingesting herbs to generate Chi internally, generating Chi in the Lower and Upper Dan Tiens through various methods, regulating the Fire Chi in the solar plexus, building up and then circulating Chi in the Conception and Governing Vessels (Small Circulation) first and later expanding the Chi to the entire body (Grand Circulation), as well as techniques which lead Chi to the marrow and brain to nourish them (Shii Soei Ching).

According to the available documents, Yi Gin Ching training emphasizes both Wai Dan and Nei Dan equally. When you train Yi Gin Ching, you should not train one and ignore the other. The Wai Dan training is considered Yang, while the Nei Dan is considered Yin. While Wai Dan Yi Gin Ching focuses on training the physical body, the Nei Dan Yi Gin Ching aims at building up Chi. Both of them must cooperate with and balance each other. When one side of the training is neglected, the balance will be lost and problems may occur. For example, many external style martial artists have emphasized only the Wai Dan Yi Gin Ching and have experienced "Sann Kung" (energy dispersion) problems. I believe that in order to avoid making this mistake, you should first understand these two subjects and study their relationship.

1. Wai Dan Yi Gin Ching

The purpose of Wai Dan Yi Gin Ching is to strengthen the physical body, which includes skin, muscles, tendons, fasciae, and bones. Though the health of the internal organs may also be improved significantly by correct training, the organs are not the primary concern. Technically, the training of the organs is handled by Nei Dan training and by the Grand Circulation, which form a combination of Wai Dan and Nei Dan practices. We will discuss this subject later.

In order to reach the goal of strengthening the physical body, many training methods were created. The popular techniques are massage, slapping, pounding, beating, and striking. In addition to these stimulation techniques, many Wai Dan exercises were created which specialize in building up the Chi in the limbs. Often, special training equipment was adapted for these exercise sets.

Normally, the first year of training focuses on the central body area, starting in the stomach area with massage, then gradually using the slapping, pounding, beating, and striking techniques. In this year you must learn Nei Dan Yi Gin Ching, which teaches you how to build up the Chi at the Lower Dan Tien, and later you must circulate it to the Conception and Governing Vessels (Small Circulation). Only after one year, after the center of the body has been trained completely, will the special Wai Dan exercises and muscular training of the limbs be started. This will last for the next two years. In these two years, the Nei Dan practice should teach you to expand the Chi which is built up at the center of the body to the limbs to complete the Grand Circulation.

The above description should give you a clearer picture of the role Wai Dan Yi Gin Ching plays in the training. You can see that the Wai Dan stimulation training described above can energize your body to a higher energy or Yang state.

2. Nei Dan Yi Gin Ching

The purpose of Nei Dan Yi Gin Ching is to build up the Chi internally at the center of the body. Later, this Chi is led to the limbs and the entire body. The reason for this is simple: in order to energize the physical body to a higher energy state for Wai Dan training, the Chi must be full and abundant. The physical body is like a machine and Chi is like electricity. Only when the machine is in good condition and the power supply is sufficient will the machine be able to perform at peak potential. One of the major goals of Yi Gin Ching training is leading the Chi to support the physical body efficiently to maintain and strengthen its health.

Another goal of Nei Dan Yi Gin Ching is to regulate the Chi in the internal organs. When you have completed the Small Circulation, you will have learned how to fill up and smoothly circulate the Chi in the Conception and Governing Vessels. The Conception Vessel is the Chi reservoir which regulates the six Yin organs, while the Governing Vessel is used to regulate the six Yang organs. When the Chi in these two vessels is full and is circulating smoothly, the twelve internal organs will be regulated effectively, and the health of the organs can be maintained and improved. Furthermore, if you have also completed the Grand Circulation, you will be able to lead and circulate the Chi in the twelve primary channels smoothly. In this instance, you may use Wai Dan exercises to enhance the health of the organs.

Usually, the Nei Dan Yi Gin Ching training begins after four months of Wai Dan Yi Gin Ching training. It normally takes three to eight months to complete the Small Circulation. However, it depends on the individual. To understand this thoroughly, you should very carefully study the Nei Dan Yi Gin Ching training, which will be discussed later. After you have completed the Small Circulation, you will start the Grand Circulation, and from there it may take you a short time or forever depending on how deep you want to dig in. When you have reached this stage you will understand that the Chi Kung field is so deep that the deeper you study, the deeper it goes.

Normally, Nei Dan Yi Gin Ching is trained through still meditation. During still meditation, both your physical and mental bodies are relaxed, your mind is calm and peaceful. Consequently, your body tends to be more Yin compared to Wai Dan training. It is only when you are in such a meditative state that you will be able to concentrate your mind on building up the Chi at the Dan Tien and directing it to the desired places.

You should be able to see from this discussion why it is so important to train both Wai Dan and Nei Dan Yi Gin Ching equally. In order to help you settle this in your mind, I conclude with the following important points:

A. Wai Dan training stimulates your physical body and energizes you, therefore it is a Yang training. Nei Dan training deals with the internal Chi field, the body is relaxed, the mind is calm and peaceful, and therefore it is a Yin training.

B. For correct and safe Yi Gin Ching training, Wai Dan and Nei Dan must be mutually coordinated to balance each other.

C. The time required for Wai Dan training is relatively shorter than that for Nei Dan training. Nei Dan training can last forever, especially when this Nei Dan is combined with the Shii Soei Ching training.

D. Wai Dan is easier while Nei Dan is harder in both theory and training.

5-5. Wai Juang and Nei Juang

Before you start your training, you must be acquainted with the terms Wai Juang and Nei Juang. These two terms refer to the results of training. Wai Juang means "external strength" while Nei Juang means "internal strength." When you have Wai Juang, you look muscular and strong externally, but it does not mean that you are strong internally. For example, a bodybuilder may look more muscular and stronger than a professional weightlifter, but he cannot necessarily lift more weight than the professional lifter. Sometimes you find people who are not strong looking, but who are able to express a great deal of strength. This is because the level of muscular strength you can exert depends on how efficiently the Chi can energize the muscles. If a person is able to lead his Chi efficiently to the muscles to energize them to a higher energy state, the power or strength generated will be greater than other people's.

Real strength means strong both externally and internally. Without internal strength, the external strength will not last long, without the external strength, the internal strength will not be able to demonstrate itself efficiently. Naturally, when a person has achieved internal strength, his internal physical body such as the organs are also strong. The internal physical body and the internal Chi are mutually related and benefited.

In Chinese martial society, the mistaken belief is often expressed that Wai Juang is Wai Dan Yi Gin Ching and Nei Juang is Nei Dan Yi Gin Ching. As a matter of fact, although they are closely related they are very different. Strictly speaking, Nei Juang can be generated from both Nei Dan and Wai Dan Yi Gin Ching. Normally, the Nei Juang generated from Wai Dan Yi Gin Ching is a local internal strength supported by the local buildup of Chi, while Nei Dan Yi Gin Ching develops a real internal strength in which the internal Chi can be stored in the Chi reservoirs and stimulated to a higher level.

To help you understand this subject more clearly, we would like to translate a portion of a Yi Gin Ching document concerning the training of Nei Juang. This article will help you to understand what Nei Juang is and why it is necessary for Yi Gin Ching training.

Nei Juang Kung

內壯功

Internal and external are opposites. Strong and weak are opposites. Comparing the strong and the weak, strong is able to last long. Comparing the internal with the external, do not ignore the external. Internal strength is able to be strong, external strength is able to be brave. Strong and also brave is really brave. Brave and also strong is really strong. Strong and brave, brave and strong, then is able to become the body even a million disasters cannot destroy. Then, (it) is the body of the metal steel.

內與外對，壯與衰對；壯與衰較，壯可久也。內與外較，外勿略也。內壯言堅，外壯言勇；堅而能勇，是真勇也．勇而能堅，是真堅也．堅堅勇勇，勇勇堅堅，乃成萬劫不化之身，方是金剛之體矣。

Nei Juang (internal strength) and Wai Juang (external strength), in many ways, are opposite to each other, yet they are mutually related to each other. Nei Juang is Yin and Wai Juang is Yang. Nei Juang relates to the Chi while Wai Juang relates to the physical body. They are like the two sides of your hand. Only when they cooperate and coordinate with each other can they be strong both internally and externally. Internal Chi is the major source of making the external body strong, which enables you to demonstrate your power. When this happens, you will be able to be brave. Brave here means the capacity to demonstrate your power. Only when you can be strong internally and brave externally have you gained a really healthy and strong body which can be like metal and stone. You must train Nei Juang. Without Nei Juang, the Wai Juang will not be strong and will not last.

When training the Nei Juang, there are three rules:
The first says: "Keep the Tao of center."
Keeping the "center" specializes in accumulating Chi. (When) accumulating Chi, concentrate on training (your) eyes, ears, nose, tongue, body, and Yi.

凡煉內壯，其則有三：
一曰："守其中道。"
守中者，專於積氣也；積氣者，專於眼耳鼻舌身意也。

There are three rules when you train Nei Juang. The most important period of training is the first 100 days. During this period, you must learn how to build the Nei Juang foundation to support further training. This article tells you the tricks of reaching this goal.

The first rule is to keep your mind at the center so that you can accumulate Chi there. "Center" means the stomach area between the solar plexus and navel. This area is where the training begins and where the Chi must first accumulate. In order to accumulate Chi in this area, your mind must always be kept there during training. In order to do this, you must restrain your eyesight, stop hearing noise generated outside of your body, not pay attention to smells, forget the sense of taste, relax your body, and control your Yi. If you can do this, your mind will not be attracted to the outside world, and you will be able to concentrate your Yi in the place you are training. Only then are you able to use your Yi to lead the Chi there and start the accumulation.

The most important (thing) when starting training is the marvelous massage, its techniques will be detailed later. When massaging, (you) should undress (the upper body) and lie down facing up. The place where the palm (should be) placed is one palm's width under the chest and above the abdomen. Named the "center." Because this "center" is the place of Chi accumulation, it must be kept (and protected) firmly.

其下手之要，妙於用揉，其法詳後。凡揉之時，宜解襟仰臥，手掌著處，其一掌下胸腹之間，即名曰中。惟此中乃存氣之地，須固守之。

This paragraph has two major points. First, the starting technique for building up Nei Juang is using massage. Second, the location in which the training should be started is between the chest and abdomen. More clearly, it is one palm's width between the solar plexus and navel. This place has been named the "center" because it is where the Chi starts to accumulate. Later, the Chi expands out to the entire body from this center. Because of this, you must learn to concentrate your mind at this center and protect it carefully.

The method of keeping (the center) is to restrain the eyesight, draw in ear correspondence, make the breathing uniform, close the mouth, relax the tired body, lock the swift Yi, do not move the four limbs, (and) one deep mind. First place your mind at the "center" place, later stop all of the miscellaneous thoughts, gradually reach a steady, concentrated mind, is named "keep" (the center). This is the correct way. Wherever the massage is, there (the mind) should be kept. Then, the entire body's Jieng, Chi, and Shen all concentrate there. (Practice) long and long to accumulate, the harmony will be enlarged to the entire area. If there are miscellaneous thoughts and the mind is quick to think of the world's affairs, (even if) Shen and Chi follow but do not condense, then the massage will be in vain, how could it be of benefit?

守之之法，在乎含其眼光，凝其耳韻，勻其鼻息，緘其口氣，逸其身勞，鎖其意馳，四肢不動，一念冥心，先存想其中道，後絕其諸妄念，漸至如一不動，是名曰守，斯為合式，蓋揉在於是，而守在於是。則一身之精氣與神，俱注於是，久久積之，自成其庚方一片矣。設若雜念紛紜，馳想世務，神氣隨之而不凝，則虛其揉矣，何益之有？

This paragraph teaches the methods of keeping your center. During massage training, you must bring your physical and mental body into a meditative state which allows you to isolate yourself from the outside world. Only then will you be able to concentrate your Yi on the training. To keep your Yi at the massage place is the secret of accumulating Chi there.

The second says: "Do not think of other places."
In man's body, Jieng, Shen, Chi, and blood cannot be independent, all listen to the Yi. (When) Yi moves, then (they) move. (When) Yi stops, then (they) stop. When you keep your mind at the center, Yi is placed under the palm. This is the correct way. If (you) allow the Yi to move around on the limbs, the condensed and accumulated Jieng, Chi, and Shen will follow, move, and disperse to the limbs. Then (the training) will become only external strength instead of internal strength. Massage without the accumulation (of Chi), the massage will be in vain. How could (you) obtain benefit?

二曰：「勿他馳想。」
人身之中，精神氣血，不能自主，悉聽於意：意行則行，意止則止。守中之時，意隨掌下，是為合式。若式馳意於各肢，其所凝積精氣與神，隨即走散於各肢，即成外壯而非內壯矣。揉而不積，又虛其揉矣，有何益哉？

The second rule of training is that after your mind has been isolated from the outside world, you should not place your mind anywhere else in your body but at the center. Your Jieng, Chi, and Shen are directed and governed by your Yi; wherever the Yi goes, they go too. Therefore, if your mind moves away from the center during training, you will lead the accumulated Chi to other places and it will never accumulate at the center. For example, if you think of your limbs during massage training, you will lead the accumulated Chi from the center to the limbs and use it. In this case, you might keep the muscles growing; however, you have also stopped the buildup of Chi in the center for future training. In this case, you have built up Wai Juang instead of Nei Juang. In fact, strictly speaking, during the first year of training, the physical Yi Gin Ching exercises are forbidden. If you massage but cannot accumulate the Chi at the center to build up the internal strength, then all of your massage training will be in vain.

Third says: "Use it (Chi) for fullness."
Whenever (you) massage and keep (the center), the Chi therefore accumulates. When the Chi is accumulated, Jieng, Shen, blood, and vessels, all move with it. (When you) keep them, they will not run wild. Massage for a long time, Chi will store within and not overflow. (When) Chi accumulates, the Li will automatically accumulate. (When) Chi is abundant, the Li will automatically be full. This Chi is what Mencius called "the greatest and most unbending, (which) fills up between the heaven and the earth, is our overwhelming Chi." If the Chi has not reached fullness, the mind runs wild away from the center. Dispersed to the four limbs, it is not only that the external strength is not complete, but also the internal strength is not strong. Then both places have gained nothing.

三曰："持其充周。"
凡揉與守，所以積氣，氣既積矣，精神血脉，悉皆附之，守之不馳，揉之且久，氣惟中蘊而不旁溢，氣積而力自積，氣充而力自周，此氣即孟子所謂至大至剛，塞乎天地之間者，是吾浩然之氣也。設未及充周，馳意外走，散於四肢，不惟外壯不全，而內壯亦屬不堅，則兩無是處矣。

After you have accumulated abundant Chi at the center, you can expand this Chi to fill up the entire body. This center is the headquarters and the "center" of Chi supply. You normally need at least 100 days (or 4 months) of training to keep this center and make the Chi accumulate abundantly. During the second 100 days, you learn how to expand this Chi to fill up the front of the body. In the third 100 days, you advance further and expand this Chi to the back. If you have done this, you have made the Chi full in the Conception and Governing Vessels and have completed the Small Circulation. It is not until the second and third years of training that this Chi is expanded to the limbs to complete the Grand Circulation When you have accomplished this, you will feel that your body has filled up with overwhelming Chi which can make you as great and strong as steel. Mencius is a great Chinese scholar and philosopher who lived after Confucius. His famous saying was: "There is a Chi that is the greatest and strongest and fills up between the heaven and the earth called overwhelming Chi." Man is considered a small heaven and earth. If you have completed your Grand Circulation, you will have filled up your body with this overwhelming Chi.

You can see that the center is the most important point in the entire training, and it is the root and source of the training. It is the key to building up the Nei Juang. If you do not follow the above three rules, then you will lose both Nei Juang and Wai Juang.

Ban Tsyh Mih Dih said: When man was just born, originally (the mind) is good (i.e., pure and clean). If attracted by emotional desires and miscellaneous ideas, then all of the original faces (purities) will be wiped out. In addition, (if this pure mind is) divided and damaged by the eyes, ears, nose, tongue, body, and Yi, the wisdom nature at the spiritual center (Lingtai) becomes obscured. Consequently it cannot comprehend the Tao. Therefore, the great teacher Da Mo faced the wall in Shaolin temple for nine years to restrain the desires of the ears and eyes. (If) ears and eyes are not attracted by the desires, the monkey (emotional mind) and the horse (wisdom mind) will automatically be locked and bonded. It resulted that Da Mo was able to acquire the real way (Tao) and return to the West (where Buddha resides), finally ascending to the state of verifying the results (of Tao)(i.e., he became a Buddha). This article was the primary mind and foundation of Da Mo, the Buddha ancestor. The real method (i.e., secret) is in the sentence of "keeping center," and its application (i.e., training methods) is in the "restrain the eye-sight" seventh sentence. If able to train following the methods, then although stupid would be bright, although soft would be strong, the world of extreme happiness will soon be ascended.

般剌蜜諦曰："人之初生，本來原善，若為情慾雜念分去，則本來面目一切抹倒。又為眼耳鼻舌身意分損，靈台蔽其慧性，以致不能悟道。所以達磨大師，面壁少林九載者，是不縱耳目之慾也。耳目不為慾縱，猿馬自被其鎖縛矣。故達磨得斯真法，始能復履西歸，而登正果也。此篇乃達磨佛祖，心印光基，真法在守中一句，其用在含其眼光又句；若能如法行之，則雖愚必明，雖柔必強，極樂世界，可立而登矣。"

Ban Tsyh Mih Dih was a Indian Buddhist priest who translated this document from Indian into Chinese. This paragraph was added by him to summarize this training. First he concluded that when a man is born, his mind is pure and simple. Because this mind becomes contaminated with emotional desires, man cannot comprehend the real "Tao." The wise part of your nature is centered in your Lingtai, which means "spiritual station" or "spiritual center," and is located in the Upper Dan Tien. In acupuncture, there is a cavity which is also named Lingtai, but it is located on the back opposite the heart.

It is said that the Yi Gin Ching and Shii Soei Ching were written by Da Mo after he meditated for nine years facing a wall. The reason he faced the wall was to restrain his eyesight and hearing. When he did this, the emotional mind (ape) and the wisdom mind (horse) were controlled. This is the reason that Da Mo was able to become a Buddha and enter the domain of the West World. West World means India, which is to the west of China. Because Buddhism was imported from India, India was considered the holy world where Buddhas reside. Only those who have attained the real "Tao" will be able to enter this holy world.

Ban Tsyh Mih Dih also points out and re-emphasizes that the trick to Nei Juang training is to keep the center, and the way to reach this goal is in the seventh sentence: "...restrain the eyesight, draw in ear correspondence, make the breathing uniform, close the mouth, relax the tired body, lock the swift Yi, do not move the four limbs, (and) one deep mind."

This document, although entitled "Nei Juang Kung," is the key to successful Yi Gin Ching training. To make sure that it is completely clear to you, we would like to conclude with the following important points:

1. Without Nei Juang (internal strength), Wai Juang training is in vain. Nei Juang is the root of Wai Juang and Wai Juang is the trunk, branches, and flowers. Nei Juang and Wai Juang are mutually related and must mutually cooperate.
2. To build up a real Wai Juang, you must build up Nei Juang first. There are three rules. These rules are: "Keep the center," "Do not think of other places," and "Use Chi for fullness."
3. Among the three rules, "keep the center" is the most important. The way to reach this is to restrain your emotions and desires.
4. Do not train your limbs until you have built up the Nei Juang at the center.

5-6. Iron Shirt and Golden Bell Cover

There are many Chinese people, especially martial artists, who mistakenly believe that the Yi Gin Ching is Iron Shirt and Golden Bell Cover training. In this section we will try to clear up the confusion.

Iron shirt in Chinese is "Tiea Bu Shan" (literally "iron cloth shirt"), and Golden Bell Cover is "Gin Jong Jaw" (literally: "metal/gold bell cover"). The training is so named because after you have completed it, your body will be so strong that most external attacks will not be able to injure you. It is as if you were wearing an iron shirt or were covered by a metal bell. The different names represent different achievements. There are two places which are considered the hardest spots to train. One of them is the eyes and the other is the groin. With proper training, it is possible to draw the testicles up into the abdomen to protect them. When an Iron Shirt practitioner can also lead his Chi to protect his entire head including his eyes, he is said to have achieved Golden Bell Cover. You can see that Golden Bell Cover is a more advanced level of Iron Shirt training.

The main differences between Yi Gin Ching training and Iron Shirt are:

1. Yi Gin Ching was created first. Iron Shirt was developed later by Chinese martial artists to toughen the body. It is based on the training theory and methods of the Yi Gin Ching.
2. Yi Gin Ching was originally created for health purposes, and it was used to strengthen the physical body and build up abundant Chi for the Shii Soei Ching training. Yi Gin Ching training is the first step

to reaching enlightenment or Buddhahood. Iron Shirt training is for martial arts defensive purposes.

3. Yi Gin Ching aims to strengthen the physical body, while Iron Shirt aims to resist external blows. For this reason, the training methods are somewhat different. For example, in Iron Shirt, developing the resistance of the vital areas or cavities is considered important, while the Yi Gin Ching does not consider this seriously.

Iron Shirt training is divided into two major styles: internal Iron Shirt and external Iron Shirt. The main differences are as follows:

1. Internal Iron Shirt training was developed mainly by the internal styles of Chinese martial artists, while external Iron Shirt was trained by the external styles.

2. Because of their different training goals, the training methods are also different. Internal Iron Shirt uses Nei Dan Yi Gin Ching as a major part of the training, while Wai Dan Yi Gin Ching is a minor part. Naturally, the external Iron Shirt training emphasizes Wai Dan Yi Gin Ching training more than the Nei Dan. In other words, internal Iron Shirt emphasizes more the buildup of Chi in the center, while external Iron Shirt training emphasizes the physical body and some local Chi.

3. Internal Iron Shirt training takes much longer to achieve its goals than external Iron Shirt training. It usually takes about three years for external Iron Shirt training, while it may take more than ten years for internal Iron Shirt training.

4. External Iron Shirt training, because it may over-emphasize the muscular training, has the risk of "Sann Kung" (energy dispersion), while there is no such problem in internal Iron Shirt training.

5. Internal Iron Shirt trains the body to be like a fully inflated beach ball, so that when someone punches you, he will bounce backward. External Iron Shirt emphasizes training and toughening the physical body.

Although there are differences between the two Iron Shirt trainings, it is well known in Chinese martial society that regardless of which approach a martial artist takes, by the time he has reached a high level he will have trained both. As with the Yi Gin Ching, you must train both Nei Juang and Wai Juang. A detailed discussion of Iron Shirt will be included in a later YMAA Chi Kung book: "Chi Kung and Martial Arts."

5-7. Training Theory

You may have already concluded a few points about Yi Gin Ching training. The following three are probably the most important:

A. Yi Gin Ching teaches ways to strengthen the physical body. Yi Gin Ching is used as the first step to reach the goal of enlightenment or Buddhahood. The second step is Shii Soei Ching, which trains your spiritual body. The Yi Gin Ching is considered Yang training, while the Shii Soei Ching is Yin training. After you have completed the Yi Gin Ching training, then you can train the Shii Soei Ching.

B. Yi Gin Ching contains Wai Dan training, which is classified as Yang, as well as Nei Dan training, which is Yin. These two must both be trained in coordination with each other.

C. Wai Juang (external strength) and Nei Juang (internal strength) are the goals of the training. Although the main training method for Wai Juang is Wai Dan Yi Gin Ching, Wai Dan is not the only way to achieve it. Similarly, although Nei Dan Yi Gin Ching is the main training method for Nei Juang, it is not the only way to achieve it.

In this section, we will discuss the Yi Gin Ching training theory by dividing it into two major categories: Wai Dan and Nei Dan.

1. Wai Dan Yi Gin Ching

The main purpose of Wai Dan Yi Gin Ching is to strengthen the physical body which includes: skin, muscles, tendons, fasciae, and bones. The basic theory of Wai Dan training is: stimulate and exercise your body until it becomes stronger. Because your body is a living object, **THE MORE YOU TRAIN AND STIMULATE IT, THE MORE IT WILL TUNE ITSELF TO FIT THE NEW SITUATION**. Therefore, the principle of the training is to create a new situation for your body to fit into gradually, and after training for a long time, both your mental and physical bodies will increase in strength as they adapt to the new conditions. Therefore, there are two major areas of adjustment or regulation - your mental body and your physical body.

In Wai Dan you are training the coordination of your mind and the functioning of your body. Since your mind controls your body's movements, you must prepare it and strengthen it if you want a stronger body. When this happens, the stronger Chi can be led by the stronger mind to the part of your body you are training. That is why, during the training, concentration is very important. Your mind must recognize the new situation and try to adjust to it. Then, this prepared mind will lead the Chi to rebuild or adjust your physical body to fit the situation.

In this section, we will discuss the training theory for each part of the body.

A. Skin

The main purpose of the Yi Gin Ching is to increase the strength of the muscles, tendons, fasciae, and bones through stimulation by massage, pounding, beating, and striking. In order to train deeper in the physical body, the power must be able to penetrate through the skin and reach the muscles and bones. If the skin is soft and tender it can be injured easily, and you will not be able to train deep.

Wai Dan skin training involves making soft skin tough. Generally speaking, your skin can be classified as Yin or Yang according to its location. Relatively speaking, Yang skin is more resistant to outside attack than Yin skin. According to acupuncture theory, under the Yang skin are the Yang Chi channels and vessels. Naturally, under the Yin skin are the Yin channels and vessels. For example, the front side of the body and the inner sides of the arms and legs are Yin areas, while the back and the external sides of the arms and legs are Yang areas.

When you train your skin, you want to make the Yin skin tough and Yang skin even tougher. The main trick of this is learning to lead the Chi to the skin to energize the skin tissue. To do this, you need to learn how to expand your Guardian Chi shield and strengthen it. When your skin is energized and the Guardian Chi is strong, you are able to train your skin so that it becomes tougher.

The mind is very important in this, because it is the mind which directs the Chi. While training, you must keep your mind on the area you are training. As your mind gets used to this, and as your concentration improves, you will be able to lead more Chi there to support the training, and you will progress faster.

It is important to remember that, while you want your skin to be able to take the training of the inside of your body, you do not want to sacrifice the sensitivity of the skin, or stagnate the Chi circulation there.

There are many methods of training the skin. However, most of the time, when you train muscles, tendons, and fasciae through different external techniques, you will also be gradually training the skin. For this reason, other than internal mind-Chi training from Nei Dan, there are no special external techniques which are designed only for skin training.

In Nei Dan training, one of the methods of strengthening the Guardian Chi and keeping the Chi circulating smoothly to the skin is to imagine that your body is like a beach ball and to learn how to expand the Chi to the skin through breathing exercises. This training is called "Tii Shyi" (body breathing) or "Fu Shyi" (skin breathing). We will discuss this subject in more detail in the next chapter.

B. Muscles and Tendons

When you train the muscles and tendons, you want to strengthen and develop them, and also increase their endurance and elasticity. The first step is to get rid of the fat which has accumulated in or around the muscles and tendons. Then you learn how to lead the Chi to the muscles and tendons for the training. When you read through the next chapter, you may discover that much of the training is actually just like today's weight lifting training. However, there are some differences. The first one is the mind. In Yi Gin Ching muscle and tendon training, the mind is the most important aspect. Without the concentrated mind, the Chi will not be led effectively to the areas being trained to energize the muscles and tendons. Second, during the training, the muscles and tendons should be as relaxed as possible. If you tense the muscles and tendons intentionally, you will not only slow down the Chi circulation in that area but you will also over-stress and over-develop the muscles and tendons. This will make your body too Yang and make your muscles and tendons lose their natural elasticity, especially when you get old. This is the general symptom of "Sann Kung" (energy dispersion). Therefore, when you are training the muscles and tendons, although some tension is necessary, you should be careful to avoid over-development. The internal (Yin) and external (Yang) must be mutually balanced.

There are many ways of training the muscles and tendons. The common training procedures are: 1. massage, 2. pounding, 3. beating, 4. Wai Dan Chi Kung exercises, and 5. exercises with equipment.

The main purpose of massage is to increase the Chi circulation in the fasciae between the muscles. Massage is also commonly used right after other training to increase the blood and Chi circulation and clear up any stagnation the training may have caused.

When you pound, you use equipment, such as a pestle, to lightly pound the muscles and tendons. This stimulates the muscles and tendons, and gradually builds up their resistance to the pounding. Naturally, you must always concentrate your mind on the area being trained so that the Chi can be led there to support the training.

Beating uses heavier tools so that the power penetrates to a deeper level of the muscles and tendons. Naturally, you must first train yourself with pounding for a long time, then change gradually to beating training.

Wai Dan exercises are the sets of special movements which were designed to train the mind and muscle/tendon coordination. The training teaches you how to lead Chi to the limbs effectively during exercise. These exercises build up the muscles and tendons to the desired state, and increase significantly the power of the muscles. These Wai Dan exercises are very common among Chinese martial artists, who use them to increase their muscular strength both internally and externally.

Exercise with equipment is commonly used to build up the muscles and tendons. Special tools such as the dumbbell and different designs of weights are used. During the training, the mind is concentrated and the muscles and tendons should be kept as relaxed as possible. Generally speaking, the muscles and tendons can be built up faster with equipment than with the simple Wai Dan exercises. However, it is easier to over-build the muscles and tendons and have an energy dispersion problem.

C. Fasciae

Fasciae training is probably the most important key for successful Yi Gin Ching training. Fasciae are everywhere in the body. They are found between the skin and the muscles, between the layers of muscles, and between the bones and the muscles. The main purpose of the fasciae is to permit the smooth movement of adjoining parts of the body such as skin and muscle, the different layers of muscle, and muscle and bone. Without fasciae, you would not be able to move as freely as you do. For example, the muscles which you use to raise your arm are different from those which you use to move the arm to the side. If there were no fasciae between the muscles, each one would interfere with the movement of the other.

Normally, as you exercise more, you will be able to move more easily, and the fat buildup in the fasciae will decrease. It is believed that when there is Chi stagnation in the body, it usually occurs in the fasciae. Therefore, if you want to keep the Chi circulating smoothly you must exercise.

In Yi Gin Ching, the fasciae must be trained. First, you use massage to increase the mobility of the fasciae and get rid of fat and other undesirable residues. You begin by training the stomach, and then expand to the chest, the back, and finally the entire body. Often, the mobility of the fasciae can be increased by simple twisting exercises. The next step is to stimulate the fasciae through pounding and beating to increase the Chi circulation and accumulation there. This training will give your muscles and tendons an internal root, and therefore internal strength (Nei Juang). Theoretically, from the point of view of today's science, the fasciae are made up of materials which are of poor electrical conductivity, while the muscles, tendons, and even bones are of material of higher electrical conductivity. In the Yi Gin Ching Wai Dan training, the fasciae are used like electric capacitors to store charges. Therefore, through special training, the fasciae are able to accumulate an abundance of Chi. This Chi is then used to nourish the muscles, tendons, bones, and skin. In order to help you understand further, we will translate the section of an ancient document which concerns the fasciae training.

The Fasciae Kung
膜功

In a man's body, there are five viscera and six bowels internally, four limbs and hundreds of skeleton bones externally; it (also) has Jieng, Chi, and Shen internally and tendons, bones, and meat (i.e., muscles) externally, and together becomes a complete body. Outside of the viscera and bowels, the tendons and bones are most important; outside of the tendons and bones, muscles are the most important. Within the muscles, blood vessels are most important. The entire body, up and down, moving, shaking, vitally moving, is mastered by the Chi.

夫一人之身，內而五臟六腑，外而四肢百骸，內而
精氣與神，外而筋骨與肉，共成其一身者也。如臟
腑之外，筋骨主之；筋骨之外，肌肉主之；肌肉之
內，血脈主之。周身上下，動搖活潑者，此又主之
於氣也。

This paragraph discusses the parts of the body, from the most internal to the most external. The most internal are the internal organs, because they are most central in the body. Chinese medicine divides them into viscera and bowels, which are respectively Yin and Yang. The five viscera are the heart, lungs, liver, kidneys, and spleen, and the six bowels are the large intestines, small intestines, gall bladder, urinary bladder, stomach, and triple burner. Sometimes the pericardium is also counted as a sixth viscera, but usually it is considered as part of the heart system.

Just as the viscera and bowels are internal, the skeleton and limbs are external. From another point of view, Jieng (Essence), Chi (energy), and Shen (spirit), which are less material, are more internal, while the physical parts, such as bones, tendons, and muscles, are more external. You need all of these parts to be a complete body.

Then it simply states that the viscera and bowels are the most internal parts of the body, that these are enclosed by the bones and tendons, and that these in turn are surrounded by muscles. In each case, the internal parts are more important than the external parts. Inside the muscles, the blood vessels are the most important because they carry blood and Chi throughout the muscles. Every part of the body is enlivened and controlled by the Chi. Without Chi, they remain dead.

Therefore, the achievement of the cultivation and training all (depends on) the mastery of cultivating and nourishing the Chi and blood. Just as heaven generates living things, nothing but follows the interaction of Yin and Yang, and hundreds of lives are born. How can it be different for a man's life! How is there any difference in cultivation!

是故修練之功，全在培養氣血者為大要也。即如天
之生物，莫予隨陰陽之所至，而百物生焉，況於人

生乎！又況乎於修練乎。

Everything you achieve through your internal cultivation and training is accomplished through cultivating and nourishing your Chi and blood. In Chinese medicine, blood is considered Yang while Chi is considered Yin. When both the blood and Chi nourish each other, everything is possible. The interaction of Yin and Yang is fundamental in all occurrences. Heaven functions through the interaction of Yin and Yang, creating all things. Similarly, all things created by this heavenly process also function themselves through the interaction of Yin and Yang. How could we function differently? If we want to change our bodies, we also have to learn how to coordinate our Yin and Yang.

However, Jieng, Chi, and Shen, the things of no shape. Tendons, bones, and meat (i.e., muscles); the body with shape.

且精、氣、神，無形之物也，筋、骨、肉，有形之身也。

Jieng, Chi, and Shen are internal, and without shape or physical substance. They are considered Yin. Tendons, bones, and muscles are external, and have shape and physical substance. They are considered Yang. Only if you cultivate the internal and train the external will you be able to coordinate them to achieve the goal of variation and change.

The method is (you) must first train those with shape to be the collaborators of those with no shape; cultivate those with no shape as the assistants of those with shape. It is one but two, and is two but one. If (you) concentrate on cultivating those with no shape and give up those with shape, it is not possible (to succeed). To concentrate on training those with shape and giving up those with no shape, it is still not possible (to achieve success). Therefore, the body with shape must acquire the shapeless Chi, mutually relying and not opposing, (this will) generate an indestructible body. If (they) oppose and do not rely on (each other), then the ones with shape will also become without shape.

法必先煉有形者為無形之佐，培無形者為有形之輔；是一而二，二而一者也。若專培無形，而棄有形，則不可。專煉有形，而棄無形，則更不可。所以有形之身，必得無形之氣，相倚而不相違，乃成不壞之體。設相違而不相倚，則有形者，亦化而無形矣。

Before discussing the fasciae training, this article again emphasizes that the internal shapeless parts (Jieng, Chi, and Shen) and the external visible parts (tendons, bones, and muscles) must rely on and assist each other. They seem to be totally separate things, but in fact they cannot be separated. This is especially true in training. But the apparent paradox works both ways. They all seem to be one, but they are actually two. If you train only tendons, bones, and muscles, which have shape, then your training will become only Wai Juang (external strength). If you train only Jieng, Chi, and Shen, which have no shape, then your physical body will be weak and the training will not last long. Therefore, the correct way is to train both and learn how to use each to assist the other.

Therefore, to change tendons, (you) must train fasciae. To train fasciae, (you) must train Chi. However, training tendons is easy and training fasciae is hard. (Though) training fasciae is hard, training Chi is even harder. First start from the extremely hard and extremely disorderly place to stabilize the foundation, (then move) toward the place not moving and shaking. Recognize the real method, cultivate the Original Chi, keep the center Chi, protect the righteous Chi, protect the Kidney Chi, nourish the Liver Chi, adjust the Lung Chi, regulate the Spleen Chi, raise the clean Chi, sink the dirty Chi, shut out the evil and unrighteous Chi. Do not be injured by Chi, do not go against Chi, do not worry, grieve, be sad and angry (which will) weaken the Chi; make the Chi clean and (then be) peaceful, peaceful and (then) harmonious, harmonious and (then) smoothly transport; (then Chi) can be transported in the tendons, connect the fasciae, until the entire body agilely moves; nowhere cannot be transported, nowhere cannot be reached. (When) Chi arrives, the fasciae will be raised, (when) Chi is transported then the fasciae expand, able to raise and expand, then fasciae and tendons together will be strong and solid.

是故易筋必須煉膜，煉膜必須煉氣；然而，煉筋易而煉膜難。煉膜難而煉氣更難也。先從極難極亂處立定腳跟後，向不動不搖處，認斯真法，培其元氣，守其中氣，保其正氣，護其腎氣，養其肝氣。調其肺氣，理其脾氣，升其清氣，降其濁氣，閉其邪惡不正之氣；勿傷於氣，勿逆於氣，勿憂思悲怒以頹其氣，使氣清而平，平而和，和而暢達，能行於筋，串於膜，以至通身靈動，無處不行，無處不到；氣至則膜起。氣行則膜張，能起能張，則膜與筋齊堅齊固矣。

This paragraph explains that the secret of Nei Juang is in the training of the fasciae. For example, to change the tendons from weak to strong, you must first train fasciae. Though training fasciae is harder than training the tendons itself, training Chi is even harder than training fasciae. The final target of fasciae training is to be able to lead your Yi to the fasciae and raise, or expand them like a beach ball. When the Chi in the fasciae is full, the tendons can be energized to a stronger state. In this case, the Chi will not be stagnant and weak anymore.

The way to train is to start from the "center" which was mentioned in the previous documents about Nei Juang. You must learn to keep your center, protect the righteous Chi (i.e., Chi which can benefit you), and regulate and nourish the Chi related to the five Yin organs. In addition, you must learn to raise up your clean Chi and sink the dirty Chi generated from the emotional mind. Therefore, you must learn to regulate your emotional mind to control anger, grief, worry, and sadness. Only then can your mental and physical bodies be clean and transparent, and the Chi be transported so that it can reach everywhere you desire.

You can see that in order to train Nei Juang, you must train fasciae. In order to train fasciae, you must train Chi. In order to train Chi, you must regulate your mind. Only when your mind is calm and peaceful can it lead the Chi to the fasciae for the training.

If (you) train tendons without training fasciae, the fasciae cannot be grown. (If you) train fasciae but without training tendons, then the fasciae have nothing to rely on. (If you) train tendons and fasciae but without training Chi, then tendons and fasciae are stagnant and cannot be raised. Train the Chi without training tendons and fasciae, then Chi is impotent and cannot be spread to circulate continuously and smoothly in the Ching and Lou (i.e., Chi channels and branches). (If) Chi cannot circulate continuously and smoothly, then tendons cannot be strong and firm. This is what is said: mutual exchange and mutual application is the Tao of interdependence. Train until the tendons are raised, (then you) must train even harder and must make the fasciae of the entire body raiseable and as strong as the tendons, then it is completed. Otherwise, (even if) tendons are strong (you) will not have the assistance (of Chi). Like if plants do not have (good) soil to cultivate, how can you talk about the completeness of the training.

如煉筋不煉膜，而膜無所生；煉膜不煉筋，而膜無所依；煉筋煉膜，而不煉氣，則筋膜泥而不起。煉氣而不煉筋膜，則氣癡而不能宣達，流串於經絡，氣不能流串，則筋不能堅固，此所謂參互共用，錯綜其道也。俟煉至筋起之後，必宜培加功力，務使周身之膜，皆能騰起，與筋齊堅，始為了當。否則筋堅無助，譬如植物無土培養，豈曰全功也哉。

If you train only tendons, though you will improve the strength of your tendons, you will not build up the abundant Chi necessary for energizing them. To do this you must train your fasciae, which are like a battery for storing Chi. The first step in training fasciae is to make them grow and raise. However, if you train only fasciae without training tendons and muscles, then even if you have an abundant Chi supply, you will have nothing to energize. If you have a machine which is in poor condition, it doesn't matter how good the power supply is, the machine still won't function well. Therefore, in order for your training to be successful, you must have good machines (tendons), batteries (fasciae), and electricity (Chi). All three must be able to support each other before the training can be said to be complete.

I would like to remind you that since tendons are the ends of the muscles, the Chinese will frequently use the words "tendons" or "muscles" to represent both tendons and muscles.

Ban Tsyh Mih Dih said: "This article said, to train Muscle/ Tendon Changing (you) must train fasciae first. To train fasciae, Chi training is the major task. However, these fasciae are not known by many people. They are not the fasciae of the fat but the fasciae of the tendons. The fat fasciae is the material in the empty cavity. Tendon fasciae is the material just outside of the bones. Tendons connect and communicate with the skeleton bones, and fasciae envelop the skeleton bones. (When) tendons are compared with fasciae, fasciae Jing (i.e., strength) is stronger than that of meat (i.e., muscles/tendons). Fasciae are located under the meat and outside of the bones; they are the material used to enwrap the bones and isolate the meat (muscles/tendons). (Because) the situation is like this, (when you) train this Kung, (you) must make the Chi connect between fasciae, protect the bones, strengthen the tendons; combined as one, then it can be said to be a complete training."

般剌密諦曰：此篇言易筋以煉膜為先，煉膜以煉氣為主。然此膜人多不識，不可為脂膜之膜，乃筋膜之膜也。脂膜，腔空中物也。筋膜，骨外物也。筋則聯絡肢骸，膜則包貼骸骨；筋與膜較，膜勁於肉，膜居肉之內，骨之外，包骨襯肉之物也，其狀若此，行此功者，必使氣串於膜間，護其骨，壯其筋，合為一體，乃曰全功。

This is the conclusion by the original translator, the Indian monk Ban Tsyh Mih Dih. In this paragraph, he re-emphasizes the importance of training Chi for fasciae training. Generally speaking, there are three places in your body where you have fasciae. The first place is right under your skin where fat also accumulates. In Yi Gin Ching practice, these fasciae are not as important. Because there is fat stored in these skin fasciae, they are considered to be an "empty cavity" which is not of much use in the training. The second place where you have fasciae is between the muscles. These fasciae are more important and useful for Yi Gin Ching training. It is in these fasciae that you learn to store the Chi for energizing the muscles and building up the physical body. However, the most important place where the fasciae training should be focused is between the bones and muscles. This training is especially important around the joints where most of the tendons can be found. It is these fasciae which can store the Chi for the marrow washing training.

In Yi Gin Ching fasciae training, you train so that the fasciae fill up with Chi, and so that the Chi can communicate and be transported smoothly between the various layers of fasciae. This will keep the Chi from stagnating, and it will connect the bones, tendons, and muscles so that they become one. When you have reached this level, you can say that you have completed the training.

You can see that fasciae training is very important. In fact, it is the foundation and center of the entire Yi Gin Ching training. It is the key to having both Nei Juang and Wai Juang. Normally, the most important period of fasciae training is the first 100 days of Yi Gin Ching training. We will discuss this further in the next chapter.

D. Bones

Bones are like the steel framework of a building. Strong bones make for a strong body. In the Yi Gin Ching, there are two goals in training the bones: first is to strengthen the structure of the bones, and second is to remove all of the causes of Chi stagnation between the Chi channels and the bone marrow. To accomplish this, you need to do certain exercises to increase the strength of the bones, and you must also train the fasciae which envelop the bones and separate the muscles. When these fasciae can be raised and filled up with Chi, the Chi will be able to support the external bone strength training and improve the structure of the bones significantly. However, the most important part of the fasciae training is removing all of the causes of Chi stagnation. This will bring an abundant supply of Chi to nourish the marrow, which will pave the way for Shii Soei Ching training.

Usually, Yi Gin Ching training involves other exercises in addition to the fasciae training for Nei Juang, and special equipment is often required. For example, a simple horse stance will increase the strength of the leg bones, especially the knee joints. Lifting weights will build up the strength of the bones in the arms, especially in the shoulder joints and elbows. Naturally, while training you must concentrate and use your mind to lead Chi to the training area to build up the Nei Juang. There are other places, however, such as the ribs and shins, where the training methods are different. For example, a metal bar or ball will be pressed down and rolled to increase the tension on the ribs. This will stress the ribs and gradually build up their strength. Naturally, the training of the fasciae around the ribs is considered critical for successful training.

2. Nei Dan Yi Gin Ching

Chinese Chi Kung has many practices which are considered Nei Dan. Here we will discuss only the Nei Dan practices related to Yi Gin Ching, specifically Small Circulation and Grand Circulation Although taking herbs orally to increase the body's Chi level is also considered Nei Dan, we will discuss that in a separate section. Before we discuss the training theory, it is very important for you to understand the purposes of these trainings.

A. Purposes of Nei Dan Yi Gin Ching

a. To build up the Chi in the body to an abundant level. This is the first step in Yi Gin Ching training. Normally, the Chi is built up at the Lower Dan Tien, and later it is used to fill up and circulate in the Conception and Governing Vessels. The Conception Vessel is responsible for regulating the Chi in the Yin organs, and the Governing Vessel regulates the Chi level of the Yang organs. In order to keep your Chi circulating smoothly and strongly in the twelve primary channels, you must increase the smooth circulation and storage of Chi in your Conception and Governing Vessels. When you have done this, it is called "Small Circulation." Small

Circulation is the key to the Nei Juang fasciae training, which is the foundation of the Wai Juang body training.

b. To lead the Chi to the extremities. After you have completed the Small Circulation, you learn how to lead the Chi to the limbs, completing the circulation of Chi throughout your whole body. This is called "Grand Circulation." At this stage, you will be able to clear out all of the stagnation in the twelve primary Chi channels, and significantly improve the health of your twelve internal organs. Normally, in the second and third years of Yi Gin Ching training you learn to extend your Chi to the limbs and start your limb Wai Juang training. At this time, Grand Circulation is critical for building up Nei Juang in the limbs.

c. To build up a firm foundation for Shii Soei Ching training. Yi Gin Ching is considered a Yang training, and generates an abundance of Chi, while Shii Soei Ching is considered a Yin training, and it uses the built up Chi to nourish the marrow and brain. If you do not have an abundance of Chi from the Yi Gin Ching Nei Dan training, you will not have enough Chi to support your Shii Soei Ching training.

You can see that the Nei Dan training is the main source of Nei Juang. Without this firm internal foundation, the Yi Gin Ching will remain only Wai Juang, and it will not last long. Next, let us discuss the general theory of Nei Dan Yi Gin Ching.

B. General Theory

Chi is the energy of the body. Without it there is no life. Without sufficient Chi the body cannot grow. In order to maintain the health and strength of the physical body, the Chi must be maintained. In order to make the body grow stronger, the Chi must grow more abundant so that the marrow will be nourished sufficiently to produce healthy blood cells. Blood cells are the main carriers of Chi. Where there is blood, there is Chi. The Chi also helps the cells carry oxygen and nutrients everywhere in the body. Chi is the original source of life and creation.

In order to make your body change from weak to strong, you must first deal with your Chi. Without a good supply of Chi, no matter how hard you train your physical body, all your efforts will be in vain. You therefore need to find the source of Chi, and find out how to increase the quantity and improve the quality.

We now know that the human body has eight Chi vessels, which function like reservoirs to regulate the twelve primary Chi channels. These channels are like rivers which transport Chi to the organs, as well as throughout the body and limbs. In addition, there are millions of small channels which branch out from the twelve primary channels. These small channels are responsible for moving Chi between the organs, to the skin, and to the marrow. The vessels (Mei), primary channels (Ching), and small channels (Lou) form a perfect Chi network to keep the body functioning normally and healthily.

In order to increase the quantity of Chi, you must find its source. It was discovered that Chi has two major sources. One is the food and air you take in. The Chi which comes from this source is considered Fire Chi. The second source is the Original Essence (Yuan Jieng) you inherited from your parents. The Chi converted from this source is considered Water Chi. The researchers examined the quality of food and air, and studied how to increase the efficiency of the conversion of Original

Essence into Chi. Since it is relatively easy to control the quality of food and air, most of the research has been directed at increasing the quantity and improving the quality of Water Chi.

After long years of study and research, it was concluded that in order to increase the quantity of Water Chi, you must imitate the way a baby breathes. When a baby breathes, its abdomen naturally moves in and out. Finally, the Chi Kung practitioners discovered that there is a spot in the lower abdomen which can store an unlimited amount of Chi, once it has been converted from the Original Essence which resides in the Kidneys. The trick of increasing the efficiency of the conversion of Original Essence to Chi is through abdominal exercises.

The spot where the Chi can be accumulated and stored is called "Dan Tien," which means "elixir field." Chinese medicine had also discovered that this is the location of a cavity where Chi could be abundantly produced. They called this cavity "Qihai," which means "Chi ocean." Since the Dan Tien or Qihai is located on the Conception Vessel and is connected with the Governing Vessel, once the Chi is produced it can be stored in these two reservoirs. These two vessels regulate the Chi in the twelve channels, which distribute the Chi to the entire body. The Conception and Governing Vessels are considered the most important of the eight vessels.

Armed with this knowledge, the Chi Kung practitioners researched how to build up the Chi and store it in the vessels. Some of the masters have been able to develop their Chi Kung to a level which is hard for the average person to understand. They concluded that in order to cultivate Chi internally, you must learn how to regulate your body, breathing, mind, Chi, and Shen. Anyone who wishes to enter the field of Nei Dan Chi Kung must train these five regulations.

Da Mo's Nei Dan Yi Gin Ching is probably the most popular training method for building up the Chi internally. It consists mainly of two major trainings: Small Circulation and Grand Circulation In Small Circulation practice, you build up Chi at the Dan Tien, and then circulate it in the Conception and Governing Vessels. Because there is some danger if it is not trained properly, Small Circulation Chi Kung was not taught to every student. Once a student has completed the Small Circulation, he then learns how to lead the Chi to the extremities through the twelve primary Chi channels, which is Grand Circulation.

You may have noticed that in Wai Dan Yi Gin Ching the stomach is considered the "center" of the training, while Nei Dan Yi Gin Ching treats the Dan Tien in the abdomen as the "center." The reason for this is very simple. Wai Dan and Nei Dan Yi Gin Ching, though related, are two independent courses of training. One is Yang and the other is Yin. If they used the same center, the Chi that each one generated would interfere with the other and affect the Chi circulation. It is better if each training builds up Chi in its own center, and later they marry.

Because many of the training theories are related to the training methods, we will discuss them in the next chapter. This subject has also been discussed in the YMAA publication: "Chi Kung - Health and Martial Arts."

5-8. Other Concerns
1. Internal Organs
The internal organs have been mentioned several times with regard to Yi Gin Ching training. The condition of your internal organs is one

of the main factors which decide your health. When you have strong organs you will be healthy, and naturally, if you have weak organs you will be weak and sickly. Therefore, during the course of training you must always consider the condition of your organs, and learn how to strengthen them. It is not uncommon for people who are training heavily to over-stress their bodies and cause failure of the internal organs. For example, if someone who has not run much decides to run twenty miles a day without building up to it, he may suffer a heart attack. It is the same with Yi Gin Ching training. You must build up and strengthen your body gradually. This will allow your internal organs to readjust and rebuild themselves to fit the new conditions.

In the course of Yi Gin Ching training you are strengthening both your physical body and your Chi body. When the Chi has become more abundant, it will flow to the internal organs. This will strengthen them, and cause them to gradually adjust themselves to the increased Chi flow. In order to make the Chi circulate more abundantly in the internal organs, you must first learn how to fill up the Conception and Governing Vessels, and then increase and regulate the Chi in the twelve organ channels.

Another common way to increase the Chi flow in the organs is to massage directly over the organs. There are also many exercises or movements which have been created to help loosen the muscles which surround the internal organs. Researchers have also studied how to use diet and certain herbs to increase or improve Chi circulation. Finally, since your emotions are closely related to the Chi circulation in your organs, you must learn how to regulate your emotional mind. Since some of these subjects have been discussed in the book "The Root of Chinese Chi Kung" and the rest will be discussed in the book "Chi Kung and Health," we will not spend much time on them here.

Herbs

Herbs have been considered an important factor in successful Yi Gin Ching training. Two main categories of herbs are used, one internal, the other external. Generally speaking, the herbs used externally get rid of bruises and increase the Chi circulation near the surface. These herbs are normally cooked in water or wine, and the juice is applied to the skin while it is warm. It is also common to soak the herbs in alcohol for a long time, and apply the alcohol solution to the skin. Massage is normally used to increase the effectiveness of the herbs. These herbs are usually poisonous, and should not be taken internally or applied to the skin when it is broken.

The internal herbs have two major purposes. The first one is to get rid of internal bruises and Chi stagnation caused by the training. The second one is to increase the quantity of the Chi, which will significantly help the Nei Juang training. Normally, if you are careful, internal injuries such as bruises will not occur. However, if somehow you have injured yourself internally, perhaps causing bruises on the inside of the ribs, then herbs must be taken internally to get rid of it. Chinese martial artists found that eating raw onions and dried Chinese radish (turnip) will often get rid of internal bruises. Naturally, eating too much of them might also be bad.

During the course of our discussion of Yi Gin Ching and Shii Soei Ching we will occasionally recommend herbal prescriptions to assist in your training. These prescriptions will be listed and briefly explained in Appendix A.

Chapter 6

Yi Gin Ching Chi Kung Training

Now that you have read the last chapter, you know the "what" and the "why" of Yi Gin Ching Chi Kung. In this chapter, we will discuss the "how." I would like to remind you that during the course of training you should always ponder and combine the theory and training; in this way, you will not become filled with doubt and lose the confidence necessary for your training. Only then will you be able to learn from the past and create for the future. Remember: it is our obligation to preserve these treasures and to continue to study and research them in a modern, scientific manner.

In the first six sections of this chapter we will discuss the important rules of training, who can train, training keys, when to train, Wai Dan training, and Nei Dan training. The seventh section will summarize the training schedule, and the last two sections will discuss a number of other related subjects.

6-1. Important Training Rules

In order to avoid injury, there are some rules which you must obey. Most of these rules are conclusions drawn from past experience. During the course of training, you should always keep them in mind.

1. It is harmful to stop midway during the training. You start with raising the fasciae through massage, pounding, beating, and striking. After they are raised, you learn how to fill up the fasciae with Chi. If you stop before you are able to complete this, the over-stressed fasciae will decay quickly, and it will be hard for them to return to their original state. It is like a balloon. After it has been inflated for a while, once you let the air out it will not return to its original elastic state. Once you start fasciae training, you must learn the techniques for keeping the fasciae filled with Chi. If you cannot do this, the fasciae will not be able to function as they originally did because they will have been injured by the training.

2. Always know "what" and "why." This will help you build your confidence, lead you to the right path, and stop your confusion and wandering. Confusion and wandering are always the main obstacles to training. If you know "what" and "why" you will not doubt, and your confidence and perseverance can be fortified.

3. Always train from easiest to hardest. Training the easy parts will give you the experience to understand the hard parts, and, most important of all, enable your body to adjust and fit the training gradually. This is the way to avoid injuries.

4. Always train from light to heavy. When you train Wai Dan Yi Gin Ching, one of the exercises involves massaging and beating the body. In this training, you should start with light power and gradually use heavier power. Naturally, in selecting the tools for the training you should start with the light ones and gradually use the heavier ones. Impatient training will only harm your body and slow your progress. One of the documents has a paragraph about massage and beating power:

Light and Heavy in Training
練功輕重法

When you start training, light (power) should be mainly used. Must use children, their strength is adequate. After one month, the Chi is gradually abundant, must use a stronger person, gradually increasing the power. Then, it is harmonious and proper. Must not (massage) too heavily and cause the raising of Fire. Must not move around and cause skin injury. Be careful, be careful.

初行功時，以輕為主，必須童子，其力平也。一月之後，其氣漸盛，須有力者，漸漸加重，乃為合宜；切勿太重，以致動火；切勿游移，或致傷皮；慎之慎之。

This paragraph explains that when you start your training, you should use children to do the massage because they do not have strong power. Later, after your body has gradually built up its strength through the training, then you should gradually increase the training power. If you do not follow this rule, you may make your body over-react and consequently raise the fire (become too Yang). In addition, you should protect your skin well because once it is injured, you cannot continue your training until it is healed.

5. Always train from shallow to deep. In Wai Dan Yi Gin Ching training, when you stimulate your physical body through massage, beating, or rolling, you should control your power and start at the skin. Over a period of time, you gradually start to penetrate with the power until you reach the muscles, fasciae, and bones. A section of the document discusses this:

Shallow and Deep in Training

練功淺深法

At the beginning of training, use massage, because (the power) is shallow. Gradually increase the (massage) power, because the Chi is getting stronger. Then, increase to heavy power, (however) still shallow. The next exercise uses pounding, then can be deep. Next use beating. Though beating still belongs to the shallow, however, the vibration caused internally belongs to the deep. Only (when) both internal and external are strong, then you have achieved (the result).

初功用擇，取其淺也；漸次加力，是因氣堅；稍為增重，仍是淺也；次功用搗，方取其深；再次用打，打外雖尚屬淺，而震入於內則屬深，俾內外皆堅，方為有得。

In the beginning of your training you use massage because the power does not penetrate far. Only after the strength of your internal Chi is built through concentration do you start the pounding training, which is more penetrating. Internal Chi (Nei Chi) is the Chi which is generated from the mind's concentration. External Chi (Wai Chi) is generated by external physical stimulation. Normally, Nei Chi comes from Nei Dan training while Wai Chi comes from Wai Dan training. Wai Chi is able to build up Wai Juang while Nei Chi is capable of strengthening Nei Juang. As the external stimulation gets stronger, the Nei Juang must also be stronger in order to resist the external stimulation. Both external and internal must be balanced and coordinating harmoniously. When you use beating or striking, although the power of the beating is still shallow, the vibration they cause can penetrate very deeply into the body

6. Always keep the training center. The Nei Dan Yi Gin Ching is different from the Wai Dan Yi Gin Ching in that you start your Chi build up and circulation internally, and gradually expand to the extremities. In Nei Dan Yi Gin Ching, the Lower Dan Tien is treated as the "center" where the Chi is built and accumulated. However, in Wai Dan Yi Gin Ching, your stomach is the "center" where your training starts. When the internal Chi is full and abundant you can gradually extend it to the chest, the back, and finally to the limbs. This training order is extremely important. It builds the Chi foundation in your body instead of in your limbs. When the Chi is built in your body it can be full and strong in the two main Chi vessels.

7. Always know the condition of your body. Don't practice when your Chi circulation is not normal. Abnormal Chi circulation may be caused by sickness, weakness, exhaustion, or emotional disturbances such as anger or extreme joy. The first 100 days of training are the most critical. In this period, while you are building up Chi at your "center," you should abstain from sex, otherwise you will lose the Chi you have accumulated. After 100 days, you should regulate your sexual life. You should also remember that you should not practice 24 hours before or after sexual activity. Many ancient documents state that you should

not practice three days before and four days after sex. I personally believe that some light training 24 hours before or after should not be too harmful. You should not practice when your stomach is full or when you are hungry. You should not practice right after drinking alcohol. You should keep away from drugs and smoking.

8. Be aware of what injuries are possible, and avoid them. This is especially important in Nei Dan, because it is possible to seriously injure yourself. Understand the theory completely, and train cautiously.

9. Do not abuse herbs. Frequently, people will start using herbs before they understand how they should be used. This can be dangerous, especially those herbs which are taken internally. Generally speaking, herbs used externally are safer than those taken internally. Herbs should only be used as prescribed by a qualified herbalist. Most minor injuries can be healed by the body itself.

10. Follow the training schedule. Do not speed up your training, because this will only harm you, and it won't help you. The condition of your body must be improved gradually. This takes time and patience. Those who wish to complete both Yi Gin Ching and Shii Soei Ching training should not start Shii Soei Ching until they have completed at least one year of Yi Gin Ching training. We will discuss this subject in Part Three.

There are a number of other general rules for Chi Kung training, which are discussed in "The Root of Chinese Chi Kung." We recommend that you read that volume before you study this book.

6-2. Who Can Train?

In this section we will discuss what kinds of people can train, and the advantages and disadvantages of training at different ages.

You must understand that in order to complete the training, you must first have enough knowledge, time, will, patience, and money. Once you decide to train, it is very important to make the commitment to finish the training, and to arrange your life so that you can finish the training. If you do not finish the program, or if you stop and start several times, you will damage the elasticity of the fasciae. Success comes from training regularly. Each day you make a little bit of progress, and each day's bit of progress builds on the previous day's. If you miss a day, you must extend the training two more days in order to make it up.

Will, patience, and endurance are the first keys to success. In order to see if you are qualified to do the training, give yourself a test first. The test is very simple: meditate at least 40 minutes once in the early morning and once in the late evening every day for at least six months. These are two of the best times for Yi Gin Ching training. Yi Gin Ching requires at least three years of continuous training every day. If you cannot even meditate for six months every day continuously, mentally and spiritually you are not ready for the training. If you were to train you would only harm your body.

You can see that it is very hard for people to train today. Every day we have to busy ourselves making money so that we can survive. If your mind is always worrying about making a living, how can you stabilize it for the training? This is why time and money are the next critical requirements for the training.

Another question you may ask is: is the training restricted to men, or may women train also? As you look through the training you will see that there is no part that women cannot do. However, since ancient times most of the practitioners of Yi Gin Ching and Shii Soei Ching have been men, almost all of the documents we have are written for men. If a woman wishes to train these arts, she will have to make a few adaptations, but if she understands the concept of the training she should have no trouble. Remember: the basic theory and principles remain the same.

The next question we will discuss is: what is the best age for training Yi Gin Ching? This is a popular subject of controversy in Chinese Chi Kung society. However, if you think carefully, the answer will become clear to you. Let us discuss this subject by considering three different age groups: from 14 to 18, from 19 to 30, and from 31 to 45.

We will not discuss training under 14 years of age or over 45, because under the age of fourteen, the physical body of the child is still weak, and the training will affect his or her normal growth; and when you are over forty-five, your muscles have already begun to deteriorate. This does not mean that people in these two age groups cannot participate in Yi Gin Ching training. They can, but they must be very careful, and know exactly what can be trained and what cannot be trained. Some training may be harmful to them. However, if they practice correctly, they will still be able to complete the training.

1. Age 14 to 18:
Advantages:
A. At this age, the physical body is growing fast. Hormone production is high, the Chi is strong and Yang is growing. Guardian Chi is easily strengthened.
B. Because Chi is strong and circulates smoothly at this age, any training injury will heal easily.
C. Because the physical body is growing, the training will tune the body as it grows. Since the body is growing into the training, the effect of the training will last longer.

Disadvantages:
A. Is is harder for them to understand and feel the Chi, and they do not have the patience for Nei Dan Yi Gin Ching training. Therefore, it is easy to achieve good results with the Wai Juang, but more difficult with the Nei Juang.
B. Once they have built their Wai Juang, if they do not train Nei Juang by the age of thirty, they will not achieve a high level of success, and energy dispersion may occur.
C. People of this age usually have weak wills and little perseverance. It is also much harder for them to control their sex drives.

To conclude, people in this age group can usually build the Wai Juang more easily, but is is harder for them to build Nei Juang.

2. Age 19 to 30:
Advantages:
A. The physical body of this group is matured, and the physical body and Guardian Chi are at their peak. Wai Juang training can be very effective, and good result can be expected.

B. Because their minds are more mature, they are more patient and it is easier for them to understand the training theory - especially the Nei Juang part. Therefore, the Nei Dan training can be coordinated harmoniously with the Wai Dan training.

Disadvantages:

A. People in this age group are creating their careers. They are busy and their time is limited. Time limitation is the main obstacle for this group.

B. At this age, people get heavily involved in social life, and many will get married. Because of this, their minds are not steady and are harder to regulate. It is also hard to abstain from sex for the duration of the training.

3. Age 31 to 45:

Advantages:

A. At this age, the career is established and the mind is more steady. This is the best group for Nei Dan training. Relatively speaking, the people in this group have stronger wills, more patience, and know what they want, and they are therefore not as confused as younger people.

B. Because of their age, they have more experience in life and their thinking is more mature. They usually understand the entire training much better than the people in the other two groups.

Disadvantages:

A. Although they have strong will, patience, steadier minds, and more extensive knowledge, their bodies, unfortunately, are not in the best condition. Their bodies are degenerating, and they are weaker than the other two groups. It is hard for them to achieve a high level of Wai Juang training.

B. Much of the time of this age group it tied up with their families.

These conclusions are general, and do not necessarily apply to any individual. Everyone has his own problems, and many disadvantages can be turned to advantages if you know how. The final conclusion is that Yi Gin Ching can be trained by anybody if he knows the "how" and "why" of the training, and if he learns to adjust his life to fit the training.

6-3. Keys to Training

Though some of these keys have been discuss in the first part of this book in the section on Kan and Lii adjustment, we would like to review them here to refresh your memory, and also add to them.

1. Internal and External Must Mutually Cooperate

In the last chapter we explained that in order to make your physical body strong, you need both external strength and internal energy support. It is like a ball which needs strong skin and air. Therefore, even in the Wai Dan Yi Gin Ching training, your mind must play a key role during the training process. Your mind must concentrate on the area being trained so that the Chi is led effectively there to energize it. You have to coordinate internal and external in order to have Wai Juang and Nei Juang, and to balance Yin and Yang.

2. Breathing Coordination

Breathing is the key and the strategy to any Chi Kung training. When you exhale, you are able to expand your Guardian Chi, leading it to the skin and even beyond. This also enables you to energize the muscles and tendons to a higher energy state. When you inhale, you allow power to penetrate into the depths of your body. Exhalation is considered Yang and inhalation is considered Yin. In Wai Dan Yi Gin Ching, you are training different depths of the muscles and tendons. Your breathing becomes, therefore, the vital key which allows you to control how deeply external force penetrates your body. If your mind and breathing are not coordinated, you will build up only Wai Juang.

3. Yi and Chi Cooperate

As mentioned, your Yi must play an important role in Wai Dan Yi Gin Ching training. Only if you can do this will you be able to lead Chi to the areas you are training to build up the Nei Juang. Not only that, when you train Wai Juang through external stimulation such as massage, beating, rolling, or exercise, the Chi will build up locally. You must use your mind to feel it, understand it, and, most important of all, learn to use it in combination with the Chi generated from the Nei Dan training. You can see that Yi and Chi must unite and become one. This exercise is called "Yi Chi Shiang Her" which means "Yi and Chi combine."

4. Shen and Chi Cooperate

Of the many people who have diligently trained Yi Gin Ching, some have seen quick progress while others progressed only slowly. What is the reason for this disparity? In addition to Chi, breathing, and correct technique, one of the most important factors is Shen. According to Chinese Chi Kung theory, Shen is the headquarters which governs the Chi. Since Yi Gin Ching is a Chi Kung training, this Chi headquarters is one of the main keys to successful practice. When Shen is raised, the Chi can be vigorous and circulate fluidly, and the Yi will be alert. Under these conditions, you will be able to feel and sense things which other people cannot. As a result, you will understand your training more deeply than other people, and your training will be faster and more effective.

5. Yin and Yang Coordinate

One of the main concerns of Chinese Chi Kung is how to adjust the Yin and Yang during training. Although Yin and Yang are not exactly the same as Kan and Lii, Yin is commonly compared to Water (Kan), lead, or the dragon, while Yang is commonly compared to Fire (Lii), mercury, or the tiger. When Yin and Yang interact properly, millions of variations can be generated. Therefore, you must learn how to adjust your Yin and Yang in the Chi Kung exercises. For example, Wai Dan Yi Gin Ching is considered Yang, while Nei Dan Yi Gin Ching is Yin. You must learn both and coordinate them properly in order to balance them. Certain parts of the Yi Gin Ching documents discuss Yin and Yang, or Water and Fire. We discussed one of these parts in the second section of the last chapter, and would like to look at another one here which is concerned with massage training techniques.

The Method of Balancing Yin and Yang in Yi Gin Ching Training

練功配合陰陽法

The Heaven and the Earth (are) one large Yin and Yang. Yin and Yang mutually interact, then millions of lives are born. Man's body (is) a small Yin and Yang. (When) Yin and Yang mutually interact, then hundreds of sicknesses are repelled. (When) Yin and Yang are mutually applied, Chi and blood will be mutually harmonized. Naturally (you) will not have sickness. (If) there is no sickness, there is strength. Its reason is clear.

天地一大陰陽也，陰陽相交，而後萬物生；人身一小陰陽也，陰陽相交，而後百病却；陰陽互用，氣血交融，自然無病，無病則壯，其理分明。

Man is considered a small heaven and earth. The head is called heaven while the lower abdomen is called the earth. If you know how to coordinate and balance Yin and Yang smoothly and harmoniously, then you will not get sick.

However, when (you) train this Kung (i.e., Yi Gin Ching), it also borrows the meaning of the Yin and Yang's mutual interaction and steals the original tricks of millions of objects in Heaven and Earth. This is the way to repel sickness.

然行此功，亦借陰陽交互之義，盜天地萬物之元機也，如此却病。

This paragraph explains that when you train Yi Gin Ching, you must also learn how to borrow the method of causing Yin and Yang to interact, and the trick of how to balance them. In other words, you must learn how to adjust your Kan and Lii.

Whoever's body is weak in Yang, mostly has illnesses of withering, weakness, feebleness, and fatigue, should use a young girl, following the methods of massage. It is because the woman is Yin externally and Yang internally. Borrow her Yang to help my weakness. This is the natural way.

凡人身中其陽衰者，多患痿弱虛憊之疾，宜用童子少婦，依法擇之；蓋以女子外陰而內陽，借取其陽，以助我之衰，自然之理也。

This paragraph talks about the massage training in Yi Gin Ching when a man's Yang is weak, either because he is old, or because, though young, his body is weak. The trick of balancing Yin and Yang here is to be massaged by a young girl. It is believed that women look weak and Yin externally, however, they are Yang and strong internally. When you are massaged by a young girl, you are able to borrow her Yang to nourish your Yin internally.

One who is strong in Yang and weak in Yin has mostly fire illnesses. You should use a young boy. It is because a man is Yang externally and Yin internally. Borrowing his Yin to suppress my Yang's abundance is also the original trick.

若陽盛陰衰者，多患火病，宜用童子少男：蓋以男子外陽而內陰，借取其陰，以制我之陽盛，亦是元機。

Yang can be strong because of sickness or youth. When Yang is strong, Yin is relatively weak. Normally, if you are not sick, your Yang is strong from the teens to around thirty. When the body is excessively Yang it is very energized and the mind is not steady. You lose your temper and get excited easily, and are impatient and uneasy. If you are like this, you should use a young boy to do the massage. The reason for this is just the reverse of the last paragraph. Males look strong and Yang externally, but they are Yin internally. Therefore, if you are massaged by a young boy, you may use his Yin to balance your Yang. To use a partner to balance the Yin and Yang in Chi Kung training is called "mutual cultivation" (Shuang Shiou).

As to those who are not sick, when training this Kung (Yi Gin Ching), then follow as convenient. If able to use a young boy and a juvenile girl to massage alternately, enabling Yin and Yang to flow smoothly, it is even more marvelous.

至於無病之人，行此功者，則從其便，若用童男少女，相間揉之，令其陰陽各暢，行之更妙。

However, those who are healthy, and whose Yin and Yang is already balanced, should try to be massaged alternately by a young boy and a girl. This will maintain the balance and harmony of Yin and Yang.

6-4. When to Train

Generally speaking, the spring is the best time of year for a beginner to start Yi Gin Ching training. There are several reasons for this:

1. In the spring, your body is gradually changing from Yin to Yang. Your body is growing stronger and stronger in Yang, so this is the best time to build up the Chi internally from both Wai Dan and Nei Dan Yi Gin Ching.

2. Yi Gin Ching training involves massaging and beating yourself, and you have to partially disrobe to do this. In the winter time, since your body and the surrounding air are Yin, you may catch cold, even though you are indoors. However, once spring comes, this is no longer a problem.

3. In the spring, the Chi and blood circulation in the body becomes stronger, more abundant, and more active. This reduces the chance of injury, and speeds up recovery when you do suffer an injury.

It is not recommended that you start in the Summer, because the environment is too Yang and your body has also adjusted to Yang. A beginner who starts at this time will find that it is too easy to build up too much Fire, which can cause problems. Theoretically, if you know how to adjust Kan and Lii skillfully, Fall is good for Nei Dan training. However, for a beginner who cannot feel or sense his body's Yin and Yang and does not know how to adjust Kan and Lii, the Nei Dan training may cause him to become too Yin.

Now let us consider the best times of day to train. In the document "Yi Gin Ching Training Secret," which was translated in the last chapter, there is a section which explains this clearly. It says:

The Tao (way) of building the foundation, begin at Tzy (midnight), Wuu (noon), between Tzy-Wuu (sunrise); or begin at Wuu-Tzy (sunset) when the variations are many, the Yin and Yang are exchanging, mutually turning and cooperating. If able (to train) day and night ceaselessly, not even a second ignored, then Heaven and man can unite. When trained for seven-seven (49 days), Chi and blood will be sufficient and abundant. When trained for ten-ten (100 days), immortality can be gradually achieved.

You can see that there are four times when it is most beneficial and advantageous to train: midnight, noon, dawn, and sunset. These four times allow you to take advantage of the change of Yin and Yang. Chi in the human body is influenced by natural timing, such as the seasons of the year and the time of day. If your body's Yin and Yang cannot follow the changes of nature smoothly, you will tend to become sick and your body will degenerate more quickly. Your body is part of nature and must fit into it smoothly and harmoniously. Most Chi Kung masters prefer to train at these four times which enable you to change your Yin and Yang in accordance with nature. It is also advisable for Yi Gin Ching. However, once you have built up a strong foundation, then you may train any time you wish.

In fact, very few Wai Dan Yi Gin Ching practitioners train four times a day. Normally, they skip the midnight practice to allow the body time to recover from the training. Another reason for this is that your body is extremely Yin at midnight. This means that your Guardian Chi is at its weakest, and it is easy for you to injure yourself. However, some practitioners claim that the midnight training is the most important. Their reasoning is this: since your body is the most Yin at that time, if you train right, the increase in strength will be greater than that of any other of the three times. It is interesting to note that in Shii Soei Ching Chi Kung, the midnight training is the most important one. We will discuss this subject further in Part Three.

You can see from the quoted paragraph that if you train for 49 days, Chi and blood will be abundant, and if you train for 100 days, you will have built the foundation for reaching Buddhahood. It is said: "Bae Ryh Jwu Ji," which means "hundred days to build the foundation." Therefore, in the first 100 days of training you must sleep well, eat nutritious meals, and most important of all, stop sexual activity completely. It is in these 100 days that you build up the Nei Juang Chi, which determines whether you will be successful in your training. If you follow the training schedule, you have a very good chance of completing the Yi Gin Ching training.

6-5. Wai Dan Yi Gin Ching Training
1. Training Equipment:

There are several documents which explain how to make the training equipment used in Wai Dan Yi Gin Ching. However, if you understand the training theory, you may design your own equipment out of materials which are more convenient or even better. For example, in ancient times many tools were made from lead, simply because lead was more available and easy to melt. However, because of the danger of lead poisoning, these tools had to be treated with herbs according to a special method before they could be used. Nowadays, you may find materials already made of stainless steel which can serve the same purposes as well or even better. In my opinion, it is easier and better to use the available implements rather than try to make equipment according to the ancient way. Therefore, we will only recommend some of the methods to make the tools. You are encouraged to design them in ways which fit your training better.

A. Rubber Ball:

A rubber ball is not very hard, but when it is pressed against the skin, the power is penetrating. You can press and roll the ball with your palm on different places such as stomach, ribs, joints, legs, or arms. This is the first step in training the skin and muscles/tendons near the skin to respond to external power. This training can also toughen the skin.

In ancient times, rubber balls weren't available, and they used a ball made from cotton thread. Different size balls were made to fit in the different areas. For example, the size of ball used to roll on the stomach is different from the size used for the ribs (Figures 6-1 and 6-2). On the ribs, a small ball is used to reach the spaces between the bones. Normally, ball rolling techniques are used in conjunction with massage.

B. Metal Ball:

A metal ball serves the same purpose as a rubber ball, but goes one step beyond. A metal ball is much harder, so when it is pressed

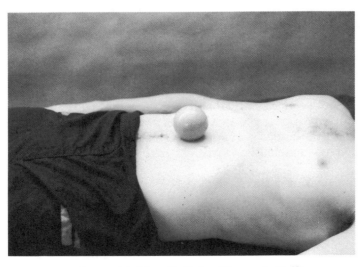

Figure 6-1. Large Rubber Ball for Stomach Rolling

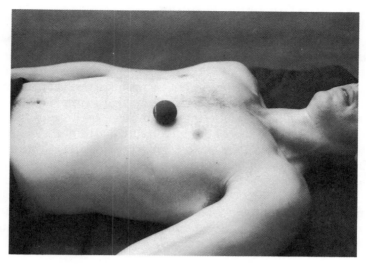

Figure 6-2. Small Rubber Ball for Rib Rolling

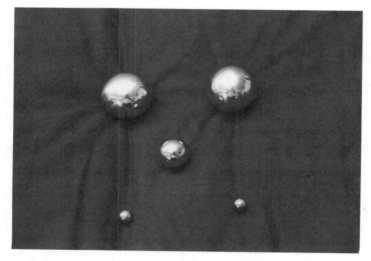

Figure 6-3. Different Sizes of Metal Balls

the power is even more penetrating than that of a rubber ball. Naturally, you must first train with the rubber ball before you begin with a metal ball. In traditional training, wooden balls were used as a bridge between the thread ball and the metal ball.

In ancient times, the metal balls was made of lead. Today, you may buy different sizes of stainless steel balls from industrial supply stores. They are clean and will not rust (Figure 6-3).

C. Wooden or Metal Bar:

After you complete the training with the metal balls, you start training with round wooden or metal bars (Figure 6-4). While metal balls focus on a small area, wooden or metal bars connect all these small areas and create a larger, stronger area. When this larger area is trained, the Chi can be built up more abundantly.

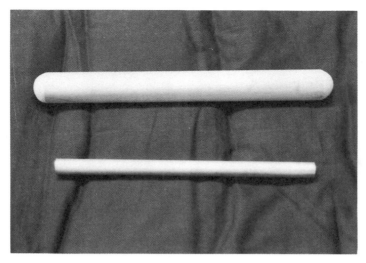

Figure 6-4. Round Bars for Rolling

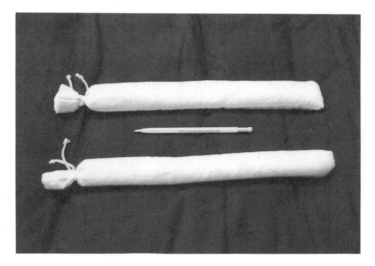

Figure 6-5. Different Sizes of Training Bags

Naturally, for different areas, different sizes of bars are used.

D. Metal Sand Bag:
The metal sand bag is used to slap the body, especially the rib area. By slapping the body, you learn to energize your muscles and fasciae with Chi and bounce the sand bag away instantly. Make several strong, long bags of different sizes, and fill them with small pieces of metal (Figure 6-5). Regular sand is often used instead of lead pellets. You slap your body with these bags, using different size bags for different areas.

E. Ball Bearing Bag:
The ball bearing bag follows the same principle as the metal sand bag, except that now the bag is filled with ball bearings (Figure 6-6). Often, round pebbles from the bottom of a stream would be used

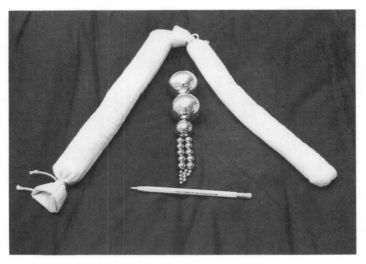

Figure 6-6. Different Sizes of Balls and Bag

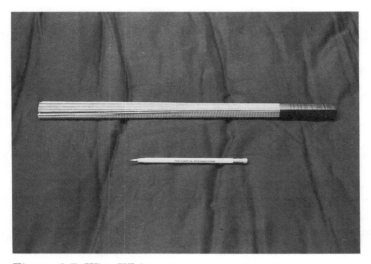

Figure 6-7. Wire Whip

instead of metal balls. It is believed that pebbles from a stream bed are more Yin and therefore more suitable for training. The size of the ball bearings can vary from very small, the size of BBs, to as large as ping-pong balls. This bag is heavier, and will train your Chi to be stronger and build up the bouncing capability of the muscles.

F. Wire Whip:

After training the body with the ball bearing bag, you then strike the entire body with a whip made of a bundle of wires. This helps to bring the Chi built up internally to the skin, and therefore increases the Chi supply or nourishment to the skin. In ancient times, the whip was usually made of bamboo or rattan. Nowadays, many Yi Gin Ching practitioners have discovered that a bundle of stainless steel wires serves the purpose much better (Figure 6-7). Three major reasons are: 1. a bundle of stainless steel wires is heavier than bamboo, and so their power is more penetrating; 2. stainless steel wires are more flexible and have a springier, more bouncing power than bamboo or rattan; 3. it lasts longer.

G. Pestle:

A "pestle" is commonly used to raise up the fasciae through pounding stimulation. It also develops the bouncing power of the muscles, which is necessary for martial arts iron shirt training. The pestle is made from heavy red oak or similar wood (Figure 6-8). Start with the most muscular areas and move gradually to the less muscular areas.

H. Mallet:

The soft areas of the body are pounded with a mallet to raise the fasciae (Figure 6-9). This is usually done after the massage training is half completed. You can buy a rubber hammer in a hardware store which may work even better.

I. Metal Disk:

Metal disks have two uses. First, because the disk is heavy, it can be used for weight training to build up and strengthen the muscles, tendons, joints, and bones. Heavier disks can be used as the training proceeds. Second, the disk can be used to grind and toughen the skin for Iron Shirt training. The traditional Metal Disk was shaped like a discus, but you may simply use the weights from a barbell set (Figure 6-10).

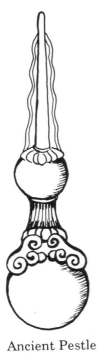

Ancient Pestle

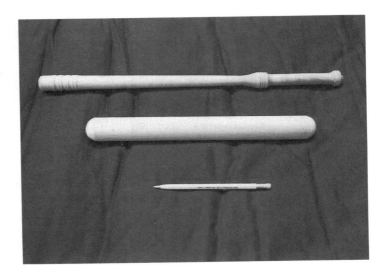

Figure 6-8. Pestle and Wood Bar

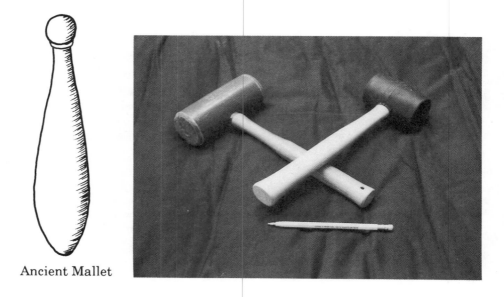

Ancient Mallet

Figure 6-9. Rubber and Wood Hammers

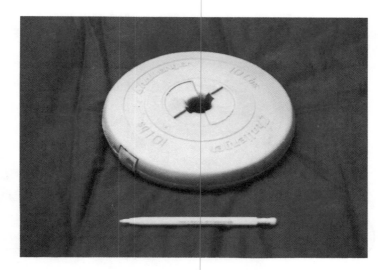

Figure 6-10. Weight from a Barbell Set

J. Metal Hammer:

The metal hammer is not used for beating exercises. It is used for weight training to build up and strengthen the muscles, tendons, joints, and bones. You can imagine that there are many ways to train with the hammer.

The above discussion is meant to give you an idea of the training equipment used. Once you understand the training, you are encouraged to design your own equipment.

2. Training Techniques
A. Massage

The Chinese character for massage is made up of two words, "soft" and "hand." This indicates that it is most important for your massage techniques to be soft. The reason for this is very simple. When a person who is being massaged feels strong, hard power against his body, he tenses up his muscles and also becomes mentally resistant. He will not be able to concentrate on the training, and the effectiveness of the training will also be decreased because of the tension.

Massage is one of the first stages of Yi Gin Ching training, and it is especially crucial during the first 100 days. Massage is started in the stomach area, which is the "center" of the training, and as the training progresses, it is expanded to cover a wider area. There are several purposes for the massage training.

a. To loosen up the fasciae between the skin and muscles, between the layers of muscle, and between the muscles and bones.

b. To get rid of fat accumulated in the fasciae.

c. To resume and increase the Chi and blood circulation in the fasciae.

d. To fill up the fasciae with Chi. Using the mind to lead the Chi to the fasciae during the massage and beating training is the key to building up Nei Juang.

e. To eliminate any bruises and Chi stagnation caused by the training.

When you massage, you should progress from soft to hard and from shallow to deep. There are many ways to massage in Chinese Chi Kung. However, in Yi Gin Ching training, the common way is to use the palm of one hand (Figure 6-11) or both hands (Figure 6-12) to push or circle the massaged area. Normally, using two palms lasts longer and the power is more penetrating. This is simply because when you use two hands, each hand needs less power than if it were being used alone. Using two hands lets the massage be softer, so your partner will be more relaxed and the power will penetrate deeper.

There are a number of techniques typically used in Yi Gin Ching massage. You should experience them carefully. After you have trained for some time, you will have enough experience to discover

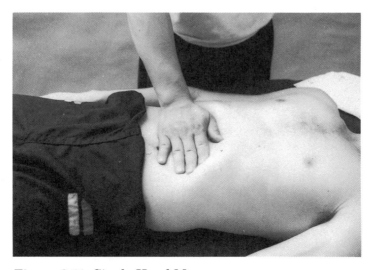

Figure 6-11. Single Hand Massage

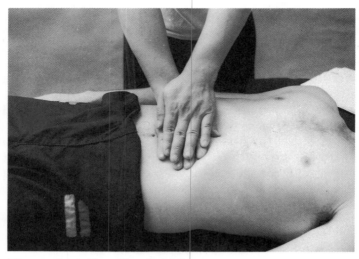

Figure 6-12. Two Handed Massage

other massage techniques which might also be effective. Remember, **WHEN YOU MASSAGE YOUR PARTNER, YOU ARE NOT ONLY SERVING. YOU ARE ALSO LEARNING**. When you massage someone, you learn about the structure of the human body, you experience the level of power which can be used for different areas, and you learn how to feel and sense the Chi built up by your partner from the training. Therefore, when you are massaging someone, you should be patient, concentrated, and always concerned with your partner's feeling. **ONLY WHEN YOUR PARTNER IS ABLE TO COOPERATE WITH YOUR MASSAGE WILL IT BECOME EFFECTIVE**.

Naturally, when you are being massaged, you should be relaxed and concentrate your mind on your partner's palm. **REMEMBER, YOUR MIND LEADS THE CHI TO THE MASSAGED AREA TO BUILD UP INTERNAL STRENGTH**. If you cannot do this, your training will be external strength only. Furthermore, when you concentrate, you will be able to feel, sense, and understand your body's condition more clearly. Before we continue to discuss the techniques of massage, we would first like to translate one of the sections about massage found in the documents.

The Massage Kung

揉功

The application of massage is to Mo Li the tendons and bones. Mo Li is what is called massage. Its methods have three sections and each section (includes) one hundreds days.

夫揉之為用，意在磨礪其筋骨也。磨礪者，即揉之謂也。其法有三段，每段百日。

Mo Li in Chinese means to sharpen, to toughen, to train, and to harden. It is just like you are sharpening a knife. It takes a long time and patience. The final purpose of massage training is to toughen the tendons and bones. However, it must start first from massaging fasciae. Only when the fasciae are raised and filled up with Chi can this Chi be used to toughen the tendons and bones. Then the training has achieved both Nei Juang and Wai Juang.

First says: Massage must have seasons.
If starting training in the early spring months, during the training (you) may catch a spring cold. It is hard to be naked, can only be undressed on the top. Must start training in the middle of the second month (Western calendar: March or April) when the weather is gradually warm, then you will be able to expose your body for the training. (When) it is gradually warm, (the Chi and blood) transport more easily and smoothly during the training.

一曰："捑有節候。"
如春月起功。功行之時，恐有春寒，難以裸體，祇可解襟；須行於二月中旬取天氣漸和，方能現身用功；漸暖乃為通便，任意可行也。

You should start training in the springtime when the weather is reasonably warm. This way you will not catch a cold. Also, at this time your body is changing from Yin to Yang, so your Chi and blood are starting to circulate more abundantly and smoothly. The Chinese year usually begins in February or March, so the second month is March or April.

Second Says: Massage must follow the fixed methods.
Man's entire body, Chi right, blood left. When massaging, the proper method starts from the body's right and pushes to the left. It is to push the Chi to the blood and make them combine harmoniously. In addition, the stomach is located on the right, massaging (the right) makes it possible to enlarge the stomach, enabling it to admit more air. Furthermore, for the massager, the right hand is more powerful, can be used without tiring easily.

二曰："捑有定式。"
人之一身，右氣左血；凡捑之法，宜從身右推向於左，是取推氣入於血分，令其通和；又取胃居於右，捑令胃寬，能多納氣；又取捑者，右掌有力，用而不勞。

In this paragraph are several points which I question or disagree with. The first one is that Chi is on the right side of the body and blood is on the left. However, according to the distribution of the Chi channels, I believe that Chi and blood in both sides should be at least almost equal and balanced. The second is that it says the stomach is on the right side of the body. However, if you look in an anatomy book, you will see that the stomach is actually more on the left side. The third is that the stomach can be enlarged from massage.

Despite this, I believe that the technique is correct since it was developed from experience rather than theory. Personally, I believe that the reason you massage from the right to the left is to follow the path of the intestines, which is also how the Chi moves internally.

Third says: Massage must have proper power and depth.
The massage methods, though done by men, should follow the methods of heavenly meaning (nature). Living things in heaven and earth, gradual and orderly without suddenness, then Chi is generated automatically. (When the time is) ripe, the things will be formed. Massage should imitate this method. Use the method of push and shake around, slowly to and fro, not heavy and not deep. Long and long (the result) automatically obtained. This is harmony and the right way. If (massage is) too heavy, the skin will be injured. Then infection and disease can be generated. (If massage is) too deep, then it injures the ligaments, bones, tendons, and fasciae. The hot swelling will be generated (internally). (You) must be careful.

三曰：" 揉宜輕淺。"
凡揉之法，雖曰人功，宜法天義。天地生物，漸次
不驟，氣至自生，候至物成，揉當法之，但取推盪
，徐徐來往，勿重勿深，久久自得，是為合式 (適)
；設令太重，必傷皮膚，恐生瘢痏；深則傷於肌骨
筋膜，恐生熱腫，不可不慎。

This paragraph makes two important points. First, your massage must start with light power and gradually become heavier. This is the natural way that all living things grow. Incorrect massage can cause injuries both externally and internally. The second point concerns the techniques of massage: push and shake around. Push can be a straight line or a circular motion. However, when you shake around, your palm adheres to the skin and vibrates gently.

Even though this article discusses several important points concerning massage techniques, there are still many unclear details which need to be discussed. We will now discuss the massage techniques which should be used for different areas.

a. Stomach:

The stomach area is considered the "center" of the training. This "center" area covers the space below the solar plexus and above the navel (Figure 6-13). Your massage training must start here. Normally, if you train three times every day, you need at least 100 days for this area.

There are three common massage methods: straight push, circular motion, and firm shake. When you are doing the straight pushing massage, you push from the right side to the left (Figure 6-14). When you are doing the circular massage, you should move clockwise to follow the large intestines (Figure 6-15). This will smooth out the Chi movement in the body.

In traditional Yi Gin Ching training, you massage this area for 90 minutes (the time it takes two sticks of incense to burn) each day at

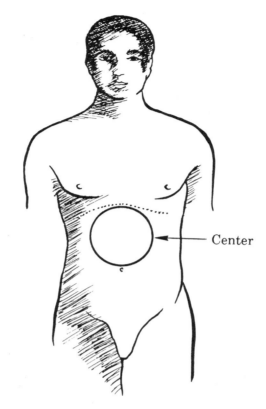

Figure 6-13. "Center" for Massage

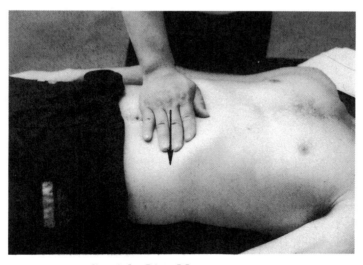

Figure 6-14. Straight Line Massage

dawn, noon, sunset, and midnight. If you cannot do it four times a day, you should keep at least the dawn and sunset training. Naturally, if you do this, the training period will be longer.

b. Ribs and Back:

After you have massaged the stomach area for 100 days, the Chi will be abundant and full. You will need another 200 days of training to extend

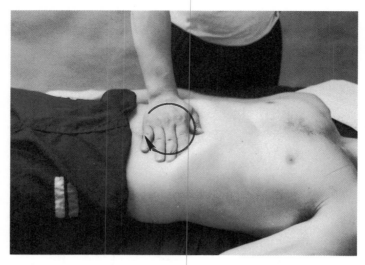

Figure 6-15. Circular Massage

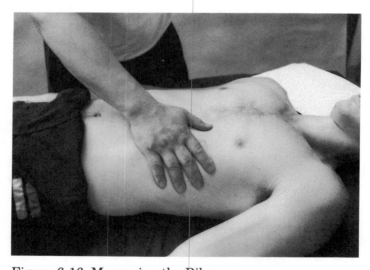

Figure 6-16. Massaging the Ribs

the Chi to the ribs both in the front of your body and the back. This will also start to fill up the Chi in the Conception and Governing Vessels.

The massage techniques for the ribs are somewhat different from those used for the stomach because you are dealing with bones beneath a thin layer of muscle.

Generally, you use straight pushing and circular techniques. The only difference is that you place your fingers in the spaces between the ribs so that your power can penetrate into them (Figure 6-16).

When you massage the lower back, you should follow the spine, pushing downward, and also push from the sides of the back to the center to nourish the Governing Vessel (Figure 6-17). When you use circular massage, circle counterclockwise (Figure 6-18).

c. Limbs:

After you have trained for at least 300 days and have completed the body, you will then extend your Chi to the limbs. Massage is not

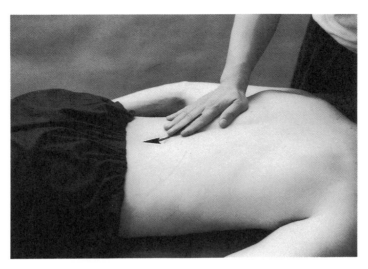

Figure 6-17. Massaging the Back

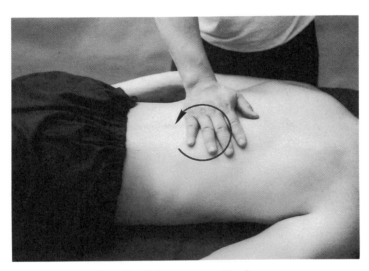

Figure 6-18. Circular Massage on Back

usually used to increase the quantity of Chi in the limbs in Yi Gin Ching. However, massage is commonly used to smooth and increase the Chi and blood circulation. Frequently, Chi and blood will accumulate and become stagnant during the training of the limbs. Massage is the main way to take care of this problem.

Straight pushing, following the fiber of the muscles from the body to the ends of limbs, is the main massage technique for the limb muscles (Figure 6-19). However, use a circular motion around the joints (Figure 6-20).

B. Rolling

Rolling is the use of different sizes of balls and bars to roll on the body with different pressures. This enables you to gradually build internal resistance to external attack. Heavy rolling training usually is not started until after 100 days of massage. The training usually

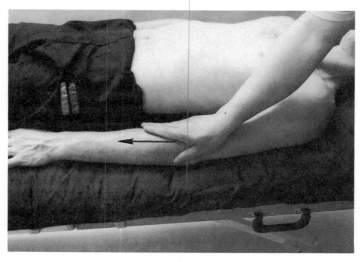

Figure 6-19. Massaging the Arm

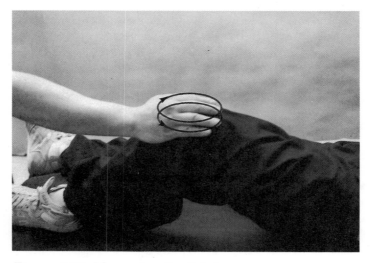

Figure 6-20. Massaging the Joints

starts in the body, and when you have completed 300 days of massage training, it is expanded to the limbs and joints.

To do this training, you or your partner press down on a ball or round bar and roll it on your body. The power will penetrate into the body, and reach into areas where other equipment cannot, such as between the ribs.

Ball rolling can be in a straight line or circular. Straight line is commonly used on the ribs and limbs (Figure 6-21), while the circular motion is usually used on the stomach (Figure 6-22).

C. Slapping

In this training, you slap your body with different size bags filled with various sizes of ball bearings, from BBs to ping-pong ball size (Figure 6-23). You gradually start slapping after 100 days of massage training. Start slapping lightly with the small BBs, and gradually increase the

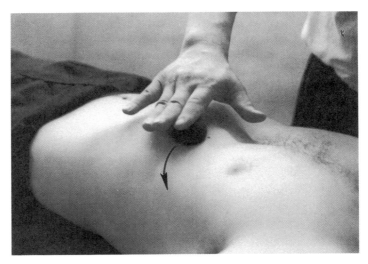

Figure 6-21. Rolling the Small Rubber Ball on the Ribs

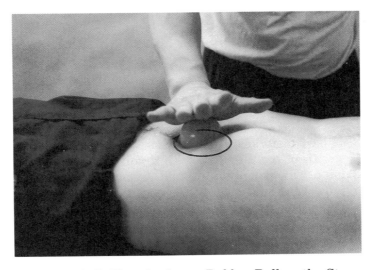

Figure 6-22. Rolling the Large Rubber Ball on the Stomach

force and the size of the bearings. Work on the body for the first 300 days of massage training, and then gradually expand out to the limbs. At the instant when the bag hits your skin, concentrate your mind on the area so the Chi moves there and energizes it, and increases the resistance.

D. Pounding and Beating

In pounding, you use a wooden mallet or similar tool to hit the muscular areas of the body, including the stomach, abdomen, waist, ribs, and ends of the ribs. This raises the fasciae. This is moderately heavy training, and should be started after 100 days of massage. Gradually increase the striking power, and later switch to beating training.

In beating, you usually use a whip made of a bunch of wires, though sometimes a solid metal bar is used. This training stiffens the muscles, tendons, and bones. It normally does not start until about 200 days of massage are completed. Since the beating power is more penetrating,

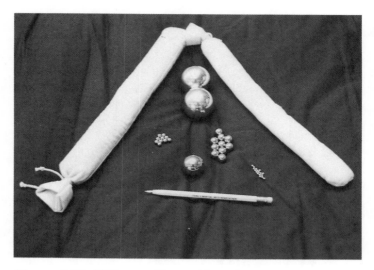

Figure 6-23. Different Sizes of Metal Balls

you must learn to lead your Chi more effectively until your internal strength is able to bounce the force away.

E. Striking

Striking training is very important for those martial artists who train Yi Gin Gin for Iron Shirt or Golden Bell Cover. In striking training, you strike your body with tools or your fists, using Jing (jerking power) so that the power enters deeper into the body. Usually, the vibration from this kind of striking makes the power reach the bone. Because the tools are made of hard materials, you cannot strike the bones or joints directly. Instead, you train the fasciae, muscles, and tendons. You start your training in the body, using your internal strength to generate a protective shield to protect the vital areas and bounce the attack away. Start with the non-vital areas, and gradually include the vital cavities. Normally, the student should be trained in this stage by a master who understands the student's capacity and can control his power.

F. Exercises

Yi Gin Ching also includes a number of Wai Dan exercise sets to train the student to use his Yi to lead Chi to the limbs to energize the muscles. Usually, these exercises are not practiced until a student has completed his first 300 days of massage and beating training. After 300 days of training the body, the student will normally develop Grand Circulation and start to train the limbs. Many different training sets were created over the last fourteen hundred years. We will introduce two of the most common sets, the fist set and the palm set, when we discuss the training of Wai Dan Grand Circulation. Other sets specifically designed for Iron Shirt training will be discussed in a later volume of this series: "Chi Kung and the Martial Arts."

6-6. Nei Dan Yi Gin Ching Training

There are many categories of Chi Kung training which are classified as Nei Dan. Theoretically, any Chi Kung practice which generates the elixir (Chi) in the body and later spreads it out to the limbs is called Nei Dan (internal elixir). Common Nei Dan practices are taking herbs internally to generate the Chi, Shii Soei Ching, and the Small Chi Circulation continuing on to the Grand Chi Circulation, which is a part of Yi Gin Ching.

In this section we will only discuss the Small Circulation and Grand Circulation, which are the major part of the training in Nei Dan Yi Gin Ching. The Shii Soei Ching will be discussed in Part Three. Although Kan and Lii Wind Chi path training is often considered part of the Small Circulation training, there are actually many other types of Chi Kung which train Kan and Lii even without completing the Small Circulation.

Small Circulation is called "Sheau Jou Tian" in Chinese, which means literally "Small Cycle Heaven" (Small Heavenly Cycle). In Chinese medical and Chi Kung society, outside of the human body there is heaven and the earth. Within the human body there is also a heaven and an earth. The head is called heaven and the lower abdomen is called earth (the Huiyin cavity is called "Hae Dii," which means "Bottom of the Sea"). When Yin and Yang interact between heaven and earth, millions of variations happen, and life is created. It is the same within a human body. When Yin and Yang interact harmoniously, the life force is generated, and health and long life can be obtained. Small Circulation is the first step in leading Yin and Yang Chi together for harmonious interaction.

Grand Circulation in Chinese is "Da Jou Tian," which means literally "Grand Cycle Heaven" (Grand Heavenly Cycle). When Chi can be expanded to the limbs, the field of the small heaven and earth is enlarged and becomes the grand heaven and earth. That is why the Chi circulation to the limbs is called Grand Circulation.

Before we discuss the Small and the Grand Circulation, you should first understand a few things:

1. There are many other non-Yi Gin Ching Chi Kung styles which also train Small and Grand Circulation. Since the major concern of any Nei Dan training is to fill up Chi in the Conception and Governing Vessels and learn how to distribute it to the twelve primary Chi channels, there were many Chi Kung styles which already had the training before the Yi Gin Ching was created.

2. Nei Dan is not the only way that Small and Grand Circulation can be achieved. In fact, many external martial artists have accomplished it simply from Wai Dan training, for example, the Wai Dan training of the Yi Gin Ching.

3. Because Small and Grand Circulation are an important part of Chinese Chi Kung, many Nei Dan training methods have been created. Despite their differences, however, the goal and theory remain the same. In my opinion, none of the methods is clearly superior to any of the others. The most important factor in successful training remains how much the practitioner understands the training theory and how much he is able to practice.

4. Small and Grand Circulation are considered the root of internal Chi, which is needed for the Nei Juang training in Yi Gin Ching. Many Chi Kung practitioners believe that only through Nei Dan Small and Grand Circulation training is one able to reach the higher levels of achievement and to build up a really firm foundation of internal Chi. Doing this involves regulating the body, breathing, mind, Chi, and Shen.

The following song about Small and Grand Circulation is also called the "Oral Secret of Nei Juang." Sometimes it is also called "Ban Tsyh Mih Dih" after the Indian monk who created it.

Song of Transporting Heavenly Circulation

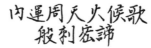

Yi Gin Ching is the secret of training Chi. (Let me) discriminate it clearly and tell you in detail. The ancestral teacher passed down this method of strengthening the body. Before midnight and after noon, you should not make a mistake. Stabilize your Chi and condense Shen to lock the emotional mind monkey. Two hands hold each other, and sit down with crossed legs. Recognize the primary source of pre-birth Tai Chi. This place is the way of enlivening the body.

易筋經，煉氣訣，分明仔細與君説，祖師留下壯身法，子前午後君休錯，定氣凝神鎖心猿，兩手搯抱趺足坐，識得先天太極初，此處便是生身路。

Heavenly circulation generally means Small Circulation. The ancestral teacher refers to Da Mo. This section of the song says that you should train the Small Circulation before midnight and after noon. It is believed that before midnight your body is reaching the extreme of Yin, so if you meditate then you will be able to maintain your Chi and keep your body from becoming too Yin (deficient). This will help you to smooth out the transition of your body from Yin to Yang at midnight. When you meditate after noon, your body is just passing the time of extreme Yang. If you meditate then, you will be able to cool down your Fire Chi faster than would happen naturally. This will prevent your body from getting too Yang. One of the main goals of Chi Kung training is to adjust your Water and Fire and maintain the Yin-Yang balance of your body as much as possible. The two times mentioned are the most important for this.

When you train, you should condense your Shen so that you will be able to control your emotional mind, which is often compared to an ape that keeps running wild. The correct posture for practice is sitting with the legs crossed and the hands folded in front of the abdomen. The Lower Dan Tien is the primary source of your life and the primary origin of Tai Chi (the interaction of Yin and Yang). The work of reinvigorating your body begins there.

Close the eyes and regulate the breathing, millions of linkages are empty. All of the thoughts are gone and (you) belong to the clean land. Chi penetrates the entire heaven and reaches the cold ground. No matter if (the spirit) exits and enters within one breath. An ocean of Chi rolls and a thousand layers of waves. This Kan Water (Water Chi) is able to cross and enter the North. The river can reverse, transport upward to Kuen Luen. White cloud toward the head and the sweet dew is generated.

瞑目調息萬緣空，念念俱無歸淨土，氣透通天徹地寒，無出無入一吸間，海氣滾滾浪千層，撞入北方坎水渡，河車逆運上崑崙，白雲朝頂生甘露。

In training, you must close your eyes to avoid being distracted by the outside world, and regulate your breathing. In this case, the millions of thoughts which link you with the outside world will be empty and your mind will be led into a calm and peaceful state, or "clean land." When you are able to reach this state, your Chi will be able to reach heaven (your head) and the cold ground (lower abdomen). Through your breathing, your Shen will be able to exit and enter your body freely. Once you are able to use your Shen to govern the Chi, the Chi can be as strong as a thousand rolling waves. Kan is one of the eight trigrams in Ba Kua, and represents Water. When you complete the Small Circulation, you are using the Water Chi generated from the Lower Dan Tien to nourish your head. Kuen Luen is one of the highest mountains in China, and here refers to the top of the body: the head or brain. When the Water Chi is led to the brain to nourish it, it feels like the top of Kuen Luen mountain has been watered, and clouds and dew are generated.

The three gates behind the back open immediately. Golden light shines into the gate of life and death. Chi must be transported abundantly and circulate to the top. (Then you will be able to) connect with heaven and lead it to return to the Shen valley. To raise and lower the Fire and Water is called for at this time. The white tiger is locked in the cave of the green dragon. (When) dragon and tiger meet, Shen and Chi are raised. Again transport six-six thirty-six. Thirty-six, few people know. The marvelous key is clearly Kan and Lii. Reverse, match, and combine (them), the marvelousness can reach the occult. (When) it comes, it is like metal steel, and (when) it is gone, it is soft like cotton.

背後三關立刻開，金光射透生死戶，氣走須彌頂上流，通天接引歸神谷，水火升降此時求，白虎鎖入青龍窟，龍虎一會神氣生，再運六六三十六，三十六，少人知，竅妙分明在坎離，顛倒配合妙通玄，來似金剛去似綿。

When you train the Small Circulation, there are three gates (or cavities) where the Chi flow is stagnant. In order to fill up the Chi and circulate it smoothly in the Conception and Governing Vessels, you must first open these three gates. This will be discussed later. Once these three gates are opened, you have opened the door to the path which moves you away from death. You have then completed the first step of the training leading you to the field of immortality.

In still meditation training, at some point when you are able to lead Chi upward to nourish the brain you will suddenly experience "lightening" in your brain. This may be caused by the extra Chi energizing inactive brain cells. Your mind perceives this as light (golden light).

When you can sense this light, your brain is highly energized. You are now able to lead this Chi to the Shen in the "Shen valley" to raise up the spirit. Since it is believed that Shen was the very origin of your life, it said that you now "return" to the Shen valley.

In Chi Kung, the Shen is believed to reside in the Upper Dan Tien (the "third eye") in the forehead. "Shen valley" has two meanings. First, physically the Upper Dan Tien is located at the exit of the valley formed by the two lobes of the brain (Figure 6-24). Some Chi Kung practitioners believe that the Shen in the Upper Dan Tien is able to sense the supernatural because of the structure of the brain. The Upper Dan Tien is located in a kind of "valley" which is able to resonant to various types of energy. Second, when you are in the meditative state, it feels like the Shen is living deep in a valley which stretches forward farther than you can see.

When you have reached the stage of seeing the lightening you will be able to control the balance of the Fire and Water. The white tiger refers to the Yang of your body, while the green dragon refers to the Yin. When these Yin and Yang meet and interact, Shen and Chi will be raised. You should train this Yin (Kan) and Yang (Lii) interaction (lightening) thirty-six times whenever you meditate. This is the key to the training. ("six-six, thirty-six" is a musical way of saying thirty-six) The tiger locked in the cave of the dragon implies that the Yang is led to meet the Yin in the Yin residence.

Da Mo passed down the herb of cultivating the body; top to the Ni Wan and bottom to the Yongquan. (When) Chi reaches the navel, the White Crane flies. When reversing the image and at the beginning of training where you are still crossing your legs, transporting (Chi), living, sitting, and lying down, you must remember, Jieng should be abundant and Shen should be complete, the Chi will naturally be round (smooth). Shen and Chi are plenty, the glow will not be extinguished. Again, it is different from other styles. If someone is able to recognize this information, (he will be able to) harden himself like gold stone and be

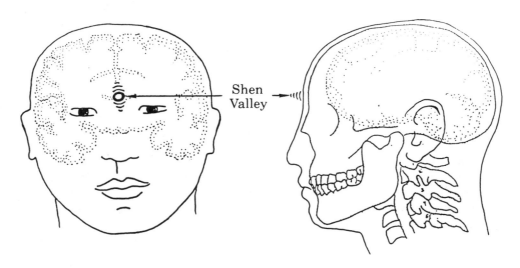

Figure 6-24. "Shen Guu" (Spirit Valley) and Brain

tough like metal. **You must be alert at every move and step. This is the real oral secret from the immortal fairy. You must remember Yi Gin Ching firmly, train your entire body like raw iron. Only then will you be able to fly your body to the golden palace.**

達磨留下修身藥，上至泥丸下湧泉，氣至臍，白鶴飛，倒像蘆芽穿膝時，行住生臥君須記，精滿神全氣自回，神氣足，光不滅，又與諸家有分別，有人識得此消息，硬如金石堅如鐵，行行步步謹提防，此是神仙真口訣，君須牢記易筋經，渾身煅煉如生鐵，只此飛身到金闕。

Ni Wan is the common name for the brain in Chinese Chi Kung society. Yongquan is the cavity on the soles of the feet. Through Da Mo's Chi Kung training you are able to build the herb (Chi) within your body from your head to the bottom of your feet. When Chi is trained at the Lower Dan Tien at the navel area, the White Crane is able to take you to the holy city. When a person has reached enlightenment or Buddhahood, his spirit can separate from his body and lightly fly away like a crane. In China, when a person dies, it is called "Jiah Heh Shi Guei," which means "to ride the crane to return to the West." The West means India, which was thought of as the residence of all of the Buddhas. This means that when he dies, his spirit has entered the holy world (west heaven).

When you are a beginner and are still "reversing the image" (looking inward to understand yourself), while meditating or carrying out your daily activities you need to remember that you must conserve your Jieng and keep it abundant and firm. You must also remember to raise your Shen to a higher level, then your Chi will naturally circulate smoothly and easily throughout your body.

1. Small Circulation

Small Circulation is commonly achieved through Nei Dan still meditation. However, there are several Wai Dan techniques which can be used to assist in the Small Circulation training. This Wai Dan Small Circulation training was normally done by practitioners of the Shaolin external martial arts, who emphasized Wai Dan training for the first few years.

Small Circulation training has two major goals. The first is to fill up the Chi in the Conception and Governing Vessels. The second is to circulate the Chi smoothly in these two vessels.

We have explained earlier that there are eight vessels in the human body which behave like Chi reservoirs and regulate the Chi level in the twelve primary Chi channels. Among these eight vessels, the Conception Vessel is responsible in the six Yin channels, while the Governing Vessel controls the six Yang channels. In order to regulate the Chi in the twelve primary channels efficiently, the Chi in the vessels must be abundant. Also, the Chi in these two vessels must be able to circulate smoothly. If there is any stagnation of the Chi flow, they will not be able to regulate the Chi in the channels effectively, and the organs will not be able to function normally.

You can see that Small Circulation is the first step of Nei Dan Chi Kung practice. Small Circulation training will help you to build up a firm foundation for further Nei Dan practices such as Grand Circulation and the Shii Soei Ching Chi Kung training.

Small Circulation Training:

In order to reach a deep stage of Nei Dan still meditation, there are five important procedures which you must learn: regulating the body, regulating the breathing, regulating the mind, regulating the Chi, and regulating the Shen. You also need to know the location of the Dan Tien and the roles which the Conception and Governing Vessels play in Chi Kung practice. These are discussed in detail in the first YMAA Chi Kung book: "The Root of Chinese Chi Kung." It is recommended that you study that book before you start practicing the exercises in this book. Since Nei Dan Small Circulation has been discussed in detail in the earlier YMAA Chi Kung book: "Chi Kung - Health and Martial Arts," we will only review the techniques here.

A. Abdominal Exercises:

You start Small Circulation training by building up the Chi at the Lower Dan Tien. This is done through abdominal exercises. You must first learn how to control the abdominal muscles again so that they can expand and withdraw. This exercise is called "Faan Torng" (back to childhood). From birth until about 8 years old, you move your abdomen in and out in coordination with your breathing. This abdominal movement was necessary for bringing in nutrients and oxygen through the umbilical cord when you were in the womb. However, once you were born, you started taking in food through your mouth and oxygen through your nose, and the abdominal movement gradually diminished. Most adults don't have this abdominal movement when they breathe. The "back to Childhood" exercise helps you to return to the type of breathing you did as a child.

Once you have regained control of your abdomen, as you continue these exercises you will feel your abdomen getting warmer. This indicates that the Chi is accumulating, and is called "Chii Huoo," or "Starting the Fire." These exercises lead the Chi which has been converted from the Original Essence in the Kidneys to the Lower Dan Tien, where it resides. The more you practice, the easier this is to do, and the more you can relax your body and feel the Chi.

B. Breathing:

Breathing is considered the "strategy" in Chi Kung. In Small Circulation, you may use either Buddhist or Taoist breathing. Buddhist breathing is also called "Jeng Hu Shi" (regular breathing) while Taoist breathing is called "Faan Hu Shi" (reverse breathing). In Buddhist breathing, you expand your abdomen as you inhale and contract it as you exhale. Taoist Breathing is just the reverse (Figure 6-25).

Generally speaking, Buddhist breathing is more relaxed than Taoist breathing. Though Taoist breathing is more tensed and harder to train, it is more efficient in expanding the Guardian Chi and in martial applications. This point can be clarified if you pay attention to the everyday movements of your abdomen. Normally, if you are relaxed or not doing a heavy job, you will see that you are using Buddhist breathing. However, if you are doing heavy work and exerting a lot of force, for example pushing a car or lifting a heavy box, then you will find that your abdomen tenses and expands when you push or lift.

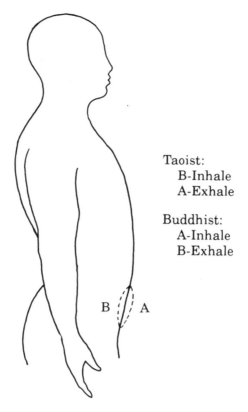

Taoist:
    B-Inhale
    A-Exhale

Buddhist:
    A-Inhale
    B-Exhale

Figure 6-25. Taoist and Buddhist Breathing

Try this very simple experiment. Put one hand on your abdomen, and hold the other in front of you. Exhale, and imagine that you are pushing something very heavy. (You exhale because exhaling is Yang, and it enables you to manifest your force externally.) When you do this you will find that your abdomen expands as you exhale. This is the way that Chi balances in Chi Kung: while one flow of Chi is outward, the other flow is inward to the Dan Tien. Weight lifters often wear a wide belt when they work out to strengthen the Chi balance in the abdomen. This enables them to lift more weight.

You can see that both Buddhist and Taoist breathing methods are totally natural ways of breathing, and which you do depends on the circumstances. Buddhist breathing is more relaxed and less aggressive, while Taoist breathing is more expressive and aggressive in demonstrating the power of Chi. It is suggested that beginners start with Buddhist breathing. After you have mastered it, you should then practice Taoist breathing. There is no conflict. After you practice for a while, you will find that you can switch from one to the other very easily.

C. Huiyin and Anus Coordination:

After you have practiced abdominal exercises for about 3-5 weeks, you may feel the abdomen get warmer and warmer every time you practice. After continued practice, the abdomen will start to tremble and shake each time after you start the fire. This means that Chi has accumulated at the Dan Tien and is about to overflow. At this time you should start to coordinate your breathing and abdominal movement with the movement of your Huiyin (literally "Meet the Yin") cavity and anus to lead the Chi to the tailbone (Weilu cavity).

The technique is very simple. If you are doing the Buddhist breathing, every time you inhale, gently expand your Huiyin and anus, when you exhale you hold them up gently. If you are doing the Taoist breathing, the movement of the Huiyin and anus is reversed: when you inhale you gently hold them up and when you exhale, you gently push them out. This up and down practice with the anus is called "Song Gang" and "Bih Gang" (loosen the anus and close the anus). When you move your Huiyin and anus, you must be relaxed and gentle, and must avoid all tension. If you tense them, the Chi will stagnate there and will not be able to flow smoothly.

The trick of holding up and loosening the Huiyin and anus is extremely important in Nei Dan Chi Kung. It is the first key to changing the body from Yin to Yang and from Yang to Yin. The bottom of your body is where the Conception (Yin) and Governing (Yang) Vessels meet. It is also the key to opening the first gate, which will be discussed next.

D. The Three Gates:

The three gates in Chinese meditation are called "San Guan." There are three places along the course of the Small Circulation where the Chi is most commonly stagnant. Before you can fill up the Conception and Governing Vessels and circulate Chi smoothly, you must open these three gates. The three gates are:

a. Tailbone (Weilu in Chi Kung and Changqiang in acupuncture):

Because there is only a thin layer of muscle on the tailbone, the Chi vessel there is narrow, and can easily be obstructed. Once you have built up a lot of Chi in the Lower Dan Tien and are ready to start circulating it, the tailbone cavity must be open, or the Chi might flow into the legs. Since you are only a beginner, you might not know how to lead the Chi back to its original path. If the Chi stagnates in the legs it could cause problems, perhaps even paralysis of the legs. This danger can be prevented if you sit with your legs crossed during meditation, which will narrow the Chi path from your Dan Tien to the legs and prevent the Chi from overflowing downward.

To prevent this kind of problem, you must know one of the important tricks which is called "Yii Yi Yiin Chi" which means "use your Yi to lead your Chi." Please pay attention to the word "**LEAD**." Chi behaves like water - it can be led by the mind, but it cannot be pushed. The more you intend to push the Chi, the more you will tense, and the worse the Chi will circulate. Therefore, the trick is to **ALWAYS PLACE YOUR YI AHEAD OF YOUR CHI**. If you can catch this trick, you will find out that the Chi can get through the tailbone cavity in just a few days.

Because there are two big sets of muscles beside the Governing Vessel, whenever there is extra Chi flowing through, these muscles will be slightly energized. The area will feel warm and slightly tense. Sometimes the area will feel slightly numb. All of these verify that Chi has been led to that point.

b. Squeeze the Spine (Jargi in Chi Kung, Mingmen in the martial arts, and Lingtai in acupuncture):

The Jargi gate is located between the sixth and seventh thoracic vertebrae, in back of the heart. If the Jargi is blocked and you circulate Chi to it, part of the Chi will flow to the heart and over-stress it. This will generally cause the heart to beat faster. If you are scared and pay attention to the heart, you are using your Yi to lead more Chi to it. This will make the situation worse and may conceivably even cause a heart attack.

The trick of leading Chi through this cavity is to **NOT** pay attention to your heart, though you should be aware of it. Instead, place your Yi a few inches above the Jargi. Since Chi follows the Yi, the Chi will pass through without too much effort.

Between the tailbone and the neck, you can easily tell when the Chi is passing through because the muscles will feel numb, tense, or warm.

c. Jade Pillow (Yuhjeen in Chi Kung and Fengfu in acupuncture):

The Jade Pillow cavity is the last gate which you must open. The cavity is so named because it is located in that part of your body which rests on a pillow, which the Chinese liked to make out of jade. There is not much muscle in this area, and so the path of the Governing Vessel is narrow, and easily constricted. This lack of muscle creates another problem. Because most of the spine is surrounded by layers of muscle, it is easy to gauge where the Chi is because of the response of the muscles. However, from the Jade Pillow up over the head there is very little muscle, and it is harder to tell what is happening with the Chi. This is especially confusing for beginners, but if you take it easy and proceed carefully, you will soon learn to recognize the new clues. For some people, when the Chi passes through the Jade Pillow cavity it feels like insects walking over their heads. Other people feel numbness or itching.

Be very conscientious when you move Chi through this area. If you do not lead the Chi in the right path, the Chi may spread over your head. If it is not kept near the surface, it may enter your brain and affect your thinking. It is said that this can cause permanent damage to the brain.

E. Breathing and Chi Circulation:

In Chi Kung, breathing is considered your strategy. Although there is only one goal, there can be many strategies. It is the same as when you are playing chess with someone. Although you both have the same goal, and want to checkmate the other's king, there are many different ways you can go about it. Chinese Chi Kung has developed at least 13 different strategies or methods of training. It is hard to say which is the best breathing strategy. It depends on the individual's understanding, the depth of his Chi Kung practice, and his training goals.

When you train using your breathing to lead the Chi, you should always pay attention to several things. The first is keeping the tip of your tongue touching the roof of your mouth. This connects the Yin (Conception) and Yang (Governing) vessels. This process is called "Da Chyau," which means "building a bridge." This allows the Chi to circulate smoothly between the Yin and Yang vessels. The bridge also causes your mouth to generate saliva, which keeps your throat moist during meditation. The area beneath the tongue where saliva is generated is called Tian Chyr (heavenly pond).

The second thing you need to pay attention to is the strength of your Yi, and how effectively it is leading the Chi. The third thing is how much is your Shen able to follow the breathing strategy? It is said:

"Shen Shyi Shiang Yi," which means "spirit and breathing mutually rely on each other." As long as the Chi can be led effectively and the Shen can be raised strongly while the body is relaxed and the mind calm, the breathing strategy is being effective.

We would like to recommend several breathing strategies which are commonly used to lead the Chi in training the Small Circulation.

a. Taoist Breathing Strategy:

As discussed earlier, Taoists use reverse breathing, whereby the abdomen draws in as you inhale, and expands as you exhale. This type of breathing reflects and augments the expanding and withdrawing of the Chi. As you exhale, the Chi can be expanded to the skin, the limbs, or even beyond the skin; while as you inhale the Chi can be drawn deep into the marrow. Reverse breathing is the natural way your body breathes when you want to get power out. The martial arts use this strategy of exhaling while the abdomen expands. The disadvantage of reverse breathing is that it is harder for beginners. When you do not do reverse breathing correctly, you will feel tension in your abdomen and a buildup of pressure in your solar plexus. This significantly affects the internal Chi circulation. To avoid this, it is highly recommended that Chi Kung beginners start with Buddhist breathing. Only when breathing this way is easy, natural, and comfortable should you switch to the Taoist reverse breathing.

There are two common ways to use the Taoist breathing to lead the Chi for Small Circulation, one with two inhalations and exhalations per cycle, and the other with one inhalation and exhalation per cycle.

i. Two Breath Cycle (Figure 6-26):

In your first inhale, lead the Chi to the Lower Dan Tien; when you exhale, lead the Chi from the Lower Dan Tien to the tailbone. As you inhale again, lead the Chi from the tailbone up along the spine to the level of the shoulders; and as you exhale, lead the Chi over the head to the nose to complete the cycle.

ii. One Breath Cycle (Figure 6-27):

On the inhale, lead the Chi from the nose to the tailbone; and on the exhale, lead the Chi from the tailbone to the nose to complete the cycle.

b. Buddhist Breathing Strategy:

The Buddhists usually use the one breath cycle, but this does not mean you cannot use a two breath cycle. As long as you follow the rules, you can experience many breathing strategies by yourself.

i. One Breath Cycle (Figure 6-28):

When you inhale, your mind leads the Chi from the nose to the tailbone; and when you exhale, it leads the Chi from the tailbone to the nose to complete the cycle.

F. When to Practice:

According to the documents, there are three times in the day which are considered the best times for practice: before midnight, dawn, and after noon (between one and two o'clock). If you cannot meditate three times a day, you should meditate in the morning and evening, and skip the afternoon session.

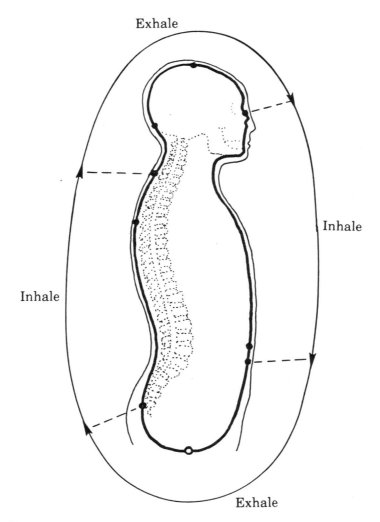

Exhale

Inhale

Inhale

Exhale

Figure 6-26. Two Breath Taoist Breathing Cycle

G. Postures for Practice:

When you practice in the morning and afternoon, it is recommended that you face the east to absorb the energy from the sun and to coordinate with the rotation of the Earth. For the evening session, you should face South to take advantage of the earth's magnetic field.

When you meditate, you should sit with your legs crossed on a mat or cushion about 3 inches thick. The tongue should touch the roof of the mouth to connect the Yin and Yang vessels.

Once you have opened up the three gates and circulated the Chi smoothly in the Conception and Governing Vessels, you should then continue meditating to build up the Chi more strongly and to learn to store the Chi in these two Chi reservoirs. Opening up the gates may take only a few months, but building up the Chi to an abundant level may take you many years of continued practice. At this stage, the more you practice, the more Chi you will accumulate. Remember: **ABUNDANT CHI STORAGE IS THE FOUNDATION OF GOOD HEALTH AND FURTHER CHI KUNG TRAINING**. It is a requirement for developing the Grand Circulation, which we will discuss next.

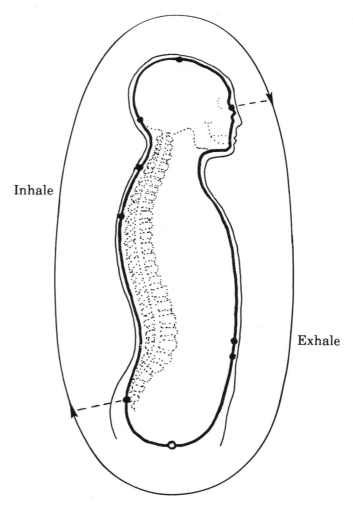

Inhale

Exhale

Figure 6-27. One Breath Taoist Breathing Cycle

2. Grand Circulation

Grand Circulation training can also be either Nei Dan or Wai Dan. In Nei Dan Grand Circulation, Chi is built up in the body and expanded out to the limbs and skin. This is usually done through still meditation.

In Wai Dan Grand Circulation, Chi is first built up locally in the limbs through special exercises. This usually involves tensing the muscles and tendons. Later, this local Chi is connected with the internal Chi of the body to complete the Grand Circulation.

A third method, and the most effective, of developing Grand Circulation is to combine both Nei Dan and Wai Dan at the same time. In this method, while you are doing the Wai Dan exercises, your mind is leading the Chi from your abdomen to your limbs. Your muscles and tendons need to be as relaxed as possible to allow the Chi to move smoothly from your center to your limbs. Many internal martial styles use this combined method to complete the Grand Circulation.

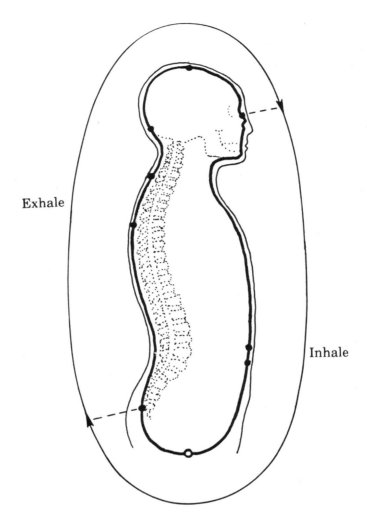

Exhale

Inhale

Figure 6-28. One Breath Buddhist Breathing Cycle

A. Nei Dan Grand Circulation
a. Five Gates Breathing:

The first step of Nei Dan Grand Circulation training is learning how to do Chi breathing through the five gates. The five gates include the head (including the Upper Dan Tien and Baihui), the two Laogong cavities in the centers of the palms, and the two Yongquan cavities on the soles of the feet. In section 4-3 we introduced the concept of five gates breathing. Here we hope to lead you to a deeper level of understanding and practice.

According to Chinese medical science, the two Laogong gates in the centers of the palms belong to the Pericardium Chi channel, and they can be used to regulate the heart Fire. Whenever the Chi in the heart is too Yang, it is led to the Laogong and released out of the body. Your heart is a very sensitive organ and its Chi level must be correct. If your heart is too Yang you can suffer a heart attack.

It is the same with the Yongquan cavities on the soles of the feet. They can be used to regulate another vital organ, the Kidney. The Kidney is classified as Water, and its Chi level is also critical for your health.

The last gate is on the head. For a Chi Kung beginner, this gate is the Baihui on the top of your head. For an advanced Chi Kung practitioner, it is the Upper Dan Tien. When an advanced Chi Kung practitioner is able to use the Upper Dan Tien for Chi breathing, it is called "Shen Shyi," or "spirit breathing." The above five gates are also commonly called "Wuu Hsin," or "the five centers."

In this training, when you inhale you lead the Chi from the five centers or gates to the Lower Dan Tien, and when you exhale you lead the Chi to the five gates (Figure 6-29). Naturally, the secret key to effectively leading the Chi inward and outward is through the coordination of the Huiyin and anus. It is very common for beginners to practice first with only the two Laogong or the two Yongquan cavities, and only later to combine them. According to my personal experience, the Taoist reverse breathing strategy can help to accomplish this training earlier and more effectively.

This training can be done lying down, sitting, or standing up. The posture is not important as long as the body is relaxed and the Chi can be led smoothly to the gates.

b. Body Expanding Breathing:

Body expanding training is also called "Tii Shyi" (body breathing) or "Fu Shyi" (skin breathing). After you have mastered the skill of five gates breathing, you should then learn body breathing. This training teaches you to lead the Chi to every pore in your skin. When you have accomplished this, you will be able to effectively lead the Chi to energize the muscles to reach their maximum power.

Since we have discussed body breathing in Chapter 4, we will only review the concept of the training here. Imagine that you are a beach ball. When you inhale you lead the Chi to the Lower Dan Tien, and when you

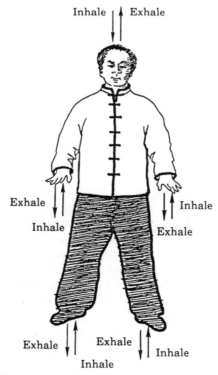

Figure 6-29. Five Gates Chi Breathing

exhale you expand the Chi to the surface of your skin so that you feel like you are inflating your body. Your posture should be easy and comfortable.

c. Yin and Yang Channels Breathing:

After you have grasped the secret of five gates and body breathing, you should enter the final stage of the Nei Dan Grand Circulation breathing. In this stage you also switch the gate on your head from the Baihui to the Upper Dan Tien. The purpose of this training is to circulate the Chi in your Yin and Yang channels through your breathing, mind, and the coordination of your Huiyin and anus.

In this training, when you inhale you lead the Chi from the inner side of your limbs (Yin Channels) to the Lower Dan Tien, and then upward through the center of your body to the Upper Dan Tien (Figure 6-30). When you do this correctly you will feel a strong Chi flow, which gathers at the Upper Dan Tien. The verification that you are doing this practice correctly will be a slight feeling of tenseness and warmth in the Upper Dan Tien.

When you exhale, relax your Upper Dan Tien and lead the Chi upward out the top of your head, and then to the external sides of your arms and legs. The Chi passes through your fingers and toes to the centers of your palms and soles. When you are doing this, the Lower

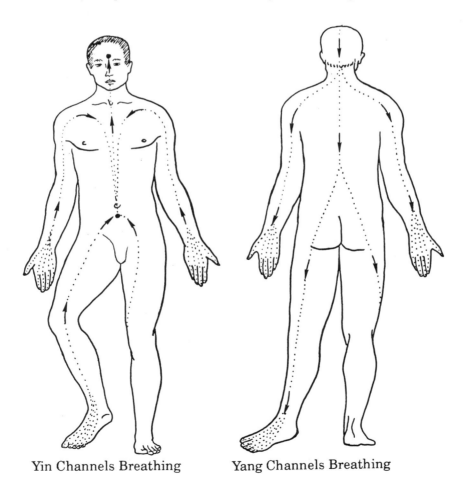

Yin Channels Breathing   Yang Channels Breathing

Figure 6-30. Yin and Yang Channels Chi Breathing

Dan Tien is expanding (reverse breathing) and the Huiyin and anus are expanding slightly. You will feel a strong Chi flow on the surface of your back and the external part of your limbs. Again, the posture is not important as long as you feel relaxed and comfortable.

B. Da Mo Wai Dan Grand Circulation

The Wai Dan Grand Circulation exercise set of Da Mo's Yi Gin Ching is well known. In later years, many other sets were created based upon the same theory and using the same format. Here, we will introduce only two sets: the Fist Set which is considered to be the original, and a Palm Set which was created later. In this training, in the beginning you tense up part of your limbs and at the same time concentrate you mind there. Chi is gradually built up in the area which you are exercising. Although Da Mo's exercises start with tensing the muscles and tendons, after you have trained for a while you should gradually start relaxing the muscles and tendons. This will allow the Chi built up in the limbs to connect with the Chi you have built up in your body through Small Circulation training.

a. Fist Set

This exercise set was originally designed for the second and third years of Yi Gin Ching training. However, because of its effectiveness, many people train it to maintain their health or increase the Chi in their arms, even without completing the first year of Yi Gin Ching training. Later on, you will learn from the Yi Gin Ching training schedule that it should not be started before the completion of the first year of training. When you practice this set, you should continue from one form to the next without stopping. You build up Chi first in the wrist, and then move sequentially to the hands, arms, and chest. If you do not follow this order, the Chi you build up will not be connected from your hands to you body. If you intend to build up the muscles in your arms and shoulders, every time you exhale you should tense up the area you are training. However, if you do not want to over-stress and build up your muscles, you should relax and build up a strong Yi to lead the Chi to the areas being trained. You should repeat each form fifty times. The entire set takes about ninety minutes to complete. Beginners may find that they feel dizzy and weak after five forms. If this happens, stop and rest. After you train for a while, you will find that you can gradually increase the number of forms, until you can finally complete the training. Alternatively, a beginner may do all twelve forms, but reduce the number of repetition. When you feel stronger, increase the repetitions until you reach 50.

Form 1   (Figure 6-31):
Hold the hands beside the body with the palms facing down and thumbs extended toward the body. Keep the elbows bent. Mentally push the palms down while exhaling, and relax them when you inhale. This form will build the Chi in the wrists, and the palms and wrists should feel warm after 50 repetitions.

Form 2   (Figure 6-32):
Without moving the arms, close your hands into fists with palms facing down and thumbs extended toward the body. Mentally tighten the fists and push the thumbs backwards when exhaling, relax when

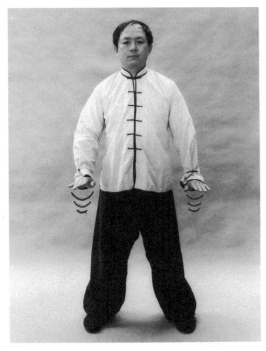

Figure 6-31. Posture #1 of the Da
Mo Fist Set

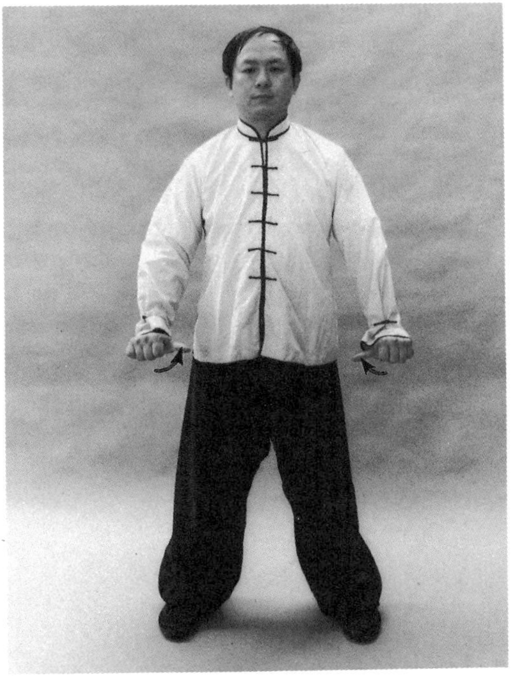

Figure 6-32. Posture #2 of the Da
Mo Fist Set

inhaling. The fists are kept bent backward to retain the energy built up in the wrists in the first form.

Form 3 (Figure 6-33):

Again without moving the arms, turn the fists so that the palms face each other and place the thumbs over the fingers, like a normal fist. Mentally tighten the fists when exhaling, relax when inhaling. The muscles and nerves of the arms will be stimulated, and energy will accumulate there.

Form 4 (Figure 6-34):

Extend the arms straight in front of the body, palms still facing each other. With the hands still in normal fists, mentally tighten them when exhaling; relax when inhaling. This will build up energy in the shoulders and chest.

Form 5 (Figure 6-35):

Extend the arms straight up, hands still in fists, palms facing each other. Mentally tighten the fists when exhaling; relax when inhaling. This builds energy in the shoulders, neck, and sides.

Form 6 (Figure 6-36):

Lower the arms so that the upper arms are parallel with the ground, the elbows bent and the fists by the ears, palms forward. Mentally tighten the fists when exhaling, relax when inhaling. This builds energy in the sides, chest, and upper arms.

Form 7 (Figure 6-37):

Extend the arms straight out to the sides with the palms facing forward. Mentally tighten the fists when exhaling; relax when inhaling. This form will build energy in the shoulders, chest, and back.

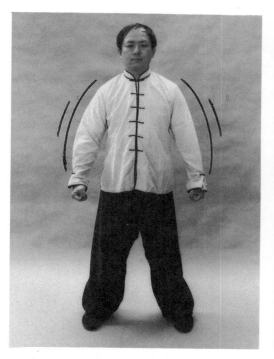

Figure 6-33. Posture #3 of the Da
Mo Fist Set

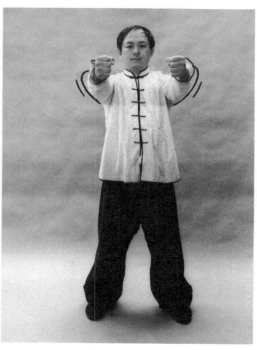

Figure 6-34. Posture #4 of the Da
Mo Fist Set

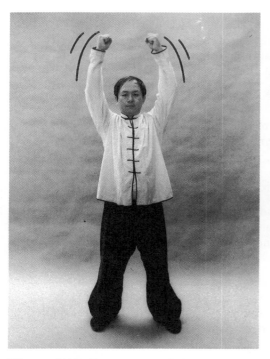

Figure 6-35. Posture #5 of the Da
Mo Fist Set

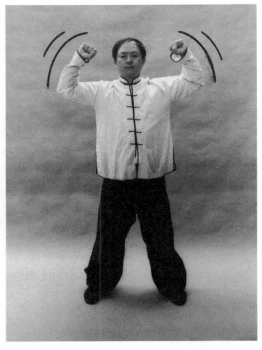

Figure 6-36. Posture #6 of the Da
Mo Fist Set

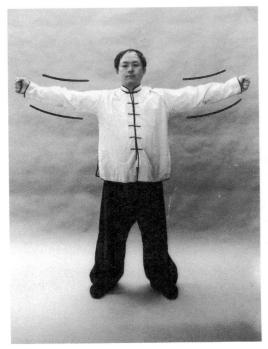 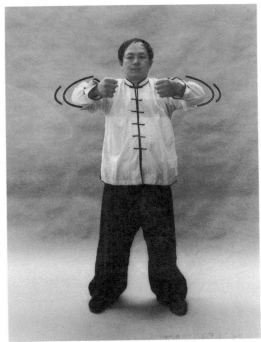

Figure 6-37. Posture #7 of the Da
      Mo Fist Set

Figure 6-38 Posture #8 of the Da
      Mo Fist Set

Form 8 (Figure 6-38):

Extend the arms straight in front of the body with the palms facing each other, but with the elbows bent slightly to create a rounded effect with the arms. Mentally tighten the fists and guide the accumulated energy through the arms to the fists when exhaling; relax when inhaling.

From 9 (Figure 6-39):

Pull the fists toward the body, bending the elbows. The fists are just in front of the face, palms forward. Mentally tighten the fists when exhaling; relax when inhaling. This form is similar to Form 6 above, but the fists are closer together and forward, so a different set of muscles is stressed. It intensifies the flow of energy through the arms.

Form 10 (Figure 6-40):

Raise the forearms vertically, Fists face forward, upper arms out to the sides and parallel with the floor. Mentally tighten the fists when exhaling, relax when inhaling. This form will circulate the built up energy in the shoulder area.

Form 11 (Figure 6-41):

Keeping the elbows bent, lower the fists until they are in front of the lower abdomen, palms down. Mentally tighten the fists and guide the energy to circulate in the arms when exhaling, relax when inhaling. This is the first recovery form.

Form 12 (Figure 6-42):

Raise the arms straight out in front of the body, palms open, facing up. Imagine lifting up when exhaling, relax when inhaling. This is the second recovery form.

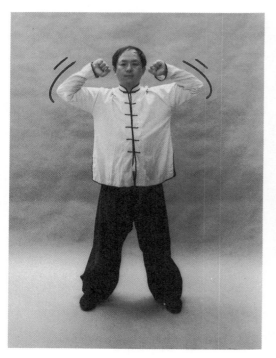

Figure 6-39. Posture #9 of the Da
Mo Fist Set

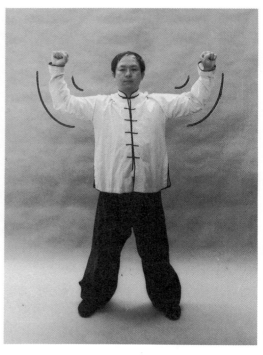

Figure 6-40. Posture #10 of the Da
Mo Fist Set

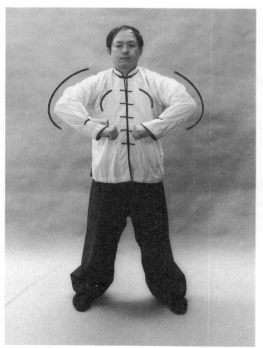

Figure 6-41. Posture #11 of the Da
Mo Fist Set

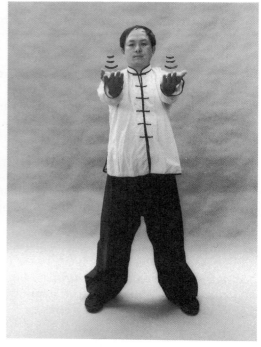

Figure 6-42. Posture #12 of the Da
Mo Fist Set

After practicing, stand a while with the arms hanging loosely at the sides. Breathe regularly, relax, and feel the energy redistribute itself for a few minutes. You can also walk around slowly until you feel comfortable.

b. Palm Set

Although the Palm Set is also considered part of the Yi Gin Ching, it was actually developed later, based on the same theory as the Fist Set. It is believed that after one has completed the training of the Fist Set, he should continue to practice the Palm Set and learn how to lead the Chi beyond his body through the palms and fingers. Simply put, the Fist Set increases and stores Chi in the body, while the Palm Set teaches you how to lead this Chi to interact with the Chi around you.

Because the Palm Set was derived from the Fist Set, all of the training rules and theory remain the same.

Form 1 (Figure 6-43):
Palms face the floor, while the fingers point out to the sides. Mentally push down when exhaling, relax when inhaling.

Form 2 (Figure 6-44):
Palms face the body, fingers pointing down. Mentally push in when exhaling, relax when inhaling.

Form 3 (Figure 6-45):
Arms are extended out to the sides, palms facing up. Mentally push up when exhaling, relax when inhaling.

Form 4 (Figure 6-46):
Bend the arms and place the hands in front of the chest, palms facing each other, fingers pointing up. Mentally push the hands toward each other when exhaling, relax when inhaling.

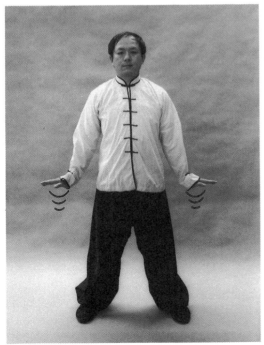

Figure 6-43. Posture #1 of the Da Mo Palm Set

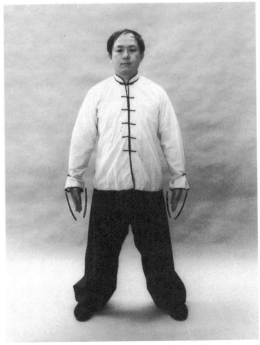

Figure 6-44. Posture #2 of the Da Mo Palm Set

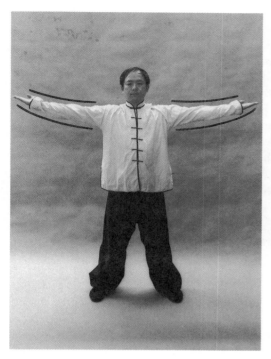

Figure 6-45. Posture #3 of the Da
Mo Palm Set

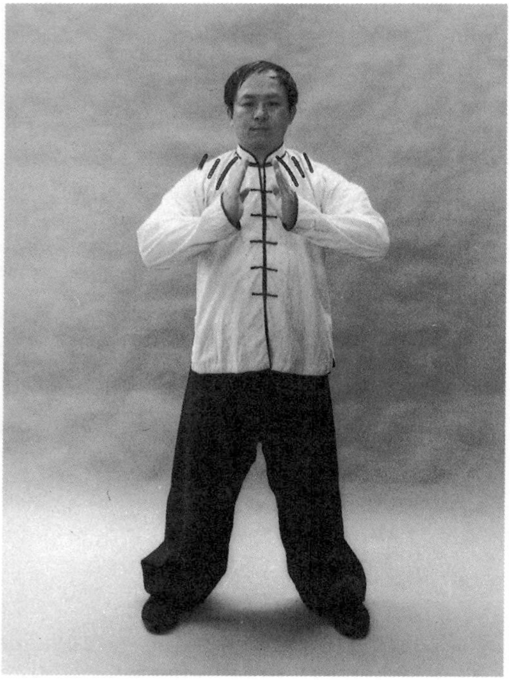

Figure 6-46. Posture #4 of the Da
Mo Palm Set

Form 5 (Figure 6-47):

Extend the arms out to the sides, palms facing out, fingers pointing up. Mentally push out when exhaling, relax when inhaling.

Form 6 (Figure 6-48):

Bend the arms and place the hands in front of the chest again, with palms touching this time, fingers pointing up. Mentally push in when exhaling, relax when inhaling.

Form 7 (Figure 6-49):

Extend the arms straight out in front, palms facing the front, fingers pointing up. Mentally push forward when exhaling, relax when inhaling.

Form 8 (Figure 6-50):

Extend the arms straight up, palms facing up, fingers pointing toward each other. Mentally push up when exhaling, relax when inhaling.

Form 9 (Figure 6-51):

Lower the hands to the front of the chest, elbows bent, palms facing up, fingers pointing toward each other. Mentally lift up when exhaling, relax when inhaling.

Form 10 (Figure 6-52):

Extend the arms straight to the front, palms facing up, fingers pointing forward. Mentally push up when exhaling, relax when inhaling.

Form 11 (Figure 6-53):

Bring the hands back to the front of the chest, palms facing down, fingers in line. Mentally push down when exhaling, relax when inhaling.

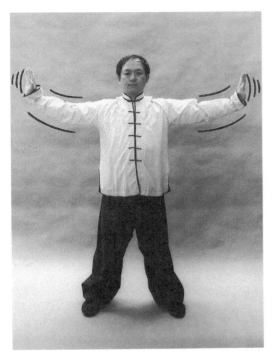

Figure 6-47. Posture #5 of the Da
Mo Palm Set

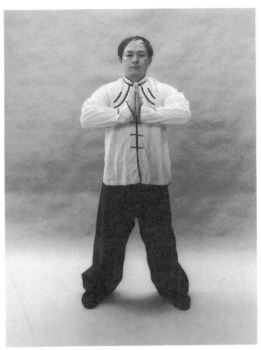

Figure 6-48. Posture #6 of the Da
Mo Palm Set

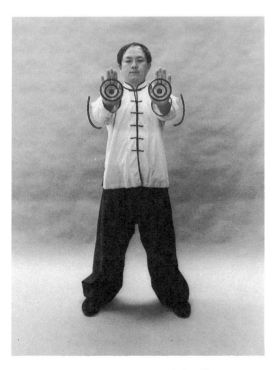

Figure 6-49. Posture #7 of the Da
Mo Palm Set

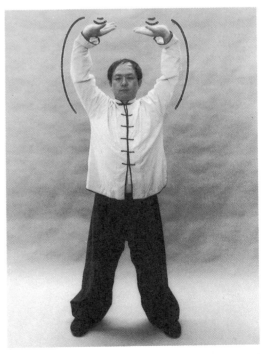

Figure 6-50. Posture #8 of the Da
Mo Palm Set

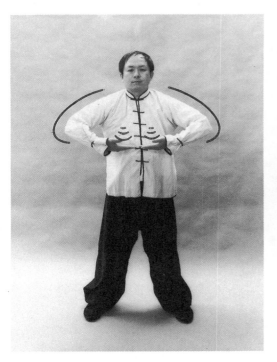

Figure 6-51. Posture #9 of the Da
Mo Palm Set

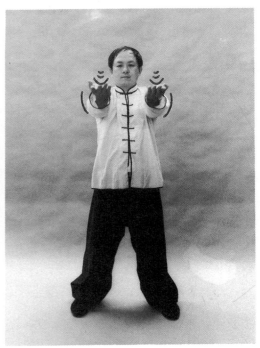

Figure 6-52. Posture #10 of the Da
Mo Palm Set

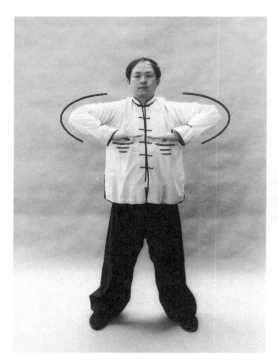

Figure 6-53. Posture #11 of the Da
Mo Palm Set

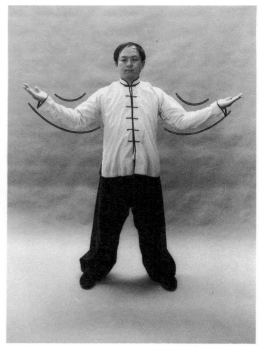

Figure 6-54. Posture #12 of the Da
Mo Palm Set

Form 12 (Figure 6-54):

Extend the arms out to the sides with the elbows bent, palms facing up and a little inward. Mentally lift upward and inward when exhaling, relax when inhaling.

Just as with the Fist Set, after practicing stand a while with the arms hanging loosely at the sides. Breathe regularly, relax, and feel the energy redistribute itself for a few minutes.

Though there are many other sets based on Da Mo's Yi Gin Ching Fist Set, many of them were created only for the purpose of maintaining health. The most famous ones are the Da Mo moving set, Da Mo Juang Chi Kung, and the Eight Pieces of Brocade. The Da Mo Juang Chi Kung will be discussed in a later volume; the other two sets have already been covered in YMAA publications. Interested readers should refer to: "Chi Kung - Health and Martial Arts" and "The Eight Pieces of Brocade."

C. Grand Circulation Through Muscle Training

The main purpose of Yi Gin Ching muscle training is to build up the muscles. As a matter of fact, many of the exercises are similar to today's weight lifting training. Usually, a weight or a special tool is held in the hands while doing certain movements. Since many books are available which extensively discuss this type of training, we will not cover them here. However, when you do these exercises, keep in mind that you must also train how to concentrate and use the Yi to lead the Chi to the areas being trained. In addition, once the body has been built to a certain point, you need to then learn how to relax and gradually increase the Chi flow to energize the muscles to a higher state. Remember, in Yi Gin Ching muscle training you must develop both your external physical body and your internal Chi body.

D. Wai Dan and Nei Dan Combined Grand Circulation

There are many available Wai Dan and Nei Dan combined Grand Circulation exercises. The theory is very simple and the training can be learned easily. Here we will introduce several typical training methods. As long as you understand the principle and theory, you may create other movements which can serve the same purpose. However, it is important for the exercises to follow the rules. First, during the movements, the muscles and tendons must be relaxed. If they are not relaxed, the Chi will not flow smoothly from the body to the limbs. Second, because it is the Yi which leads your Chi, when you create a new movement you must make sure that the movement also develops your Yi. Remember, only when your Yi is strong can your Chi be led strongly. For example, you may imagine that you are pushing a car. The intention of pushing the car is the Yi which can lead the Chi to the palms. Third, you must coordinate your breathing, mind, and Shen. If you follow these three rules, you will be able to effectively lead Chi to your limbs. Here we will offer several examples for your reference.

a. Pushing Forward:

Inhale and lift your hands up to your chest (Figure 6-55), then exhale and push forward with your palms (Figure 6-56). Imagine that you are pushing something heavy, but keep your body relaxed. When you inhale, withdraw your abdomen to store the Chi at the Lower Dan Tien. When you exhale, expand the abdomen to lead the Chi to the hands and legs.

-159-

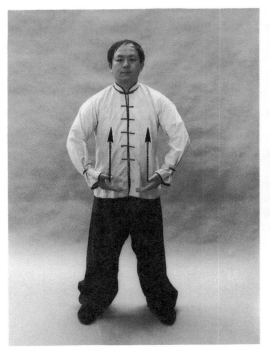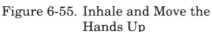
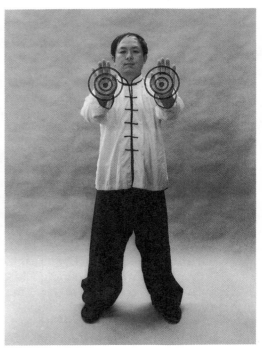

Figure 6-55. Inhale and Move the
Hands Up

Figure 6-56. Exhale and Push the
Hands Forward

b. Pushing Sideward:

Inhale and lift your hands up to your chest (Figure 6-57), then
exhale and push to both sides with your palms (Figure 6-58). When
you inhale, withdraw your abdomen and store the Chi at the Lower
Dan Tien. When you exhale, imagine that you are pushing something while your body is relaxed. While you are exhaling, the
abdomen expands and leads the Chi to the extremities.

c. Squeezing a Ball:

Imagine that you are holding a ball with both hands. When you
inhale, withdraw your abdomen and move your hands apart as if you
were stretching a spring (Figure 6-59), and when you exhale, lead
your Chi to the limbs and squeeze your hands together as if you were
squeezing a ball (Figure 6-60).

6-7. Yi Gin Ching Training Schedule

Yi Gin Ching training usually lasts for three years. It is called "San
Nian Yeou Cherng" (three years of accomplishment). The most important period is the first 100 days. It is said: "Bae Ryh Jwu Ji" (a
hundred days of building the foundation). In this 100 days, the training must be continuous, and you must abstain totally from sexual
activity. In this time, Chi is built up in the body through massage,
slapping, pounding and beating Wai Dan training. In the second 100
days, in addition to Wai Dan training you should also start the Nei Dan
Yi Gin Ching to build up the Chi in the body internally. When you have
completed 300 days of training the body, you should start developing
Grand Circulation and train your entire body for two more years.
According to the documents, after you have completed 300 days of Yi
Gin Ching training, you should also start the Shii Soei Ching training.

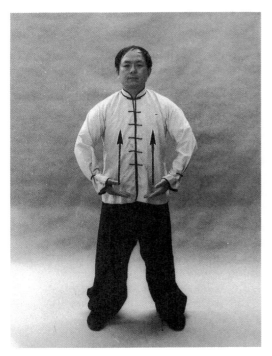

Figure 6-57. Inhale an Move the
Hands Up

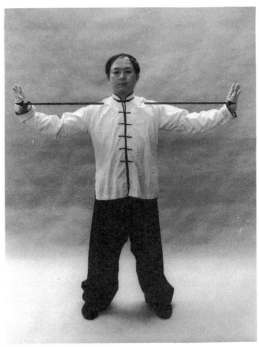

Figure 6-58. Exhale and Push
Sideways

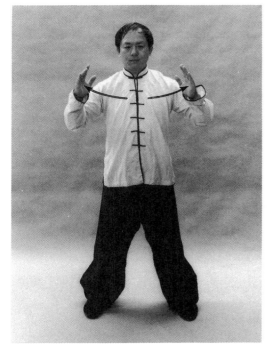

Figure 6-59. Inhale to Pull Spring
Apart

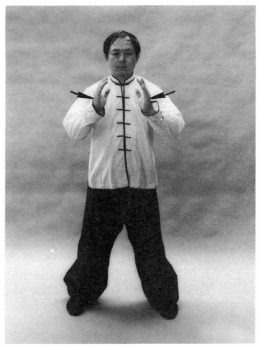

Figure 6-60. Exhale to Squeeze a
Ball

In this section, we will list the traditional training procedures. If you find that you cannot keep up the training schedule, you should adjust the training period. Remember: **TRAINING RIGHT IS MORE IMPORTANT THAN TRAINING FAST BUT WRONG**.

1. First Year:

This schedule for the first year of training was found in the document "The Real Manuscript of Yi Gin Ching." It is said that this document was found hidden in a wall of the Shaolin temple, and was originally written in an Indian language. Later it was hand carried by a Shaolin priest to Ermei mountain, where an Indian priest named Ban Tsyh Mih Dih translated it. This document was again edited by White Clothes Ocean and Mountain Traveler. After many hundreds of years of transmission, the final document was revealed to the public in the Harn Fen Lou (Tower of Fragrance Manuscripts). At the beginning of the document were several prefaces, which we have translated in Part One. The document continued with some training theory, part of which has been translated in Part Two of this book, and the schedule for the first year of training. Unfortunately, although the document explains that at least three years of training are required, only the first year of training was found. Therefore, the schedule for the second and third years will be laid out based on my personal understanding of the theory and training principles. I will also draw from many other training sources.

The original document then discusses Shii Soei Ching Chi Kung. Part of the text translated in Part Three of this book also originates with this document.

Several of the available documents list herbal prescriptions to assist with the first year Small Circulation training and the second and third year Grand Circulation Yi Gin Ching training. Because I have not had the chance to experience these herbs, I am unable to offer you any suggestions as to which prescription from which source is the best. I believe that any of them should be effective, since they have been used for the last thousand years. The prescriptions will be listed in Appendix A.

A. From First to Fourth Month 第一個月練功法
a. First 30 Days (Massage Kung)

When starting the massage, select young boys, take turns to massage. One (reason) is (because) the power is weaker, the massage and push will not be hard. Another (reason) is (because) the youth's blood and Chi are strong and abundant.

初擇之時，揀擇少年童子，更迭擇之。一取力小，擇推不重；一取少年血氣壯盛。

Because each training takes at least 90 minutes, you will normally need several boys for the massage. When one is tired, the other can take a turn. A child's strength is not strong, but his Chi and blood are strong and abundant, so you can use their Chi to nourish you and make the training more effective.

Before massage, take an herb pill. When the herb is dissolving, start the massage. Massage and the herb power transport and train together, then (you are) able to obtain marvelous results.

未揉之先，服藥一丸，約藥將化時，即行揉法。揉與藥力，一齊運行，乃得其妙。

Before massage, you should take an herb pill. This herb pill is supposed to bring up the Chi level of your body internally, and enable you to build up the Nei Juang (internal strength) more easily. The prescription for this herb pill is included in Appendix A.

During the massage, take the upper clothes off and lie down face up. Under the heart and above the navel, properly position your center. Press the palm and start from the right to the left massage. Slowly massage to and fro, should (be) uniform. Not too light, (don't) leave the skin. Not so heavy as to reach the bones. Do not move around randomly. Then, it is the right way.

揉時，當解襟仰臥，心下臍上，適當其中。按以一掌自右向左揉之，徐徐往來，宜均勻，勿輕而離皮，勿重而着骨，勿亂動游擊，斯為合式(適)。

It is important to keep your "center" under the solar plexus and above the navel. Remember that the purpose of massage is to first get rid of the fat accumulated in the fasciae, next to loosen them up, and finally to raise these fasciae. Since there are many layers of fasciae in the area of your center, you must start with light power and gradually increase the power until the massage reaches the deeper layers of the fasciae. When you massage, you should not be rough. The power should not be so heavy as to injure the bones. Also, when you massage, the massaging hands should be firm, the power should be uniform, and the hands should not rub on the skin. Also, the massaging hand should stay in contact with the skin.

During the massage, the heart (i.e., mind) should look internally, place your Yi and keep it on the "center." Do not forget and do not assist. (If) the Yi does not stray externally, then Jieng, Chi, and Shen all adhere and gather under the palm; (this) is the way. After time is matured, if (you) have mastered the "keeping center," massage and push are all uniform and clean. During the massage, even able to fall sleep. When you awaken, keep the "center" (again). Do this each time for about two sticks of incense.

當揉之時，心宜內觀，着意守中，勿忘勿助，意不外馳，則精、神、氣，皆附注一掌之下，是為如法。火候，若守中練熟，揉推勻淨。正揉之際，竟能睡熟，更為得法，愈於醒守也。如此行時，約略一時，時不能定，則以大香二炷為則。

When you are massaged, you must first regulate your mind and keep it at the "center." When you do this, you should not forget the center, but you must not concentrate your mind at this center forcefully. This would make you tense and the Chi circulation would stagnate. The trick is to place your mind under the palm which is massaging you. After you have trained for some time, you will have grasped the trick of how to keep your mind there. Gradually, you will be able to relax and even fall asleep. When you wake up, keep the center again. It takes about 90 minutes to burn two sticks of incense. This was a common way of measuring time in the old days when there were no clocks.

Morning, noon, and evening, total train three times. Train every day and become routine. If the boys used are fire-abundant, then only train morning and evening two times. (Because it is) afraid too positive and cause other problems. After training, sleep quietly for a while. After you wake up, do your daily work without disturbance. (If) there are no boys for massage, you may massage yourself.

早、午、晚，共行三次，日以為常。如少年火盛，只宜早晚二次，恐其太驟，致生他虞。行功即畢，靜睡片時，清醒而起，應酬無礙。無童子可行功時，可自捧之。

In one of the documents which was mentioned in Part One, it stated that you could train four times a day, but this paragraph tells you that you should train three times, in the morning, noon, and evening. You must train the massage every day for the first 30 days without fail. The purpose of the massage is to loosen up the fasciae and fill them with Chi. If you skip even a single time, the training will fall behind and you will need to double your effort and extend the training period to catch up. If the boys who massage you are very Yang and their power is too strong, then massage twice a day. After massage, rest for a while until your mind and body have recovered from the training. If there are no boys available to massage you, you can do it by yourself. Naturally, it is better if you have someone else to massage you, simply because you are able to relax more and concentrate your mind on feeling and sensing more effectively.

To summarize the first 30 days of training according to this document:

i.   Only massage training is involved.
ii. Herb pills are recommended.
iii. Only the "center" is massaged. The center is located under the solar plexus and above the navel.
iv. Mind is an important factor for successful Nei Juang training. You should not force your mind to the center because it will become tense.
v.   If possible use young boys or girls to do the massage. If you do not have them to help you, you can do it by yourself.
vi. Massage 90 minutes each time. If you do not have so much time for training, you should extend your training period proportionally.
vii. Massage from the right to the left with appropriate power.

b. Second 30 Days　第二個月練功法
　　　　　　　　　　　（揉搗功）

After one month of primary training, Chi has condensed and accumulated, the stomach (area) feels expanded and enlarged. Beside the stomach, the two tendons are raised, each has a width of more than an inch. Use the Chi to grab, hard like wood or a stone, then there will be verification. Between these two tendons, from the heart to the navel, soft and sinkable, this is (where) the fasciae are. (When trained) they are better than the tendons. (If) the palm cannot reach them, (they) cannot be raised. Then, this time you should massage the areas one palm's distance to the side of the one palm (i.e., center) massaged before. Massage and expand the area, following the same method, massage slowly. Amidst the soft area, should use the pestle to pound deeply. Longer, the fasciae will be raised to the skin and strong as the tendons, all not soft or sinkable, then it is the completeness of the training. When you train the massage and pounding, also allow two sticks of incense. Three times a day as routine. Then, there is no worry of too much Fire.

初功一月，氣已凝聚，胃覺寬大；其腹兩旁，筋皆騰起，各寬寸餘，用氣擊之，硬如木石，便為有驗；兩筋之間，自心至臍，軟而有陷，此則是膜，較勝於筋，掌揉不到，不能騰起也。此時應於前所揉一掌之旁，各揉開此掌，仍如前法，徐徐揉之，其中軟處，須用木杵深深搗之，久則膜皆騰起，浮至於皮，與筋齊堅，全無軟陷，始為全功。此揉搗之功，亦准二香。日行三次以為常，則可無火盛之虞矣。

After 30 days of massage training, the tendons on the sides of your stomach should be raised. It should feel like your stomach is enlarged. When you push or grab these tendons, they should feel as hard as stone. This is verification that the tendons are raised. Then you must locate the fasciae and raise them also. They are located in the lower area between the two tendons, and they will feel soft. Massage is usually not powerful enough to reach these fasciae, so you should use a pestle or wooden mallet to pound and raise them. In the training period when you are doing this, you should also extend the area you are massaging out to the sides, one palm's distance from the center. Again, pound the soft spots with a wooden mallet or pestle. In this period, you should train until there are no areas that are soft or "sinkable" (where your hand can penetrate deeply).

In summary, the second 30 days of training involve:
i.   Verifying the first 30 days of training by determining that the tendons on the sides of the stomach are raised and quite firm.
ii. Extending the massage one palm's distance out from the "center."
iii. Pounding the soft and "sinkable" spots with a pestle or wooden mallet until the fasciae are also raised.

-165-

c. Third 30 Days 第三個月練功法

In this third 30 days, the massage extends out even further, and pounding and beating become the main training. It is said in the document:

(When) training has completed two months (60 days), the sunken places in the area are slightly raised up. Then use the wooden mallet to pound lightly. The massaged place one palm away from the center, should pound the same way. Again, beside the two tendons one palm away, pound them with the same method. Should train for two sticks of incense. Train three times a day.

功滿兩月，其間陷處，至此略起，乃用木槌輕輕打之。兩旁所揉，各寬一掌處，都用木槌如法搗之。又於其旁，至兩筋梢，各開一掌，如法揉之。准以二香為則，日行三次。

The third 30 days of training follows the same methods of massage, pounding, and beating, and expands the area one palm's distance farther than the last period.

d. Fourth 30 Days: 第四個月練功法

This is the last step in the massage training of the center and its neighboring areas. You now expand the training area to the waist.

The training has completed three months, (the area) three palms away from the center, all use the mallet to beat; (the area) two palms away, first pound and then beat. Train three times a day, allow only two sticks of incense. After the training has passed 100 days, then Chi is full, tendons are strong, fasciae are springing up (to the surface) means the training has been achieved.

功滿三月，其中三掌，皆用槌打。其外二掌，先搗後打。日行三次，俱准二香，功逾百日，則氣滿筋堅，膜亦騰起，是為有驗。

In the fourth 30 days of training you are still following the same methods of massage, pounding, and beating, and you expand the area to three palms away from the "center." This should bring the area you are training to your waist.

B. From Fifth to Eighth Months:

In this period, the training is extended to the chest, sides of ribs, and lower abdomen areas. In fact, you may say that for this four months you are focusing your training on the front side of your body. In this period, in addition to Wai Dan training, you should also start Nei Dan Yi Gin Ching Small Circulation training, which will help you to build up Nei Juang to a significant level.

a. Wai Dan:

The document has two sections about this period's training:

1. The Internal and External Training
of the Two Tendons
兩肋內外功

(When) the training has passed 100 days, the Chi is already full and abundant. Like water in the stream already reaching the level of the ground and to the top of the dam. If banks are slightly broken, then it floods out, no hiding place cannot be reached as it no longer stays in the streambed. At this time, you must not use the Yi to lead it into the limbs. Other than massage, should not use the mallet to strike or pestle to pound. If you lead it (even) slightly, then (it will) enter into the limbs, and become external bravery and (it will) no longer return. (In this case, the Chi) transporting in the bones and meat will not become internal strength.

功逾百日，氣已盈滿，譬之澗水，平岸浮堤，稍為決道，則令放他之，無藏不到，無復在澗矣。當比之時，切勿用意引入四肢。所揉之外，切勿輕用槌打杵搗。略有引導，則入四肢，即成外勇，不復來歸。行於骨肉，不成內壯矣。

Each month in the Chinese calendar has 28 days, instead of 30 or 31 days as in the western calendar. Therefore after four months of training, you have trained only 112 days. After you have trained constantly for this period, you should have accumulated Chi in your stomach area and expanded it to your waist. At this stage, the Chi should feel as full as water lapping over the top of a dam, and if there is even the slightest hole it will flow out unstoppably. This is the most important stage of the training. You must protect the accumulated Chi as you would a tiny baby. Be restrained with your sexual activity and do not lose the accumulated Chi. This is the time when you can lead the Chi deep inside your body where it can become Nei Juang.

You must remember when you have reached this stage not to do heavy external exercises, or lift weights, or pound or beat the limbs. If you do any of this, you will lead the accumulated Chi to the limbs and it will become Wai Juang, and it will not return back to the center of your body for Nei Juang training. The next section teaches how to lead the accumulated Chi deeper in the body to build up Nei Juang.

The method of (leading) inward, use small pebbles and place them in a bag, start from the heart mouth (solar plexus) to the ending of the ribs. Pound it closely, also use massage, and again use the beating. Like this for a long time, then the accumulated Chi will follow (the path) and enter the bones (ribs). (If you) have done this, then (Chi) will not overflow, and finally become internal strength. Internal and external, two divisions divide here. Must be extremely careful and discriminate. If there is a misuse, and if you are careless in using the different training postures (i.e., methods), then (the Chi) will rush to the external and never again return into the internal. Be careful, be careful.

其入內之法，以小石盛於袋中為一石袋，自從心口至兩脅梢骨肉之間，密密搗之，兼用搓法，更用打法，如是久久，則所積盈滿之氣循循入骨，有此則不外溢，始成內壯矣。內外兩歧，於此分界。極當辨審，倘其中稍有夾雜，若輕用引弓弩拳捧撲等勢，則空趨行於外，永不能復入內矣：慎之慎之。

To lead the Chi inward into the body, slap from the "center" (stomach) of your front body with a bag filled with small pebbles. Start from the solar plexus and work out to the sides of the ribs. Also, use massage, pounding, and beating. When you are training this, remember always to start from the solar plexus and move out to the sides of the body, not the other way around. The correct method will move the Chi properly so that it enters the ribs. This is the beginning of leading the Chi into the body to build up the Nei Juang.

In Yi Gin Ching training, it is believed that this period is the most critical. You are building up the Nei Juang (Yin) to balance the Wai Juang (Yang). If you do not understand the theory and use the wrong training methods, once the accumulated Chi is misled to the limbs, you will not be able to build up the Nei Juang in your body. Therefore, until you have completed the training of this period, you should not do other heavy external exercises or do Wai Dan or Nei Dan Grand Circulation practice which might cause the Chi to flow into the limbs.

2. The Training Method

第五六七八個月練功法

(When) the training has passed 100 days, (from) the heart down to the sides to the ends of the ribs, already used the bag of stones to strike, and massage. This place is the junction of the bones and meat, and the internal strength and external strength are divided at this place. (If) not led and guided to the sides, then the accumulated Chi will enter into the gaps between the bones (ribs). Chi moves along the path of the striking. Striking should start from the heart mouth (solar plexus) to the neck. Again strike from the tendon ends to the shoulder. When complete, repeat from the beginning. Must not reverse the striking path. Three times a day, and in total allow six sticks of incense to burn, and do not stop. Like this for 100 days, then Chi is full on the front of the chest, the Conception Vessel is full and abundant (with Chi), then achievement has been half accomplished.

功逾百日，心下兩旁至脅兩脅之梢，已用石袋打而且搓矣。此處乃骨肉之交，內壯外壯在此分界，不於此處導引向外，則其積氣向骨縫中行矣。氣循打處逐路而行，宜自心口打至於頸，又自肋梢打至於肩，週而復始，切不可逆打。日行三次，共准六香，勿得間斷；如此百日，則氣滿前胸，任脈充盈，功將半矣。

This section is very similar to what has been discussed previously, only now you are to continue the massage, pounding, and beating training until you have covered the front side of the body.

You can see from the last two sections that the second period of Wai Dan Yi Gin Ching training involves the same techniques as the first period, but they are now used over the entire front of your body. The most critical point in this period is learning how to create the Nei Juang from the Wai Dan training.

In this period it is customary to also learn the Small Circulation from Nei Dan Yi Gin Ching. We will discuss this next.

b. Nei Dan

In order for your Yi Gin Ching training to be successful, you must also practice Nei Dan. There are several reasons for this.

1. Nei Dan training will give you a firm root and plenty of internal Chi to support the Wai Dan training. Internal Chi (Nei Chi) means the Chi generated internally from Nei Dan training, and external Chi (Wai Chi) is from external stimulation or from Wai Dan practice. Without this internal Chi foundation, your Wai Dan Yi Gin Ching training will remain at the Wai Juang stage.

2. Nei Dan training is Yin relative to Wai Dan training, which is Yang. Without Nei Dan training, the body can become too Yang and lose its Yin-Yang balance. This can cause problems with overheating and energy dispersion.

3. Nei Dan Yi Gin Ching is more effective in filling up the Chi in the Conception and Governing Vessels, and later directing this Chi to the channels. While the Wai Dan training focuses on the physical body, Nei Dan Yi Gin Ching concentrates on the Chi supply.

Depending on the individual, it normally takes from 90 days to many years to complete the Small Circulation. It is best to complete the Small Circulation before you start the second year training. You will then be able to work on Grand Circulation, whereby you expand the Chi circulation in the limbs, concurrently with your expanded Wai Dan training. If you follow the schedule in the documents, you will have only eight months to complete the Small Circulation. If this is insufficient for you, it is advisable to continue with the Wai Dan training until you achieve success. Then, when you do start training your limbs in the second year of the program, you will have plenty of internal Chi to support the Wai Juang limbs training.

Traditionally, with a disciple learning the Yi Gin Ching from a master, there was no problem completing Small Circulation. If you do not have a qualified master, you should take it easy and not rush. Rushing is not the natural way to learn Chi Kung.

C. From the Ninth to the Twelfth Month: 第九、十、十一、十二月練功法

These last four months are the final stage of the 300 days, or one year, of Yi Gin Ching training of the body. You now start training your back and the Governing Vessel with Wai Dan, and at the same time continue training your Nei Dan Small Circulation.

a. Wai Dan

For this period, the document says:

Train until 200 days, the front chest Chi is full and Conception Vessel is full and abundant, then should transport to the spine on the back to fill up the Governing Vessel. The Chi before has reached the shoulder and the neck, now from the shoulder to the neck, follow the same striking method, also use the massage technique. Top to the Jade Pillow, center to the Jargi ("Squeeze the Spine" cavity), and bottom to the Weilu (Tailbone). Strike everywhere, complete and repeat from the beginning. Must not reverse (the path). The soft places beside the spine, use the palm to massage, again use the mallet or pestle to strike as wished. Every day allow six sticks of incense to burn, and train three times. Either upward or downward, either left or right, massage and strike in a cycle. Like this for 100 days, Chi is full on the back spine, able to prevent a hundred sicknesses, and the Governing Vessel is full and abundant. Whenever you finish one cycle of striking, use the hand to massage thoroughly, (this will) make the Chi uniform.

功至兩百日，前胸氣滿，任脈充盈，則宜運入脊後，以充督脈。從前之氣，已至肩頭，今則自肩至頭；照前打法，兼用搓法：上循玉枕，中至夾脊，下至尾閭；處處打之，週而復始，不可倒行；脊旁軟處，以掌搓之，或用趟杵，隨便搗打。日進六香，共行三次；或上或下，或左或右，搓打週遍，如此百日，氣滿脊後，能無百病，督脈充盈。凡打一次，用手遍搓，令其勻潤。

Once you have completed the second period of Wai Dan Yi Gin Ching training, the Chi should be full in the Conception Vessel and the front of the body. Then you start your training on your back and the Governing Vessel. Generally speaking, you are using the same methods as before. Massage, pound, and beat until the Chi on the back is also full.

b. Nei Dan

In this period, you should continue your Nei Dan Small Circulation training. If you have completed Small Circulation, do not start Grand Circulation. The Wai Dan training is still working on your body, and Grand Circulation would lead the Chi to the limbs, depriving the Governing Vessel of its Chi supply just when you are training it. If you have completed your Small Circulation, continue to practice it and increase the Chi supply.

However, if you have not completed the Nei Dan Small Circulation training by the end of this period, do not start the next period. Instead, continue your Nei Dan Small Circulation, and at the same time, keep up your Wai Dan training to build up the external Chi to a higher level.

2. Second Year

By the end of the first year of Yi Gin Ching training, you should have completed the Wai Dan training for the body and the Nei Dan Small Circulation training. The Chi should now be full and abundant in your body, both internally and externally. You should remember that you should not start the second year's training until you have completed both the Wai Dan and the Nei Dan training of the first year. This will enable you to develop both Nei Juang and Wai Juang.

The second year of Yi Gin Ching training has several goals:

A. To expand the Chi you have built up in your body to the limbs through both Wai Dan and Nei Dan training. This will complete the Grand Circulation, opening up all twelve primary Chi channels and consequently benefiting the internal organs.

B. To toughen the muscles, tendons, and bones of the limbs. This training is especially important for martial artists since the limbs are so heavily involved in fighting.

C. To increase the working power and efficiency of the muscles. It is in this stage that you learn how to build up a stronger Yi. This is important for both health and martial arts, since it is the Yi which leads the Chi. When the Yi is strong, the Chi will circulate smoothly, and you will be more resistant to illness. For the martial artist, when the Yi is strong it will be able to lead more Chi to the muscles, energizing them to a higher level of efficiency and power.

D. To start softening the body. Physical training stresses your body and makes it tense, and it will become more Yang. After you have completed the training of your physical body, you should start gradually strengthening your internal Chi and making your body soft and relaxed again. If you do not do this, the muscles and tendons will remain tensed. This excessively Yang condition will speed up the deterioration and aging of your body. As you get older, your over-stressed muscles and tendons will lose their elasticity and flexibility more quickly than normal, and you may suffer from "Energy Dispersion." Therefore, in this period you should train with the goal of regaining the natural flexibility and elasticity of your muscles and tendons. At the same time, continue to train the fasciae with your internal Chi to increase their ability to accumulate Chi. You want to be like a strongly inflated beach ball. Internally, your Chi should flow smoothly without stagnation; and externally, nobody should be able to attack you without being bounced back.

E. Most important of all, in this period you also start Shii Soei Ching training. You must learn to be relaxed and soft both internally and externally before you can lead Chi deep inside to the marrow. If you continue to tense your body, Chi will stagnate in the muscles and tendons, and this will prevent the Chi from being transported to the surface of the body and deep into the marrow.

You can see from this list that the second year of Yi Gin Ching training is designed to soften your body while toughening your limbs. As mentioned at the beginning of this section, there are some herbal prescriptions listed in Appendix A which can be used to assist in the training of this period. In this period of Grand Circulation training, the training can again be divided into Wai Dan and Nei Dan.

a. Wai Dan
i. Body:

Continue the beating training. However, the training starts to focus on softening the physical body and using the abundant internal Chi to bounce the beating away. Gradually, you will find that you are able to bounce the strikes away strongly without tensing your muscles and tendons.

ii. Limbs:

Again, use massage, pounding, beating, and striking to treat the limbs from the shoulders to the hands and from the hips to the feet. At the same time, use the Yi Gin Ching exercise set. Start with the Fist Set until you are able to complete the entire training. Then continue to train for another three months. After training the Fist Set, then train the Palm Set for another six months. If you also wish to build up your muscles and tendons, then you may use weights or training equipment to enhance and speed up the training.

b. Nei Dan

i. Continue to build up the Chi and circulate it in the Conception and Governing Vessels.
ii. Learn to lead the Chi to the limbs, especially the Laogong cavities in the palms and the Yongquan cavities on the soles of the feet. These four cavities are the gates through which the internal Chi can communicate with the surrounding Chi. While you are training this, your entire body should remain relaxed. Use your mind and breathing to lead the Chi.

3. Third Year

The goals of the third year of training are:

A. To continue to build up the Chi internally to support the Shii Soei Ching training. In this year you gradually transfer the emphasis of your training from Yi Gin Ching to Shii Soei Ching. Yi Gin Ching is Yang compared to Shii Soei Ching, which is considered Yin. In this stage, you gradually give up the external Wai Dan Yi Gin Ching training, and gradually replace it with the Nei Dan Yi Gin Ching training. You continue building up the Chi in the Conception and Governing Vessels and the limbs for Shii Soei Ching training. This will continue to build up the Yang which is required for the Yi Shii Soei Ching training.

B. To soften the muscles and tendons in the limbs. In this period, Nei Dan Yi Gin Ching gradually replaces the Wai Dan Yi Gin Ching. The muscles and tendons will start to soften and not be tensed continuously, which was the case when you were emphasizing the Wai Dan Yi Gin Ching training. This will prevent the problem of "Energy Dispersion."

C. To expand the Chi to the surface of your body or beyond. This training is called "Tii Shyi" (body breathing) or "Fu Shyi" (skin breathing). In this period you are also learning how to lead the Chi to every cell of your body. In addition, you should also train the Yin and Yang Chi channel breathing which was discussed in the previous section. When you have reached this stage, your body can then be transparent to the Chi, and you have built up a firm foundation for the Shii Soei Ching. You will now be able to grow a "baby Shen" and finally reach the domain of enlightenment.

In three years you have completed the Yi Gin Ching training. For the rest of your physical life you should maintain the growth of Chi with Nei Dan Yi Gin Ching, and use this Chi to wash your marrow and nourish your brain. Without Yi Gin Ching as a foundation, the Shii Soei Ching training will not be effective.

6-8. Other Considerations

By this time, although you understand the theory and the training methods of Yi Gin Ching, there are probably still some concerns or questions remaining. As I said at the beginning of Part 2, there are still many pieces of the puzzle waiting for you to figure out how to put them together. I am quite sure that many unclear parts of this Yi Gin Ching puzzle will start showing up after you have accumulated some experience through your training.

Here, we would like to translate one section from the document which discusses what to do if your body becomes too Yang from the Yi Gin Ching training. This technique can be very useful anytime you feel your body is too Yang.

Decreasing the Fire Kung
退火功

When you train the massage in the beginning (of training), (it) can enhance the Fire from outside, (if you) take herbs internally, and (again) there is Chi accumulated in the center, (when) these three Chis get together, then the (internal) Fire will start automatically. When the internal Fire starts to move, the ears buzz and the cheeks swell. When this joined Fire transports (in the body), the body will have poison rash and flushed fainting. (When the) internal Fire is burning, the Yang Fire (sperm) is lost at night, you dream and think about the different strange appearances, various different changes (i.e., switching from one nightmare to another). If you have these illnesses, cross the legs and sit facing east. The two hands hold firm, or place the hands beside the waist and inhale the air to fill up the abdomen. Hold the breath like this for three, seven, or nine times. The more the better. Tightly hold up the grain path (i.e., anus), then expel the air finely. Stop for a while, again inhaling the clean air to the abdomen, repeat the method.

初行揉法，外能助火，內服丹藥，中有聚氣，三氣相合，自有生火竅，凡內火一動，或耳鳴腮腫，相火遊行，身有毒疹紅暈。內火發燒，陽火夜逸，夢思異境，種種不一之變，如有此症，盤膝面東正坐，兩手握固，叉腰吸氣，滿入腹中，閉氣三息，或五息、七息、九息，以多為益，緊提穀道，細細吐之，少停一時，又吸清氣滿腹內，照前法行之。

In the beginning of Yi Gin Ching training you massage to generate Chi externally, and take Yang herbs to increase the internal Chi. When these two Chis meet the Chi which you already have in your body, these three Chis may form a strong Chi and make your body too Yang. There are a number of symptoms which indicate that this has happened, such as a buzzing in the ears, red face, dizziness, or a red rash. You may also have nocturnal emissions, and find that your mind is not steady and you dream and daydream about many strange things. If you have these symptoms, you should learn how to cool down the Fire in your body. You do this by sitting crosslegged facing the east, with your hands clasped in front of the abdomen or held on the sides of the waist. Calm your mind. Inhale deeply into the abdomen and hold the breath as long as possible, let the air out slowly. Repeat three times, five times, seven times, or nine times as necessary. The more you do this, the more you will be able to lead the Chi inward and cool your body down and become more Yin. It is very important that when you are training this, you hold up your anus and Huiyin cavity. This is the trick to leading the Chi inward to the marrow. We will discuss this subject in the Shii Soei Ching section later. "Grain path" refers to the anus.

6-9. Conclusion
Before we end this discussion of Yi Gin Ching training, I would like to translate an article written by the Taoist Tzyy Ning Tao Ren, which offers you an idea of what this ancient master thought about the Yi Gin Ching training.

Postscript to the Yi Gin Ching
By Tzyy Ning Tao Ren

易筋經跋
紫凝道人

I read the translated meaning of the Yi Gin Ching, (and) repeated three more times. I saw the moral cultivation and achievement within, threaded together by one theory. Can't help but say with a sigh when I cover the scroll: "(What) greatness this classic has hidden! (It is) the precious raft to the path of the real immortal and fairy." However, from ancient times to today, there are many who look for the Tao, but for generations (we) cannot even see the one who can enter the Tao. It is not because the Tao is too high to be reached, it is just like entering the water without knowing how to row the boat, ascending the mountain without knowing the path. Though one desires to reach the other shore and ascend to the top, it is difficult. Therefore, the Buddhist family uses wisdom as the choice in entering the door. Even Lao Tzyy also said that if only the knowing is reached, then (the mind) can be calm and steady.

余讀易筋經譯義，為之三覆，見其中之德性功業，
一以貫之，未嘗不掩卷而嘆曰："大哉斯經之所蘊乎

，真仙佛兩途之寶筏也。"然古今求道者甚眾，而入
道者累世不一見也，非斯道之不可仰企也，是猶入
水而不知行船，登山而不知循徑，欲以臻彼岸躋絕
頂也難矣；故佛家以智慧為入門，即老氏亦曰知止
則泰定。

In summary, in order to achieve effectiveness, you must first
trace back the methods of training. If you cannot acquire the
methods, then during the process of training, (you will be) confused and won't be able to distinguish (the correct way). If
training comes first and understanding comes afterwards, then
you will have lost sight of the beginning and be looking for the
end. The training should be done later, for if you are rashly
moved to start too soon, then there is a problem in advancing
with skipping steps. (Since this is so), how can you blame it all
on the difficulty of entering the Tao, and say that this is why no
successor has been found in the accumulated generations.

總言欲奏其効，必先溯洄其功之法也。使不得其法
，則於行功之次第，茫然莫辨，如功之宜行於前者
，或昧焉行之於後，則有舍本圖末之失。功之宜施
行於後者，或貿焉行之於前，則有躐等而進之患。
又何怪夫入道之難，而累世不一見哉。

Therefore, in order to measure the cold or warmth of heaven and
earth, (you) must deliberate and investigate the weather. To see
the fullness and void of the sun and the moon, (you) must inspect
and pay attention to the light. Because (we) worry about
whether the tools are too long or too short, wide or narrow, light
or heavy, sharp or round, (and it is) hard to obtain the proper
size, then (we) make rules to standardize the sizes. Consider
there is high and low, when you apply (them), then (you know
the) advantages and disadvantages. Then (we are) afraid to lose
the advantageous ones. Think to select the most refined and the
best, again worry the herb must have the proper amount. When
it is used to wash and train, is afraid men lose the control.
(Therefore), for them, the prescriptions shown to be the standard.
(If there are) slight differences, are detailed.

是經天地之寒暑，必參之而稽其候。於日月之盈虛
，必察之而著其光。應夫器之長短、廣狹、輕重、
尖圓，難於中節也，為之定其規制。應夫則有高下
，用有利弊，恐取之失其美也。為之精其選要，又
慮夫藥之有定數。洗練有定法，恐人之失其制也，
為之列方而示以準則，纖毫有所必詳。

As to the entire body, up and down, internal and external, left
and right, front and back, no gap, skin and fasciae, tendons and

bones, blood and Chi, Ching and Lou, such kinds, all these things are explained in detail and completeness about the training's shallow and deep and sequence. When you open the scroll and read, (it will all be) clear as your palm and fingers. Following the order and pursuing it, you can enter the holy domain peacefully, and still have enough room to spare. Therefore, from this, the Chi is abundant and the Li is strong. The bones are sturdy and the fasciae are tough. Marvelous men and women are able to use this holy scholarship and martial result (i.e., bodily strength) to do the great business such as raising up the heaven and lifting up the earth (i.e., raising the spirit and improving the body), can be obtained (as easily as) dropping your hands. What (we) are talking about is the training of natural personality and moral achievement, (there is) no other way but using the single (theory) to connect them.

至於周身之上下內外左右、前後、無間、皮膜、筋骨、血氣、經絡之類。更無不貫惡夫功之淺深次第，使人開卷一覽，瞭如指掌，循其序而求之，可以平入聖境，而綽有餘裕矣。由是而氣盈力健，骨勁膜堅，以文武神聖之奇男女，作掀天揭地之大事業，可垂手而得之。非所云性功德業，一以貫之哉。

After this (stage), the more you advance, the more you refine the achievement. Then entering the water it will not wet, entering the fire it will not burn. The heaven and the earth (i.e., nature) cannot damage (you), the cold and hot cannot harm (you), I can build up my one life without limit like heaven. Think about what the great teacher Da Mo said, use this (Yi Gin Ching) as the foundation to become the Buddha and immortal, it isn't false. Gentlemen in later (generations), then believe it and excel in studying it. Therefore, complete the great achievement, and acquire the complete effectiveness. Therefore, (they) did not shame this inheritance by holy men which is to lead men into the Tao. (Because of this) I cannot but also place my heavy expectations (on you).

繼此功愈醇而愈進，則入水不濡、入火不焚、天地不能為之害，寒暑不能為之賊，可以命自我立，與天無極矣。想昔達磨大師所言，基此作佛成仙之語，為不誣。後之君子，於是經信而好之，所以服其全功，收其全劾，庶不負聖聖相傳，引人入道之意，余不能無厚望云爾。　　　　　　　　　　紫凝道人跋

PART THREE

MARROW/BRAIN WASHING CHI KUNG
(Shii Soei Ching)

Chapter 7

Theories and Principles

7-1. Introduction

As discussed in Part One, the Shii Soei Ching includes two main practices which enable you to extend the length of your life and perhaps even reach the goal of enlightenment. The first is leading sufficient Chi to the bone marrow to keep it clean, healthy, and functioning properly, the second is leading the abundant Chi to the brain to nourish it.

Although religious Chi Kung training had been kept secret for more than a thousand years, most of it was eventually more or less revealed to the public. However, in the case of the Shii Soei Ching, greater efforts were taken to preserve its secrecy, and it was generally believed to have been lost. It was not until this century that information on it was published and people were openly instructed. However, documentation on the Shii Soei Ching is still scarce, especially when compared with the wealth of information available on the Yi Gin Ching and other forms of Chi Kung. In Part One we discussed the reasons why many Chi Kung practices were kept secret for a long time. Now let us analyze why the Shii Soei Ching was kept more secret than any other Chi Kung practice. Generally speaking, there are several reasons for this:

1. The Shii Soei Ching training theories are much harder to understand than those of the Yi Gin Ching or any other Chi Kung training. Usually, only the monastery disciples or priests, who had reached a high level of understanding in Chi Kung, were taught.
2. The exercises are difficult and the final goal is hard to achieve. People who practice the Yi Gin Ching or other forms of Chi Kung can see results much more quickly, generally after one to three years of training. However, with the Shii Soei Ching, it may take more than ten years of correct training.
3. In order to reach a high level of Shii Soei Ching, your mind must be calm and peaceful. This requires separation from the emotional disturbances of everyday life, and perhaps even becoming a hermit. This is very difficult for most people to arrange.
4. In order reach a high level of Shii Soei Ching training, you must first train Yi Gin Ching to build up sufficient Chi. Though many

people omit this first step, and achieve some results in increasing their longevity, they have great difficulty in reaching the final goal of enlightenment.

5. In Shii Soei Ching training, the sexual organs are stimulated to increase the quantity of Water Chi (Pre-birth or Original Chi) and improve the efficiency of the Essence-Chi conversion. This was difficult to teach in the conservative Chinese society, and only trusted disciples learned the secrets.

Although a great number of the secrets of Shii Soei Ching training have been revealed to the public, it is still just as difficult, if not more so, to reach the final goal. Many questions still remain. For example, how do we define enlightenment? How can we explain enlightenment from the scientific point of view? How is it possible for people practicing part of the Shii Soei Ching to hibernate like some animals do? How can the spirit leave the physical body? In order to solve these kinds of questions, we must encourage those people who have the knowledge to open their minds and share it with us. At the same time, we must remain humble, open minded, and use the limited knowledge of modern science to aid us in our research. Unfortunately, I have not heard of anybody who has reached enlightenment and yet stayed part of lay society, rather than secluding himself away somewhere.

Before you make a serious commitment in Shii Soei training, you should analyze your intentions and goals. You can be confident and firm only if you understand the purpose of your training, and you have to set goals before you can reach them. Traditionally, there are three different goals for Shii Soei Ching training. The first is health and longevity. The second is to improve martial ability, and the third is enlightenment or Buddhahood. This book will go into the first goal in detail, but will discuss the third only superficially, because of the scarcity of documentation. The second goal will be discussed in a later volume: "Chi Kung and Martial Arts." Most people are probably interested primarily in the first goal, that of health and longevity. To reach this goal, you must understand the theory and training methods. However, the greatest requirement is patience and perseverance. Although the training is hard, you will find it very challenging, and you will gradually come to better understand the meaning of your life.

During the course of your study, you must clearly understand the differences between the Yi Gin Ching and the Shii Soei Ching. You must also know how they relate to each other for Kan and Lii adjustment. As mentioned earlier, if you wish to reach a higher efficiency in your training, you should first complete some level of the Yi Gin Ching training before you start the Shii Soei Ching. Although many people omit this first step and build up Chi solely by stimulating the sexual organs, their Chi will not have sufficient foundation and they will achieve only limited success. The biggest problem with this "quick" approach is that these people have not learned to regulate their minds, which is an important result of Yi Gin Ching training, and when they stimulate their sexual organs they also increase their sexual desire. The regulated mind is the main key in leading Chi to the marrow and to the brain. If you start Shii Soei Ching training without the necessary self-control, you may be caught up in the world of sexual fantasy.

Part of the required training for Buddhists is using the mind and certain techniques to lead Chi to the marrow and the brain. This is the main method the monks use to suppress their sexual desire. Because leading Chi to the brain raises the Shen, it is part of the enlightenment training for both Buddhists and Taoists. Although Shii Soei Ching originated with the Buddhists, it has divided into Buddhist and Taoist styles. Since more Taoist training documents are available, we will focus mainly on their training, and discuss the Buddhist methods only for purposes of comparison.

This chapter will focus on Shii Soei Ching theories and principles. To increase the depth of your understanding of the training, we will first review the relationship of the eight vessels to the training. This will be followed by a discussion of the general theories of Shii Soei Ching. The next section will summarize the training concepts, and the last section will discuss the four steps in the training process.

Once you have grasped the keys and the general concepts of the training, Chapter 8 will discuss the training methods. That chapter will first look at a number of important considerations, such as who can train, and will list the rules of the training. The fourth section will offer translations of and commentary on the available documents about Shii Soei Ching training methods. Finally, we will discuss the four major training procedures individually in the following four sections.

7-2. The Eight Vessels and Shii Soei Ching Chi Kung

I would like to begin with a review of a few important points concerning the purpose of Chi Kung training.

1. In order to keep your body healthy and have a long life, you must learn how to adjust Kan and Lii so that the Yin and Yang in your body are balanced and interact harmoniously. The Yang side is your physical body and the Yin side is your mental and spiritual body. These two bodies are mutually related, and they are connected by the Chi. Therefore, Chi is the center and the root of the entire body's health.

2. In order to understand how Chi can affect your body's Yin and Yang, you must first understand the Chi circulatory system. There are twelve primary organ-related Chi channels, which are considered to be like rivers which distribute Chi to the entire body. There are also eight Chi vessels, which are like reservoirs which store Chi and regulate the Chi which is circulating in the twelve primary channels. There are also millions of small Chi branches which circulate Chi from the primary channels out to the skin or beyond and also into the marrow to keep it clean.

3. In order to keep the Chi circulating smoothly, the Chi in the vessels (reservoirs) must be kept full and abundant. Shii Soei Ching teaches you how to accomplish this. You need to know how these vessels work, how they connect to the twelve primary channels, and how the eight vessels relate to each other.

In one of the documents, there is a section which says:

Transport (the Chi through) the marvelous meridians (i.e., the 12 primary channels), get through the eight vessels, every part of the body will meet the (Chi) source. The more you refine

your training, the more you will advance, (you will) enter the door to the large Tao.

This section clearly tells you that the way to advance in the Tao is to learn how to transport Chi through the twelve channels and the eight vessels. This means that the Chi in all of the channels and vessels must be circulating smoothly so that they can mutually support each other.

Imagine that the Chi in your body is like water running through a network of many rivers (primary channels) and streams (small Chi channels) to nourish your body. In order to keep the water running smoothly, the rivers and streams must be clear and without stagnation. You need to insure that there is plenty of water so that the flow will be continuous and smooth. This requires that the reservoirs which store and regulate the flow in the rivers and streams be kept full.

Unfortunately, although there are many documents which discuss the eight vessels, there is still a great deal about them which is not understood. This is why these vessels are commonly called "mysterious vessels" (Chyi Ching Ba Mei). They are also sometimes referred to in English as the "extraordinary vessels." In this section we will draw upon the available documents first to summarize briefly the purpose and functions of each vessel, and then we will discuss how they relate to each other and how they connect to the Chi channels and regulate them. If you wish to have a deeper explanation, please consult any of the acupuncture books which discuss this subject.

The Eight Extraordinary Vessels
1. The Governing Vessel (Du Mei)(Figure 7-1)
The Governing Vessel includes four courses and is the confluence of all the Yang channels, over which it is said to "govern." Because it controls all the Yang channels, it is called the "Sea of Yang Meridians." This is apparent from its pathway because it flows on the midline of the back, a Yang area, and in the center of all Yang channels (except the Stomach channel, which flows in the front). The Governing Vessel governs all the Yang channels, which means that it can be used to increase the Yang energy of the body.

Since the Governing Vessel is the "Sea of Yang Meridians" and it controls or governs the back, the area richest in Guardian Chi (Wey Chi), it is also responsible for the circulation of the body's Guardian Chi to guard against external evil influences. The circulation of Guardian Chi starts from Fengfu (Gv-16), and moves down the Governing Vessel to the Huiyin (Co-1).

According to Chinese medical science, Guardian Chi is Yang Chi, and therefore represents the "Fire" of the body. Its quick and ubiquitous circulation keeps the Fire going in the body and controls the loss of body heat. Guardian Chi is also inextricably linked with the fluids that flow outside the channels, in the skin and flesh. Consequently, through the breathing (under control of the Lungs), Guardian Chi is responsible for the opening and the closing of the pores, and also controls the sweat.

The Governing Vessel is also responsible for nourishing the five ancestral organs, which include the brain and spinal cord. This is one of the ways in which the Kidneys "control" the brain, as is said in Chinese medicine.

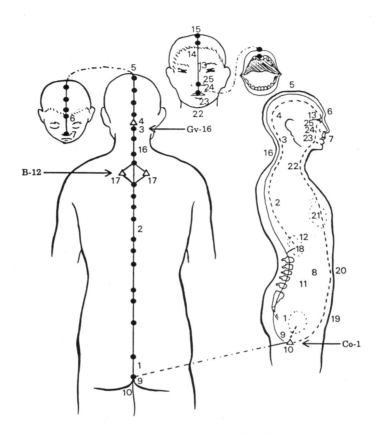

Figure 7-1. The Governing Vessel (Du Mei)

Because of their importance to health, the Governing Vessel together with the Conception Vessel are considered the two most important Chi channels to be trained in Chi Kung, especially in Nei Dan. Training related to these two vessels includes: 1. How to fill them with Chi so that you have enough to regulate the twelve channels, 2. How to open up stagnant areas in these two vessels so that the Chi flows smoothly and strongly, 3. How to effectively direct the Chi to nourish the brain and raise up the Shen, 4. How to effectively govern the Chi in the twelve channels, and nourish the organs, 5. How to use your raised Shen to lead the Guardian Chi to the skin and strengthen the Guardian Chi shield covering your body.

In Nei Dan Chi Kung training, when you have filled up the Chi in these two vessels and can effectively circulate the Chi in them, you have achieved the "Small Circulation." In order to do this, you must know how to convert the Essence stored in the Kidneys into Chi, circulate this Chi in the Governing and Conception Vessels, and finally lead this Chi to the head to nourish the brain and Shen (spirit).

This vessel intersects Fengmen (B-12) on the Bladder channels and connects with the Conception and Thrusting Vessels at the Huiyin (Co-1), Yang Linking Vessel at the Yamen (Gv-15) and Fengfu (Gv-16), and Yang Heel Vessel at Fengfu (Gv-16).

2. The Conception Vessel (Ren Mei)(Figure 7-2)

Ren in Chinese means "direction, responsibility." Ren Mei, the "Conception Vessel," has a major role in Chi circulation, directing and being responsible for all of the Yin channels (plus the Stomach channel).

This vessel includes two courses which nourish the uterus (one of the five ancestral organs) and the whole genital system. It is said in the Nei Ching that the Conception and Thrusting Vessels contain both blood and Essence (Jieng), and both flow up to the face and around the mouth.

It was described in the Su Wen that both the Conception and Thrusting Vessels control the life cycles, which have been traditionally considered to last 7 years for women and 8 years for men. It is the changes taking place in these vessels at those intervals that promote the major alterations in our lives.

In addition, the Conception Vessel also controls the distribution and "dispersion" of Guardian Chi all over the abdomen and thorax via numerous small Chi branches (Lou). This vessel also plays an important role in the distribution of body fluids in the abdomen.

As mentioned previously, in Chi Kung society this vessel and the Governing Vessel are considered the most important among the Chi channels and vessels, and must be trained first. It is believed that there is usually no significant Chi stagnation in the Conception Vessel. However, it is important to increase the amount of Chi you are able to store, which also increases your ability to regulate the Yin channels.

This vessel intersects Chengqi (S-1) on the Stomach channel and connects with the Governing Vessel at Yinjiao (Gv-28) and Huiyin (Co-1), the Yin Linking Vessel at Tiantu (Co-22) and Lianquan (Co-23), and the Thrusting Vessel at Huiyin (Co-1) and Yinjiao (Co-7).

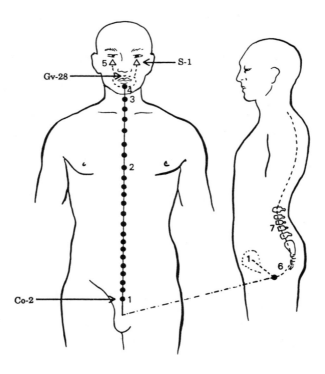

Figure 7-2. The Conception Vessel (Ren Mei)

3. The Thrusting Vessel (Chong Mei)(Figure 7-3)

This vessel includes five courses. One of the major purposes of the Thrusting Vessel is to connect, communicate with, and mutually support the Conception Vessel. Because of this mutual Chi support, both can effectively regulate the Chi in the Kidney channel. The Kidneys are the residence of Original Chi and are considered one of the most vital Yin organs.

The Thrusting Vessel is considered one of the most important and decisive vessels in successful Chi Kung training, especially in Shii Soei Ching. There are many reasons for this. The first reason is that this vessel intersects two cavities on the Conception Vessel: Huiyin (Co-1) and Yinjiao (Co-7). Huiyin means "meeting with Yin" and is the cavity where the Yang and Yin Chi are transferred. Yinjiao means "Yin Junction," and it is located slightly above the Qihai (Co-6)(called the Lower Dan Tien in Chi Kung). It is the cavity where the Original Chi (Water Chi, or Yin Chi) interfaces with the Fire Chi created from food and air. The Thrusting Vessel also connects with eleven cavities on the Kidney channel. The Kidney is considered the residence of Original Essence (Yuan Jieng), which is converted into Original Chi (Yuan Chi).

The second reason for the importance of the Thrusting Vessel in Chi Kung training is that it is connected directly to the marrow of the

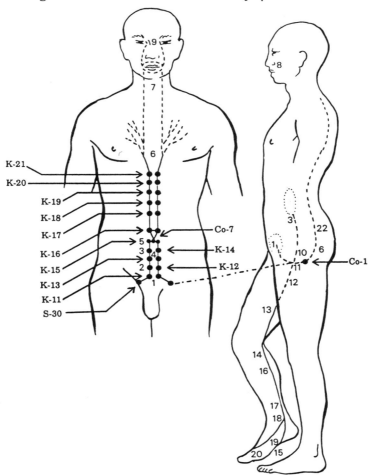

Figure 7-3. The Thrusting Vessel (Chong Mei)

spinal cord and reaches up to the brain. The main goal of Shii Soei Ching Chi Kung is to lead the Chi into the marrow and then further on to the head, nourishing the brain and spirit (Shen).

And finally, the third reason is found in actual Chi Kung practice. There are three common training paths: Fire, Wind, and Water. In Fire path Chi Kung, the emphasis is on the Fire or Yang Chi circulating in the Governing Vessel and therefore strengthening the muscles and organs. The Fire path is the main Chi training in Yi Gin Ching Chi Kung. However, the Fire path can also cause the body to become too Yang, and therefore speed up the process of degeneration. In order to adjust the Fire to a proper level, Shii Soei Ching Chi Kung is also trained. This uses the Water path, in which Chi separates from the route of the Fire path at the Huiyin cavity (Co-1), enters the spinal cord, and finally reaches up to the head. The Water path teaches how to use Original Chi to cool down the body, and then to use this Chi to nourish the brain and train the spirit. Learning to adjust the Fire and Water Chi circulation in the body is called Kan-Lii, which means Water-Fire. You can see from this that the Thrusting Vessel plays a very important role in Chi Kung training.

This vessel intersects the Kidney channel at Henggu (K-11), Dahe (K-12), Qixue (K-13), Siman (K-14), Zhongzhu (K-15), Huangshu (K-16), Shangqu (K-17), Shiguan (K-18), Yindu (K-19), Tonggu (K-20), and Youmen (K-21), and the Stomach channel at Qichong (S-30). It also connects with the Conception Vessel at Huiyin (Co-1) and Yinjiao (Co-7), and the Governing Vessel at Huiyin (Co-1).

4. The Girdle Vessel (Dai Mei)(Figure 7-4)

The major purpose of the Girdle Vessel is to regulate the Chi of the Gall Bladder. It is also responsible for the Chis horizontal balance. If you have lost this balance, you will have lost your center and balance both mentally and physically.

From the point of view of Chi Kung, the Girdle Vessel is also responsible for the strength of the waist area. When Chi is full and circulating smoothly, back pain will be avoided. In addition, because the Kidneys are located nearby, this vessel is also responsible for Chi circulation around the Kidneys, maintaining their health. Most important of all for the Girdle Vessel is the fact that the Lower Dan Tien is located in its area. In order to lead Original Chi from the Kidneys to the Lower Dan Tien, the waist area must be healthy and relaxed. This means that the Chi flow in the waist area must be smooth.

This vessel intersects the Gall Bladder channel at Daimai (GB-26), Wushu (GB-27), and Weidao (GB-28).

5. The Yang Heel Vessel (Yangchiao Mei)(Figure 7-5)

While the preceding four vessels (Governing, Conception, Thrusting, and Girdle) are located in the trunk, this and the next three are located in the trunk and legs. (In addition, each of these four vessels is paired.) For millions of years, man has been walking on his rear legs, which do much more strenuous work than the arms do. I believe that it was because of this that, as evolution proceeded, the legs gradually developed these vessels to provide Chi support and regulate the channels. If this is true, it may be that, as time goes on

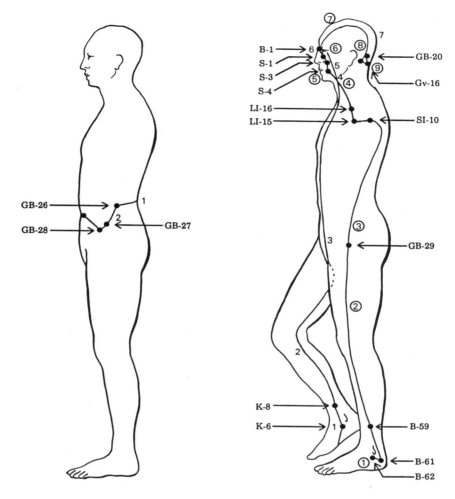

Figure 7-4. The Girdle Vessel
(Dai Mei)

Figure 7-5. The Yang Heel Vessel
(Yangchiao Mei) and
The Yin Heel Vessel
(Yinchiao Mei)

and man uses his legs less and less, in a few million years these vessels will gradually disappear.

The Chi filling this vessel is supplied mainly through exercising the legs, which converts the food Essence or fat stored in the legs. This Chi is then led upward to nourish the Yang channels. It is believed in Chi Kung that, since this vessel is also connected with your brain, certain leg exercises can be used to cure headaches. Since a headache is caused by excess Chi in the head, exercising the legs will draw this Chi downward to the leg muscles and relieve the pressure in the head.

Most of the training that relates to this vessel is Wai Dan. Wai Dan Chi Kung is considered Yang, and specializes in training the Yang channels, while Nei Dan Chi Kung is considered relatively Yin, and emphasizes the Yin channels more.

This vessel intersects the Bladder channel at Jingming (B-1), Fuyang (B-59), Pushen (B-61), and Shenmai (B-62), the Gall Bladder channel at Fengchi (GB-20) and Juliao (GB-29), the Small Intestine channel at Naoshu (SI-10), the Large Intestine channel at Jianyu (LI-15) and Jugu (LI-16), and the Stomach channel at Chengqi (S-1), Juliao (S-3), and Dicang (S-4). It also connects to the Governing Vessel directly at Fengfu (Gv-16) and communicates with the Yang Linking Vessel through the Small Intestine channel at (SI-10), the Yin Heel Vessel through the Bladder channel at Jingming (B-1), and the Conception Vessel through the Stomach channel at Chengqi (S-1).

6. The Yin Heel Vessel (Yinchiao Mei)(Figure 7-5)

The Yin Heel Vessel intersects with the Kidney channel at Zhaohai (K-6) and Jiaoxin (K-8), and the Bladder channel at Jingming (B-1). It communicates with the Yang Heel Vessel through the Bladder channel (B-1). This vessel connects directly to the brain. One of the main sources of Chi for this vessel is the conversion of the Kidney Essence into Chi. It is believed in Chi Kung society that the other main Chi source is the Essence of the external Kidneys (testicles). In Shii Soei Ching Chi Kung, one of the training processes is to stimulate the testicles in order to increase the hormone production and increase the conversion of the Essence into Chi. At the same time, you would learn how to lead the Chi in this vessel up to the head to nourish the brain and spirit (Shen). With this nourishment, you would be able to reach Buddhahood or enlightenment. From a health and longevity point of view, the raised spirit will be able to efficiently direct the Chi of the entire body and maintain your health.

7. The Yang Linking Vessel (Yangwei Mei)(Figure 7-6)

This vessel intersects the Bladder channel at Jinmen (B-63), the Gall Bladder channel at Benshen (GB-13), Yangbai (GB-14), Head-Linqi (GB-15), Muchuang (GB-16), Zhengying (GB-17), Chengling (GB-18), Naokong (GB-19), Fengchi (GB-20), Jianjing (GB-21), and Yangjiao (GB-35), the Triple Burner channel at Tianliao (TB-15), and the Small Intestine channel at Naoshu (SI-10). It also directly connects with the Governing Vessel at Yamen (Gv-15) and Fengfu (Gv-16), and communicates with the Yin Linking Vessel through the Stomach channel at Touwei (S-8), and with the Gall Bladder channel through the above intersecting cavities.

You can see from these connections that the Yang Linking Vessel regulates the Chi mainly in the Yang channels: the Urinary Bladder, Gall Bladder, Triple Burner, Small Intestine, and Stomach channels. This vessel and the Yang Heel Vessel have not been emphasized much in Chi Kung, except in Iron Shirt training where these two and the Governing Vessel are trained.

8. The Yin Linking Vessel (Yinwei Mei)(Figure 7-6)

This vessel intersects the Kidney channel at Zhubin (K-9), the Spleen channel at Chongmen (Sp-12), Fushe (Sp-13), Daheng (Sp-15) and Fuai (Sp-16), and the Liver channel at Qimen (Li-14). It connects directly to the Conception Vessel at Tiantu (Co-22) and Lianquan (Co-23), and communicates with the Yang Linking Vessel through the Stomach channel and the Gall Bladder channel. This vessel is not trained much in Chi Kung.

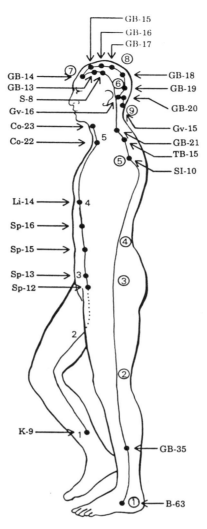

Figure 7-6. The Yang Linking Vessel (Yangwei Mei) and The Yin Linking Vessel (Yinwei Mei)

The Connection of the Vessels

From the above information you can see that, except for the Girdle Vessel which must connect to other vessels through the Gall Bladder channel, the other seven Chi vessels are connected to each other either directly or through gates in the channels. These gates are usually used by the vessels to regulate the Chi flow in the channels. The vessels provide mutual support for each other whenever the Chi level in any one vessel is low. Therefore, in Chi Kung practice, you may just choose a few vessels (usually the Conception and Governing Vessels) in which to store the Chi generated from your training, and this Chi will flow automatically to the other vessels.

Figure 7-7 shows how the vessels are connected to each other. A solid line is use when there is a direct connection between the vessels, and a dotted line is used if the connection is through a channel by way of the Chi gates. A study of the diagram leads to several important conclusions:

1. The Huiyin cavity (Co-1) is the main intersection point for three major vessels: Governing, Conception, and Thrusting. Naturally, this cavity will become the key point in adjusting the Chi flow

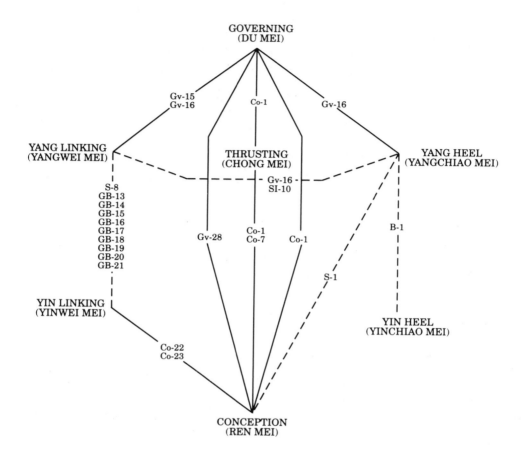

Figure 7-7. The Connections Among the Vessels

among these three vessels. The Huiyin is one of the key cavities called "Shyuan Guan," or "Magic Gate." In Chinese Chi Kung, especially Nei Dan, it is believed that when this cavity is adjusted accurately, the Kan and Lii can be effectively controlled and the body's Yin and Yang can be regulated.

2. The Thrusting Vessel is connected with the Conception Vessel not only at Huiyin (Co-1) but also at Yinjiao (Co-7). Yinjiao means "Yin Junction" and is believed to be the place where the Yang and Yin Chi meet. Yinjiao is located slightly above the Lower Dan Tien or Qihai (Co-6), which is the residence of the Water Chi. In Chi Kung, it is through this cavity that the Chi's Kan and Lii can be adjusted and, consequently, the body's Yin and Yang can be regulated.

3. There is another cavity which is also called Yinjiao (Gv-28). Although the pronunciation is the same, it is a different word from the Yinjiao (Co-7) mentioned above. The Yinjiao (Gv-28) is the place where the Governing and Conception Vessels connect. Not much attention is paid to this cavity in Chi Kung practice.

4. The cavity Fengfu (Gv-16) in the Governing Vessel behind the head is the intersection of the Governing, Yang Heel, and Yang Linking

Vessels. Therefore, the Chi in these three vessels is mutually supported through this cavity.

5. The Yin Linking Vessel connects directly with the Conception Vessel, and they regulate each other.

6. The Yang Linking and Yin Linking Vessels do not connect to each other directly, however, they communicate to each other through the Stomach and Gall Bladder channels.

7. The Yang Heel and Yang Linking Vessels, although they connect to each other through the Governing Vessel, also use the Small Intestine channel to communicate with each other.

8. The Yang Heel Vessel and Conception Vessel communicate with each other through the Stomach channel. The Yang Heel Vessel also communicates with the Yin Heel Vessel through the Bladder channel.

Now let us put the connections of the eight vessels to the twelve primary Chi channels together in a diagram, shown in Figure 7-8. We can see more clearly from this picture how the Chi vessels regulate the Chi channels. In this diagram, the top line lists the six Yin channels while the bottom line lists the paired Yang channels. For example, the Heart channel is Yin and its paired Yang channel is the Small Intestine. The center line, of course, lists the eight vessels. We can draw a number of important conclusions from this diagram:

1. You may be surprised to see that none of the vessels are connected to the Heart, Pericardium, or Lung channels. If you think carefully, you will realize something. The Heart and the Pericardium are the two most vital organs in the body, and the Chi level must be very accurate. If they were connected to the vessels, an excessive amount of Chi might flood into them when the body reacted to an emergency, and cause a serious malfunction. Therefore, I believe that the Chi level in these two channels is regulated through their paired Yang channels (Small Intestine and Triple Burner), which are connected to the Yang Linking and Yang Heel Vessels. Since paired channels balance each other, when the Chi level in one is too strong or too weak, the other channel will regulate it. Therefore, the Chi level in the Heart and Pericardium channels is regulated indirectly by the Yang Linking and Yang Heel Vessels.

    Then, if you wonder why there is no connection between the Lung channel and any of the vessels, you should again think of the function of the Lungs. The Lung is the organ which absorbs air Chi. It is a Chi supply center for the body, and so there is never a problem with its being deficient in Chi. Furthermore, its Chi level can again be regulated through its paired Yang channel, the Large Intestine.

2. The Thrusting, Yin Linking, and Yin Heel Vessels are directly connected with the Kidney. The Kidney is the residence of the Original Essence. Whenever the Chi in these three vessels is low, the Original Essence in the Kidney will be converted into Original Chi to supply them. In Shii Soei Ching training, the Thrusting and Yin Heel are the two main vessels. In the training, Chi is led from the Yin Heel Vessel upward through the Kidney channel to the Thrusting Vessel and finally to the brain.

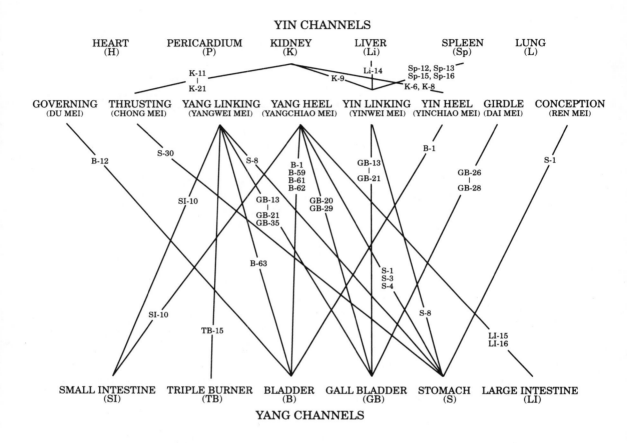

Figure 7-8. The Connections of the Eight Vessels to the Twelve
Primary Channels

7-3. Theories

In this section we will discuss the fundamental theory of Shii Soei Ching Chi Kung. We will discuss it in two parts. The first part will be on how the Shii Soei Ching nourishes and cleans the marrow, and the second part will be on how it washes the brain.

Shii Soei Ching and the Marrow

Before we discuss how Shii Soei Ching cleans the bone marrow, we would first like to review the relationship between marrow and your health. Then we will discuss the relationship between the Shii Soei Ching training and the marrow.

1. Marrow and Health
A. Marrow is a factory for blood cells.

To understand how marrow relates to your health, you must first understand the role that marrow plays in your life. We know today that marrow is a living factory which manufactures most of your red and white blood cells. To work efficiently, this factory needs an abundant supply of Chi. When you are young and still growing, The Chi supply is sufficient and the marrow produces a large amount of fresh, healthy blood cells to supply your body's needs. The blood cells carry nutrition and oxygen throughout your body, and are the main source of your body's nourishment. When you have healthy blood cells, your body will function properly and continue to grow. Your body is just like a car: it needs good fuel to keep running smoothly. Once you get older and the Chi supply becomes deficient, part of the marrow becomes fat. The marrow starts to function more slowly, and it produces an ever greater percentage of unhealthy blood cells. As these circulate in your body, your organs and muscles start to degenerate.

According to Chinese medicine, the blood cells are also the main carriers of Chi. The Chi in the blood cells not only keeps them alive, but it also is carried to every part of the body. It is believed that the reason an injured child can heal himself much faster than an adult is because the Chi in his marrow is more abundant. You can see that you must supply plenty of Chi to your marrow both to keep it functioning and to supply adequate Chi for the blood cells.

B. Marrow is the reservoir of your Chi.

According to updated body bioelectric research, it is believed that the marrow might be a plasma which is able to store an abundance of electrical charges. If this is true, then the marrow acts like a battery which not only produces blood cells, but also regulates Chi like the vessels. This means when the Chi in the marrow starts to be deficient, the body starts to age and deteriorate.

You can see from this discussion that the first step in maintaining your health and increasing your longevity is to learn how to increase the Chi circulation to your marrow to re-activate the marrow which is degenerating. This will prevent the marrow from changing into fat. Naturally, you must have plenty of Chi before you can do this. Next, let us see how the Shii Soei Chi Kung can wash the marrow.

2. How Shii Soei Ching Cleans the Marrow

There are two requirements for cleaning the marrow in the Shii Soei Ching training. First, you must have a lot more Chi than you normally need. If you do not have this surplus of Chi, you will not have enough to clean the marrow. Second, you must learn the methods of leading the Chi to the marrow. Even if you have produced a sufficient level of Chi, if you do not know how to use it, the abundant Chi may make your body too Yang and make your body degenerate faster than normal. We have already mentioned earlier that in order to increase your Chi level, in addition to Yi Gin Ching training, you must also learn how to obtain more Chi from other methods, such as stimulating the sexual organs. This training will increase your Chi level, but it will also make your body Yang. Shii Soei Ching is the training which teaches you how to use this abundance of Chi and make your body more Yin in order to balance the Yang. Increasing the Chi level through Yi Gin Ching has been discussed in Part Two, and sexual stimulation will be discussed later. Here, we will focus on how the Chi can be led to the marrow. The discussion will be divided into spine marrow, limb marrow, and rib marrow.

A. Spine Marrow:

Cleaning the spine marrow is probably the most important part of the Shii Soei Ching. Because the spine marrow connects to the brain, when you train to lead the Chi up to the head from the lower part of your body, you are also cleaning the spine marrow. This will be discussed later in "How Shii Soei Ching nourishes the brain."

B. Limb Marrow:

Generally, there are two main techniques for cleaning the bone marrow in the limbs. However, these techniques can also be used for other parts of the body. If you understand the theory and the principles, and then you can apply this understanding to other places.

a. Bone Breathing

Bone breathing technique is classified as Nei Dan Shii Soei Ching. In Chi Kung, it is believed that there are two ways the Chi can be led into the marrow in bone breathing. One way is through the joint area of the bones. Since the center of the joint is the weakest part of the bone, it is believed that the Chi can enter here most easily (Figure 7-9). The other way is to lead the Chi into the bones laterally through the millions of small Chi channels (Figure 7-10). It is believed that the fasciae between the bone and the muscles is the key to marrow nour-

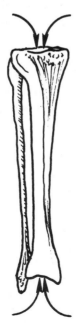
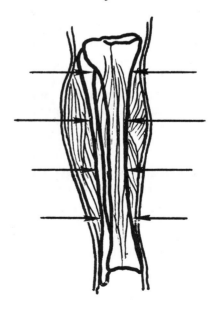

Figure 7-9.   Chi Entering the Bone Through the Joint

Figure 7-10.   Chi Entering the Bone Laterally Through the Small Chi Channels

ishment. The more Chi you are able to store in these fasciae, the more you will be able to supply to the marrow.

In bone breathing you learn how to use your Yi and inhaling to lead Chi from the primary channels deep into the marrow. We have explained in Part One how you use your Yi and breathing for the Kan and Lii adjustment. Inhaling is the Kan which enables you to lead the Chi deep into your body and make your body Yin. This is the reason why you must first build up your Chi and make your body Yang before Shii Soei Ching training.

In the bone breathing training, your mind must be calm, steady, and able to sense the Chi very deeply in your body. As you practice deep inhalation in coordination with holding up your Huiyin and anus, you will be able to lead the Chi gradually deeper and deeper until it reaches the marrow. The training is as hard as you would expect. You need to have reached a very high level of Chi Kung practice before you can sense this deep in your body.

b. Beating Stimulation

The second method for bringing Chi into the marrow is the beating exercises. This is a well known Wai Dan exercise to increase the effectiveness of the Chi exchange in the marrow. You use a pestle or bunch of steel wires to strike the bones, joints, and muscles to increase the potential of the fasciae for storing Chi. You start hitting lightly and gradually increase the force. The beating increases the Chi circulation between the bone marrow and the skin through stimulation (Figure 7-11). You should not use too much power, or you may injure yourself.

You can see that the second method is easier. However, the first method is considered to be more effective. Nei Dan Marrow Washing has been considered a vital key to longevity and enlightenment.

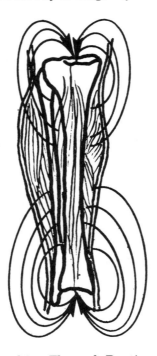

Figure 7-11. Bone Breathing Through Beating Stimulation

C. Rib Marrow:

You use the same methods to clean the rib marrow that you used to clean the limb marrow. However, it is much harder to lead the Chi to the rib marrow with Nei Dan bone breathing than it is to lead it to the limbs. The Wai Dan beating methods remain effective since the ribs are very close to the surface of the skin. It is therefore recommended that you continue the beating even after you have completed the Yi Gin Ching training.

Shii Soei Ching and the Brain

Before we discuss this subject, we would first like to review how your brain relates to your health:

1. The Brain and Health

A. Your brain is the center of your whole being. It generates ideas which govern your thoughts, your spirit, and the Chi field of your body. When your brain degenerates, you age and lose the normal functioning of your body.

B. Your brain is the main source of the EMF which is necessary for the circulation of Chi. If you are able to concentrate to a higher degree, the EMF will be stronger and the Chi flow which is led by the brain will be stronger and smoother.

C. When your brain is healthy, you can raise your spirit to a higher level while keeping it at its center. When this happens, your mental and physical body can be energized and the spirit of vitality can be raised. Raising the spirit of vitality is the key to a long life.

D. When the brain cells are activated to a higher level, you may increase your sensitivity to nature and events happening around you. This will increase your wisdom and your understanding of nature. The average person uses approximately 30-35% of his brain. If you can learn to increase the percentage of your brain that you use, you will become smarter, govern your body's Chi more efficiently, and raise your spirit significantly. All of these are factors in health and longevity.

Let us then summarize how we increase the functioning of our brains to a higher level. This will provide you with the key to the following discussion of Shii Soei Ching.

2. How the Shii Soei Ching Nourishes the Brain and Raises the Shen

In Chi Kung, the top of your head (Baihui) is also called "Guu Shen," which means "Valley Spirit," while the Upper Dan Tien (the third eye) is also called "Shen Guu," which means "Spirit Valley." From the structure of the brain (Figure 7-12), you can see that the two brain lobes form a deep valley on the top of your head. From the top of your head the heaven Chi is able to reach the center of your brain. It is believed that the Baihui or Guu Shen is the place or gate where the body's Chi communicates with the heaven Chi. With the nourishment of heaven Chi, you will grow wiser and more clever. Again, please notice the area of your third eye or Upper Dan Tien where your Shen resides: you can see that the Shen resides at the entrance to the valley formed by the two lobes of the brain. I personally believe that this valley structure

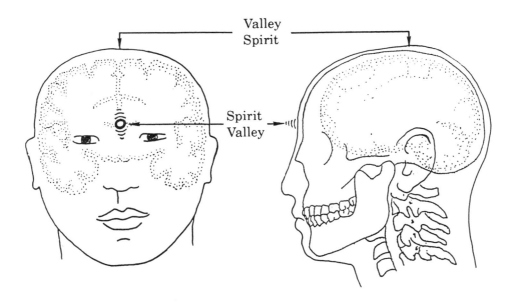

Figure 7-12. "Valley Spirit" (Guu Shen) and "Spirit Valley" (Shen Guu)

forms a resonant chamber for energy, which allows us to correspond to and sense nature more clearly and easily.

Chinese Chi Kung practitioners believe that if you keep leading Chi to the Upper Dan Tien you will be able to completely open up the third eye, which will give you a much greater sensitivity to the world around you. This process is called "Kai Chiaw," or "Opening the Tricky Gate." Modern science has found that bone is a semi-conductor. Therefore, once you have plenty of Chi or bioelectricity you can activate the bone in the area of the third eye so that it becomes a conductor.

You can see from this brief discussion that, in order to increase the efficiency of your brain and open the gate of the Upper Dan Tien, you must first have plenty of Chi. The next step is to learn how to lead this Chi to your head correctly. Next, we will consider some of the Chi Kung practices which teach you how to nourish your brain.

A. Increase the Oxygen Supply to the Brain.

In order to keep the brain functioning properly, you first have to provide it with plenty of oxygen. Modern science tells us that a brain cell needs more than ten times as much oxygen as any other cell in the body. That means that when there is an oxygen deficiency in your body, your brain will be the first organ to sense it, and you will feel dizzy. If the condition persists, the brain cells will be damaged before any other cells. When people get old, their inhalations usually become shorter and shorter, and their bodies run short of oxygen. This may account for the fact that memory loss is one of the first symptoms of aging.

In Chi Kung, training the breath is a vital requirement. It is called "Tyau Shyi," or "regulating the breath." The goal of regulating your breath is learning how to increase the oxygen input while keeping the body relaxed. In advanced Chi Kung training, you must also learn how to reduce the waste of oxygen during meditation. This is done by leading your mind into a very deep and relaxed meditative state.

B. Activate More Brain Cells.

We normally use only 30-35% of our brain cells, which means we are wasting 65-70% of our brains. This is like having a big computer, but only using a third of it. Through Chi Kung it is possible to increase the percentage of your brain that you use. This will enable you to feel what ordinary people cannot feel, sense what ordinary people cannot sense, and see and judge the future more clearly. When your brain has reached the higher stages of sensitivity, it will be able to act like a radio station and communicate with the energy of nature and other human brains. Theoretically, it is very simple to reach this goal. If you increase the amount of Chi or bioelectricity going to your brain, you will activate more brain cells. It is believed that once the unused cells have been activated, they will remain activated.

Since a brain cell requires more than ten times as much oxygen as other cells, it is reasonable to assume that they will also need at least ten times as much Chi. If this is correct, then you will need to know how to generate a large quantity of Chi in your body.

It is believed that, as you activate more brain cells, you will increase the energy level of your brain. Naturally, this will increase the sensitivity of your brain, and also raise your spirit. When people reach the higher levels, as they meditate they will generate a large electrical charge in their brains. This will react with the atmosphere around their heads, creating a halo effect which may be visible in the dark.

Once you are able to lead your spirit to a higher level, you will be able to use it to govern your Chi circulation more effectively. This is the main key to longevity.

In order to generate plenty of Chi to nourish and activate the brain, you must learn how to conserve your Chi, how to increase its production, and also how to interact the Yin (Water) and Yang (Fire) Chi in the Huang Ting cavity (Figure 7-13). In Taoist Chi Kung the Huang Ting is considered the place where the elixir embryo can be generated. Normally, if it is done correctly in Shii Soei Ching, it will take 100 days of storing Chi in the Huang Ting (called "100 days of building the foundation") and ten months of increasing the Chi level to the necessary high level ("ten months of pregnancy") before you are able to lead the Chi to the head and grow the "holy baby" at the Upper Dan Tien. Growing the holy baby ultimately means gradually activating the brain cells until they have reached a high enough energy level. In Shii Soei Ching training, this stage is called "three years of nursing." Once your brain and spirit have reached this stage, you start learning how to lead the spirit to separate from your physical body.

C. Train the Concentration to Purify the Peaceful Mind.

Modern science says that at least twelve ideas pass through your brain every second, although we are normally only aware of a few of them. Your mind is seldom concentrated enough for you to be aware of what you are thinking and reduce the unnecessary thoughts. Most people can only do this under hypnosis. This explains why, when you are hypnotized, your mind is able to sense situations to a higher level than you normally could. Meditation is a type of self-hypnosis which

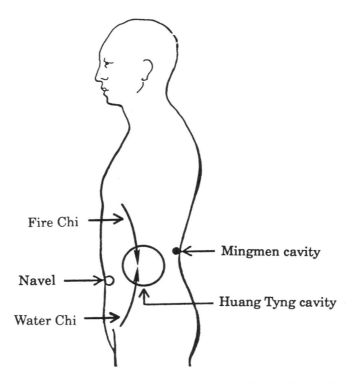

Figure 7-13. Interaction of the Yin (Water) and Yang (Fire) Chi in the Huang Ting Cavity

trains you to lead your mind to a higher meditative state and reach a higher level of concentration. It is believed that the greater your concentration, the higher you can raise your spirit. You can see that, in addition to increasing the Chi to activate the brain cells, you must also learn how to concentrate and how to use the activated cells efficiently. Only then can your spirit be raised.

D. Train to Feel and Sense Yourself and Nature.

After you have been nursing your holy spiritual baby for three years, the baby learns to be independent. Then you must educate the baby. This stage is called "nine years of facing the wall," and means nine years of education for the baby Shen. The goal is returning this spirit to its very origin (before its birth into a human form), and learning to feel and sense nature. This teaches the baby to again be an independent life form. I have not found any document which teaches why and how you do this. I believe that this is because the people who have reached this stage do not bother to write it down because they are in an emotionally neutral state.

7-4. Training Concepts

In this section we will discuss the general theory and principles which are used to approach the heart of the Shii Soei Ching training. You should understand that it does not matter whether you follow the Taoist or Buddhist approach, you must follow these fundamental theories and training procedures. This section will help you build up a firm understanding of the training which will be discussed in the next chapter.

After fourteen hundred years of Shii Soei Ching training, it is believed that in order to reach the final goal of enlightenment or Buddhahood, you must follow four necessary steps:

A. Refining the Essence (Semen) and Converting it into Chi (Liann Jieng Huah Chi) - One Hundred days of Building the Foundation (Bae Ryh Jwu Ji)

B. Purifying Chi and Converting it into Shen (Liann Chi Huah Shen) - Ten Months of Pregnancy (Shyr Yueh Hwai Tai)

C. Refining Shen and Returning it to Nothingness (Liann Shen Faan Shiu) - Three Years of Nursing (San Nian Buh Ruu)

D. Crushing the Nothingness (Feen Suory Shiu Kong) - Nine Years of Facing the Wall (Jeou Nian Miann Bih)

You can see that the Tao of reaching enlightenment or becoming a Buddha requires years of training. It includes four basic stages of conversion training, which includes the formation of "Baby Elixir"(100 days of foundation) which is commonly called "Sheng Tai" (holy embryo) or "Ling Tai" (spiritual embryo), 10 months of nourishing and growing, three years of nursing, and finally educating this baby spirit until it grows stronger and becomes independent. In Taoist and Buddhist Chi Kung training, it is believed that in order to reach the final goal of enlightenment and Buddhahood, you must first build up an independent spiritual energy body. After your physical body is dead, this spiritual body will continue to live eternally and will not reenter the path of reincarnation.

After the Shii Soei Ching was revealed to laymen, a change took place in the training. Because the final goal of enlightenment or Buddhahood was not the main reason laymen practiced, and because the final step of training was hard to understand and to reach, many Shii Soei Ching practitioners who were looking only for longevity considered that there were only the first three steps of training, and ignored the final step. For this reason, there are very few documents which can lead you to this final step. We will now discuss these four training stages in more detail.

A. Refining the Essence (Semen) and Converting it into Chi (Liann Jieng Huah Chi) - One Hundred Days of Building the Foundation (Bae Ryh Jwu Ji)

In China, Taoists always visualize the achievement of enlightenment first in terms of forming a Spiritual Embryo (Ling Tai) or Holy Embryo (Sheng Tai), and then its feeding, nursing, and education until it can be independent. For many Shii Soei Ching practitioners who are looking only for longevity, this spiritual baby is considered a "Baby Elixir" which will lead them to longevity. It is believed that the healthy and harmonious interaction of Yin and Yang Chi is necessary to form this spiritual baby. Yin is considered the mother while Yang is considered the father. In order to make this happens, Yin (Water) and Yang (Fire) Chi must be abundant, and both the father (Yang) and mother (Yin) must be strong enough to balance each other. In order to obtain abundant Yang Chi and Yin Chi in your body, you must learn the methods of building up these two Chis. In order to make Yin and Yang interact harmoniously, you must also learn how to adjust Kan (Water) and Lii (Fire). Therefore, in this stage, you are leading both Yang and Yin Chi to the Huang Ting cavity (Figure 7-13) and causing them to interact harmoniously. This process has commonly called "Kan and Lii."

From the scientific point of view, what you are doing is storing electric charges in the Huang Ting, which can be considered a battery. When you have stored enough Chi you can activate more brain cells and consequently raise your spirit to a higher level. You can see that the "holy embryo" is formed and matured in the Huang Ting, and then it is led to the brain where it grows up.

How can the Huang Ting be used for storing Chi and carrying the embryo? Let us analyze the Huang Ting. This cavity is also called Yuh Hwan Shiuh (Jade Ring Cavity). The name Jade Ring is first used in the Torng Ren Yu Shiuh Jen Jeou Twu (Illustration of the Brass Acupuncture and Moxibustion), by Dr. Wang Wei-Yi. The Taoist book Wang Luh Shyh Yu said: "In the Illustration of the Brass Acupuncture and Moxibustion it was recorded (that) within the body's cavities of viscera and bowels, there is a Jade Ring (Yuh Hwan), (but) I do not know what the Jade Ring is." Later, the Taoist Chang Tzyy-Yang explained about the place which the immortals use to form the elixir: "The Heart is on the top, the kidneys are underneath, spleen is on the left, and the liver is on the right. The life door is in the front, the closed door is in the rear, they are connected like a ring, it is white like cotton with an inch diameter. It encloses the Essence and the refinement of the entire body. This is the Jade Ring."(*1) The life door in the front means the Chi door is open in the front, and naturally it is closed in the rear. That means that if you intend to lead the Yin and Yang Chi here for interaction, you should access this cavity from the front.

From the point of view of Chinese medical science, the Huang Ting is connected with the Conception and Thrusting Vessels through Yinjiao (Co-7). In addition, through the Thrusting Vessel it is again connected with the Governing Vessel at the Huiyin (Co-1). Because of these connections, it is able to store a great amount of Chi. Furthermore, the Huang Ting is located between the solar plexus (Middle Dan Tien), which is where the Yang (Fire) Chi is stored, and the Lower Dan Tien, where the Yin (Water) Chi is stored. It is therefore the center where Yin and Yang can interact. In addition, we know from the Yi Gin Ching training that the fasciae in the Huang Ting area is able to store an abundance of Chi. This increases the amount of Chi available to the "holy embryo."

In Yi Gin Ching training you generate Chi by converting the Original Essence in the internal Kidneys. However, this process does not provide enough Chi for the Shii Soei Ching training. To remedy this lack, more Essence must be drawn from the external Kidneys (testicles) by stimulating them, and converted into Chi.

From the standpoint of modern medicine, part of the health benefit of Shii Soei Chi Kung comes from its use of self-stimulation to increase the production of hormones. Hormones are secretions of the endocrine glands, which include the testicles. They are complex chemical com-

(*1) 王錄識餘云："銅人針灸圖，載臟腑一身俞穴有玉環，余不知玉環是何物。"張紫陽玉清金華祕文，論神仙結丹處曰："心上腎下，脾左肝右，生門在前，密戶居後，其連如環，其白如綿，方圓徑寸，密裹一身之精粹，此即玉環。"

pounds which are transported by the blood or lymph, and they have powerful and specific effects on the functions of the body.

Hormones can stimulate activity, thinking, growth; they are directly related to the strength of your lifeforce. They determine the length of a person's life, and whether he is healthy or sickly. They stimulate your emotions and lift your mood, or they depress you physically and emotionally. Traced back far enough, hormones are the very original source which stimulates man's thinking and ideas, and even generates the enthusiasm for energetic activity. If you know how to generate these hormones and use them properly, you can energize yourself to a degree quite impossible for the ordinary person.

Many important hormones can now be produced synthetically. However, you must understand that taking synthetic hormones is like taking vitamins: it is an unnatural and discontinuous process. When you generate a hormone within your own body, it is natural and continuous. In addition, when you produce the hormones yourself, your body is able to tune into and adjust to the gradual increase in production. However, if the hormones come from outside of your body, your body is subject to an abrupt change. This can produce side effects. Many hormones can be obtained from certain foods. However, these hormones will not be able to provide enough Chi to fill up the vessels. The Taoists say: "Food is better than medicine for increasing health. Using Chi to improve health is better than eating food (Yaw Buu Buh Ru Shyr Buu, Shyr Buu Buh Ru Chi Buu)(*2).

You can see that Shii Soei Chi Kung is a way of stimulating the growth of hormones in the body. These hormones are then used to increase the quantity of Chi, which in turn is used to nourish the brain and raise the spirit of vitality.

You can only develop a healthy spiritual baby when you have sufficient Chi. To form the embryo, you will need at least one hundred days of proper diet, accurate Kan and Lii adjustment, correct stimulation of the sexual organ to increase the Essence (semen), and abstinence from sex in order to build up a strong Chi body combining Yin and Yang. In Shii Soei Chi Kung, the process of refining Essence (semen) and converting it into Chi over the first one hundred days is considered the laying of the foundation. The process is called "hundred days to build the foundation" (Bae Ryh Jwu Ji). The spiritual embryo will be healthy only if it has this foundation.

The testicle Essence (semen) is one of the main sources of human energy. When a person's semen is full, his vital energy is high and his lifeforce is strong. When a man loses the balance between the production and the loss of his semen, his emotions will also lose their balance. This will cause his mental body to be depressed, resulting in the speedy degeneration of his physical body. When a person has normal semen or hormone production, he will have enough Essence to stimulate his growth, thinking, and daily activities. According to the Shii Soei Ching, part of this Essence is converted into Chi and then transported to the brain. This Chi will stimulate the brain to do the thinking and energize the body for activity. When a man's semen production is insufficient, his brain will not obtain enough Chi nourishment and the

_____

(*2) 藥補不如食補，食補不如氣補。

-202-

spirit will be weakened in its governing of the Chi circulation in the body. This will result in sickness.

Therefore, the first step in Shii Soei Ching training is to increase the semen production and learn to convert this semen into Chi faster and more effectively than the body normally does. With the average mature man, the supply of semen will fill up naturally without any stimulation. It usually takes two to three weeks to replenish the supply of semen once it is empty. Whenever the semen and sperm are full, a hormone stimulates the brain and generates sexual desires. This hormone can sometimes energize a man and make him impatient, depressed, and inclined to lose his temper.

You should understand that the time needed for the semen to replenish itself varies from individual to individual. For example, if someone has sex frequently, his semen will be replenished faster. However, if a man refrains from sexual activity for a period of time, his testicles will start to function more slowly. If a man has sex too often, his semen level will be low most of the time, and this will affect the conversion of hormone into the Chi which is transported to the brain. In addition to this, the four Chi vessels in the legs receive most of their Chi from the conversion of semen. If you have too much sex you will find that your legs become weak because the Chi in these vessels is deficient. It is therefore advisable to control your sexual activity.

When a boy is growing, his body produces semen during his sleep from midnight until morning. This is because Chi circulation starts in the head (Baihui) and circulates down the front of the body, following the Conception Vessel, and reaches the Huiyin cavity in the perineum at midnight. (The Huiyin and Baihui, which are connected by the Thrusting Vessel, are both major points of Chi flow at midnight). When this Chi circulation reach the Huiyin, it will stimulate the genitals and interact with the Original Chi from the Dan Tien and generate semen Chi (Jieng Chi).

Young boys usually have erections when they wake in the morning. This starts quite soon after birth. Of course, at this age boys cannot generate any sperm, and they do not have any sexual urge. Chinese medical society believes that once a boy is formed, his testicles continuously generate semen. This interacts with the Yuan Chi (Original Chi) which resides at the Dan Tien and generates Semen Chi (Jieng Chi), which is transported to the brain (including the pituitary gland) to stimulate the boy's growth. When a boy's Yuan Chi is healthy and strong, the interaction of semen and Yuan Chi will also be effective and the boy will grow normally and be healthy. Once the boy reaches his teens, his testicles will also start to generate sperm. Normally, more is produced than is needed for growth, so his Chi is full and abundant, and he is therefore healthy and strong.

It is interesting to note that, starting at midnight when you are sleeping and your entire body is relaxed, the Semen Chi from the testicles will naturally start to nourish the brain and rebalance its energy. It is this rebalancing which generates dreams.

In Shii Soei Ching training, there are two general methods for stimulating semen production. One is Wai Dan, and uses physical stimulation, and the other is Nei Dan, and uses mental stimulation. The more the groin is stimulated, the more semen will be produced and the longer this organ will function normally. You must also learn how to convert this semen into Chi more efficiently than is normally done automatically by your body. If you do not effectively convert the excess semen into Chi, lead it to the brain, and spread it out among the twelve channels, the abundant semen will cause your sexual desire to increase and your emotions to lose their balance.

Theoretically, the method of Essence-Chi conversion is very simple. You lead the Chi from the four vessels in the legs upward to the Huang Ting cavity and also to the brain. This causes the Chi in these four vessels to become deficient, and more Essence must be converted to replenish the supply. In this case, you are "digesting" or "consuming" the extra Essence which is generated. The process of leading the Chi upward is called "Liann Chi Sheng Hwa," which means "train the Chi to sublimate." Because the Chi is an energy form, when it is led upward, it is like the water molecules sublimated upward from ice. When the Chi is led upward and used to nourish the brain, it is called "Faan Jieng Buu Nao," which means "return the Essence to nourish the brain."

In the beginning you might not be able to convert the semen into Chi efficiently. However, the more you practice the better it will become. Generally speaking, there are two major styles of semen conversion: Buddhist and Taoist. Buddhists emphasize mainly the Nei Dan conversion process, which is generally much slower than that of the Taoists, who in addition to the Nei Dan also train Wai Dan conversion. Buddhist priests are not allowed to get married. However, they still have sexual desires, which occur naturally because of the body's production of hormones and semen. In order to eliminate their desire, they found the way of converting the semen into Chi and using this Chi to energize the brain and reach Buddhahood. In Nei Dan conversion training, the Yi and the breathing are the keys to leading the Chi upward. With the coordination of the posture and some controlling movements at the Huiyin and anus, the Chi can be led upward to the Huang Ting and brain. We will discuss these training methods in detail in the next chapter.

In addition to the Nei Dan practice, the Taoist have also discovered several Wai Dan conversion methods. The theory remains the same - leading the Chi in the vessels of the legs upward to the Huang Ting and brain. Generally speaking, Wai Dan methods are faster. As mentioned previously, the Taoists use primarily Wai Dan methods of testicle stimulation to increase the semen production and Wai Dan Essence-Chi conversion. The exercise for stimulating semen production is called "Gau Wan Yunn Dong" (Testicle Exercises) or "Chyr Lao Faan Ji Yunn Dong" (Slowing the Aging and Return the Functioning Exercises). Remember, only when you have enough semen will you be able to convert it into Chi more effectively than the average person can. The more semen you have, the more Chi you can convert.

B. Purifying Chi and Converting it into Shen (Liann Chi Huah Shen) - Ten Months of Pregnancy (Shyr Yueh Hwai Tai)

It is said that after 100 days of the first stage of building the foundation, the spiritual embryo is formed in the Huang Ting. This is the seed from which the baby grows. Now, in this second stage, you will need ten months of pregnancy (28 days for each Chinese month). In this ten months you must continue to provide purified Chi for the baby, just like a mother supplies nutrition and oxygen to the embryo. In these ten months you must train to convert the semen into Chi more efficiently while the spiritual embryo is continuously growing bigger and bigger. If the conversion process is insufficient, the baby will either die before its birth, or else it will be born unhealthy, and it may not continue to grow well. In this stage, you are growing the embryo into a complete baby so that it has its own life.

Theoretically, in the previous stage you learned how to lead the Yin and Yang Chi to the Huang Ting and make them interact harmoniously. The spirit embryo was formed from this interaction. In this stage, you are continuing to build up your Chi in the Huang Ting. Normally, it will take you ten months of Chi building to reach a high level of storage. Only then, in the third stage of the training, will you have enough Chi to activate the extra brain cells and increase the functioning of the brain. When you have done this, you will be able to raise up your spirit to a higher level.

When you are carrying the spirit embryo, you must also do one important thing. When an embryo is forming, the spirit in this embryo is also growing. Therefore, in this second stage of training, in addition to the Chi nourishment, you also need to lead your spirit to this embryo. It is like a mother whose spirit and concentration must be in the embryo while it is growing in order to obtain a spiritually healthy baby. In this stage, the mother's habits and what she thinks will be passed on to the baby.

This means that in this stage, with the mother's help, the spirit embryo will also grow its own spirit. That is why this stage is called "Purifying the Chi and converting it into Shen." Remember, only when the embryo has its own spirit can it be born as a healthy, whole being. The Taoist Li Ching-An said: "Shen and Chi combine to originate the super spiritual quality. Hsin and breath are mutually dependent to generate the holy embryo."(*3) That means that in order to grow a holy embryo you must first learn to combine your Shen and Chi in the Huang Ting. Only then will the holy embryo have a supernatural, spiritual quality. Hsin is your emotional mind, and the breathing is the strategy of the training. Only when you concentrate all of your emotion and coordinate it with your breathing in this holy embryo will it be able to grow and mature.

Many Chi Kung practitioners believe that once the embryo is formed, it should be moved upward to the Upper Dan Tien to grow. As a matter of fact, it does not matter where your embryo grows. First you must have plenty of Chi, then you must learn how to use this Chi to nourish the embryo, and finally, you must help the embryo to build up its own spirit. As long as you are able to store an abundance of Chi to activate and energize your brain cells and raise up your spirit, where the embryo grows is not important.

C. Refining Shen and Returning it to Nothingness (Liann Shen Faan Shiu) - Three Years of Nursing (San Nian Buh Ruu)

After you have carried the spiritual embryo for ten months, it is mature enough for birth. This means that the Chi you are storing in the Huang Ting is strong enough, and your Shen has helped this embryo to build up its own Shen. In this third stage of training you lead this embryo upward to the Upper Dan Tien to be born. According to the experience of many people, the Upper Dan Tien (called the third eye in the Western world) is the place where you can sense and commu-

---

(*3) 李清菴詩云：「神氣和合生靈篤，心息相依結聖胎。」

nicate with the natural energy and the spirit world. As mentioned earlier, this place is called "Shen Guu" (spirit valley) in Chi Kung. This is because the physical structure of this place looks like the entrance to a deep valley formed by the two lobes of the brain. Another reason is that when you sense or communicate with the natural energy it seems to be happening in a deep valley which is able to reach the center of your thinking and also far beyond what you can see.

According to science today, we understand less than 10% of the functions of the brain. This means that the brain contains many mysteries which today's science still cannot explain. I believe that the valley formed by the two brain lobes is the key to the length of brainwaves. Energy resonates in this valley, and is transmitted outward like waves from the antenna of a radio station. I believe that the Upper Dan Tien or third eye is the gate which allows our thoughts to be passed to others, and allows us also to communicate with nature.

If a person can activate a larger percentage of his brain cells through Chi Kung, he will probably increase the sensitivity of his brain to a wider range of wavelengths. He may be able to perceive more things more clearly, and he may have a greatly heightened sensitivity to natural energy. He may even be able to sense other people's brain waves, and see what they think without oral communication. At this level, when your Chi is abundant and your concentration very high, it is also possible to use your mind and Chi to cure people.

If my hypothesis is right, then the biggest obstacle to advancing your training, once you are able to lead the Chi to activate the brain cells, is learning how to open the gate of the Upper Dan Tien. Physically, beneath the skin is the skeleton, and underneath it is the frontal sinus. Both the skeleton and the skin can absorb much of the energy which is emitted from or received by the brain. This is why this gate is considered closed. We now know that the bones are semi-conductors. This means that if enough electric current passes through it, an area can be activated and become a conductor. In higher stages of spiritual Chi Kung this gate is called "Shyuan Guan," which means "tricky gate." When the Chi is condensed in this gate to open it up through concentration, the process is called "Kai Chiaw," or "opening the tricky gate." According to the Chinese Chi Kung society, once this gate is opened, it remains opened.

Another gate is located on the top your your head. It is called "Baihui" in acupuncture or "Ni Wan Gong" in Chi Kung. This gate is also called "Guu Shen," which means "Valley Spirit." This is another place where your brain can communicate with natural energy. However, Chinese Chi Kung does not consider it the spiritual center, and simply considers it a gate which is able to exchange Chi with nature. This gate is commonly used to absorb heaven Chi (from the sun and stars) and earth Chi (Earth's magnetic field) to nourish the body.

If you are able to understand this discussion, then you will not be confused by the third stage of Shii Soei Ching training. In the third stage, you lead the abundant Chi to the brain to activate more of the unused brain cells and increase the brain's working efficiency. In addition, you are using the abundant Chi through concentration, focusing, and meditation to activate the bone cells of the Upper Dan Tien and open the gate. This means that the spirit baby is born in the Upper Dan Tien.

After you have opened this gate and have given birth to the spirit baby, you must nurse it. Nursing means to watch, to take care of, and to nourish continuously. This process in Shii Soei Ching is called "Yeang Shen," or "to nurse the Shen." You can see that in this stage you are continuously nursing the baby as it grows stronger and stronger. In other words, you are increasing the Chi there so that you can sense nature more easily. When you have reached this stage, because you are leading your spirit to feel nature, it will gradually get used to staying with the natural energy and it will slowly forget the physical body. Since the natural spirit cannot be seen, it is nothingness. Nothingness also refers to the absence of emotional feelings and desires. This is why this stage of training is called "Refining Shen and Returning it to Nothingness." Since your spirit body originated from physical and emotional nothingness, in this training, you are returning to nothingness. The Buddhists call this "Syh Dah Jie Kong," or "Four Large are Empty." This means that the four elements (earth, fire, water, and air) are absent from the mind so that you are completely indifferent to worldly temptations.

When your spirit baby is born, you will need to nurse it for at least three years. Just like a real baby, it needs to be protected and nurtured until it can be self-sufficient. The spiritual baby needs to stay near the mother's body to stay alive, so if it travels, it cannot go too far. It is just like a two or three year old baby gradually familiarizing itself with its new environment. Normally, when you have reached this stage, you have approached the first step of enlightenment or Buddhahood.

D. Crushing the Nothingness (Feen Suory Shiu Kong) - Nine Years of Facing the Wall (Jeou Nian Miann Bih)

At this stage you begin to see the spiritual world as the more real one. Crushing nothingness means destroying the illusion which connects the physical world with the spiritual plane. According to Buddhism, your spirit cannot separate from your physical body completely because it is still connected to the human world by emotional feelings and desires. Only if you are able to free yourself from all of these bonds of human emotions and desires will your spirit be able to separate from the physical body and be independent. Nine years of meditation gives your spirit the time to experience the natural energy world and to learn to live independently. When the nine years are up, your spirit will be twelve years old, and it will be able to separate from your physical body, and continue living even after your body dies.

The final target of a monk is to reach enlightenment or become a Buddha. In order to become a Buddha, he must continue to develop his Shen until it can be independent, and can exist even after the physical body dies. When a monk has reached this level his Chi will be able to energize his brain so strongly that it interacts with the energy (electrical charges) in the air, and generates a glow around his head. In fact, this glow or halo may even occur in earlier training stages. This glow around the head is frequently shown in pictures of the Buddha, especially when he is shown meditating in the dark. This is identical to the glow, or halo, shown in pictures of Western saints. I believe that if these pictures were drawn according to what people saw, it shows that the people represented had reached enlightenment.

In order to reach this level, the spirit baby must grow stronger and be neutral. It is called "nine years of facing the wall." When you face the wall, you will not be tempted by many things, and you will be able to calm down more easily. In this nine years of meditation your spirit baby learns how to live in the natural energy and continue to grow even when the physical body is dead.

This stage is called "Liann Shen," or "train the spirit." At this time your spirit receives its education from the natural energy. Of course, this normally takes more than twelve years. In fact, the Buddhists believe that it usually takes many lifetimes. You strengthen your Baby Shen in every lifetime, and if you continue to train, one day you will be able to reach the level of enlightenment. However, there are also many Buddhists and Taoists who believe that the entire training depends on the individual's understanding. They believe that if a person could really understand the training process, he would be able to reach enlightenment in virtually no time at all. I am inclined to agree with these people. I have found that in virtually every area of endeavor, if a person knows the principles and studies them, he will find ways to reach the goal in a far shorter time than those who do not think and ponder about what they are doing.

To conclude this section, I would like to point out that what this book can teach you is how to do the first two stages of Shii Soei Ching Chi Kung training, which can give you a long and healthy life. There are many documents about the first two stages of training, but there is very little written about the last two stages of enlightenment training. However, I believe that if your desire is sincere and you keep your mind on the target, you will understand what you need to do in order to reach the next higher level. Remember: **NO ONE CAN UNDERSTAND YOU BETTER THAN YOURSELF**.

7-5. Wai Dan and Nei Dan Shii Soei Ching

In Part Two, we have explained the general differences between Wai Dan and Nei Dan training. In this section, we would like to clarify how the Wai Dan and Nei Dan theory applies to the Shii Soei Ching.

According to the theory, any external training methods which cause Chi buildup or redistribution is called Wai Dan. This implies that in Wai Dan Shii Soei Ching it is mostly physical stimulation which causes the generation and distribution of Chi. However, if the generation and redistribution of Chi are caused by the concentrated mind in coordination with the breathing, these methods are classified as Nei Dan Shii Soei Ching. Here, we will briefly list some of the Wai Dan and Nei Dan practices for your reference. The detailed training methods will be discussed in the next chapter.

Wai Dan Shii Soei Ching:
Stage 1: Refining the Essence (Semen) and Converting it into Chi (Liann Jieng Huah Chi)
A. Physical stimulation of testicles and penis to increase Essence production.
B. To absorb Chi from or give it to the training partner in "Double Cultivation" in order to reach a new balance of Chi in the body. This also includes the methods of exchanging or absorbing Chi with a sexual partner in order to increase the Chi level in the body.

Stage 2: Purifying Chi and Converting it into Shen (Liann Chi Huah Shen)

A. Hanging weights from the groin in order to lead the Chi upward to the Huang Ting and the head.
B. Using finger pressure on the Huiyin to control the gate which leads Chi to the Fire path or the Water path.
C. Holding up the groin with hands to lead the Chi upward to the Huang Ting and the head.
D. To increase the Chi circulation in the marrow through beating stimulation.

Stage 3: Refining Shen and Returning it to Nothingness (Liann Shen Faan Shiu)

A. Beating the heavenly drum to clear the mind and increase the concentration.
B. Massaging or tapping the Upper Dan Tien to strengthen the focus of power there.

Stage 4: Crushing Nothingness (Feen Suory Shiu Kong)
No information about Wai Dan practice for this stage.

Nei Dan Shii Soei Ching:

Nei Dan Shii Soei Ching uses the Yi in coordination with the breathing to lead the Chi to the places being trained. To reach this high level of Nei Dan practice, a practitioner normally must have understood and experienced some level of the five necessary steps of Nei Dan Chi Kung cultivation. These five steps are: 1. regulating the body, 2. regulating the breathing, 3. regulating the mind, 4. regulating the Chi, and finally 5. regulating the spirit. Before you begin Nei Dan Shii Soei Ching training, you should have mastered the training of regulating the body, breathing, and the mind, and have some experience in regulating the Chi and spirit. Regulating the Chi and spirit are the main targets of training in Nei Dan Shii Soei Ching. In volume 1 of the YMAA Chi Kung series: "The Root of Chinese Chi Kung," we discussed these five training steps in detail. If you are not clear on this subject, you should review the pertinent sections of that book.

Here we will discuss some of the available Nei Dan Shii Soei Ching training. We know that when we reach the third and fourth stages of the spiritual training, Nei Dan Shii Soei Ching becomes the vital key to success. Unfortunately, we will not be able to offer a very deep discussion, since documents on these stages are very scarce. Despite this, I believe that those practitioners who wish to reach the final stages of enlightenment will be able to understand their next steps without further guidelines. If you cannot understand the training, then I believe you are not ready to enter that stage.

Stage 1: Refining the Essence (Semen) and Converting it into Chi (Liann Jieng Huah Chi)

A. Breath pumping Chi training. With breathing and the guidance of the Yi, Chi can be led to the groin to stimulate the production of semen.
B. Cavity Breathing training. Cavity breathing includes the breathing of the Huang Ting cavity and the Huiyin cavity. This technique also uses the Yi and the coordination of the breathing to lead the Chi to

these two cavities. This will clear up stagnation and increase the efficiency of the Essence-Chi conversion.

Stage 2: Purifying Chi and Converting it into Shen (Liann Chi Huah Shen)

A. Shen Breathing. Shen breathing in this stage concentrates on the spirit baby in the Huang Ting. This is to help the baby obtain its own spirit and guide it the right way.

B. Bone Breathing. In this stage, you are also using the Yi and breathing coordination to lead Chi to the spine and bone marrow to clean them and keep them functioning properly.

Stage 3: Refining Shen and Returning it to Nothingness (Liann Shen Faan Shiu)

A. Shen Breathing. This Shen breathing trains the baby's spirit, which resides in the Upper Dan Tien. The spirit baby must have its own spirit to be independent.

B. Shen focusing training. In this stage, you must nourish your spirit and make it grow. In addition, you must also learn to focus the spirit into a tiny point to make it strong until the "tricky gate" is opened. Naturally, mind regulation training is a vital key to success.

C. Separating the spirit and the physical body training. Once the gate is opened, you lead the spirit away from your physical body. However, this baby spirit cannot move too far from your physical body.

Stage 4: Crushing the Nothingness (Feen Suory Shiu Kong)

A. Shen Training. In this stage, you are educating your spirit and leading it further and further away from your body.

B. Hibernation training. In order to enable your spirit to leave your physical body, you must be able to meditate very deeply. The heart beat must slow down, and oxygen usage must be reduced to the minimum. Only when your physical body has reached this Yin stage will the spirit be able to leave. Hibernation training is necessary for this. It is said that once a monk has reached this level, his spirit is able to leave his physical body for several months and later come back to his body and wake it up again.

To conclude this section, we would like to remind you that in order to reach a high level of Shii Soei Ching, both Nei Dan and Wai Dan training are important. One is internal and the other is external training. One is Yin and the other is Yang. Both must mutually assist and balance each other. As mentioned before, Yi Gin Ching and Shii Soei Ching training are one and should not be separated. Yi Gin Ching training is Lii while Shii Soei Ching training is Kan. If you do them together, you will be able to balance the Yin and Yang in your body.

Chapter 8

Shii Soei Ching
Chi Kung Training

8-1. Introduction

The last chapter should have given you a foundation in the theory and principles of Shii Soei Ching Chi Kung training. Even though some of the theory and principles are deep, and most people find them hard to understand, many of the training processes are simple. In ancient China, a student was normally first taught the How of the training. The Why he would only learn later, if at all. Most of the time the reasoning behind the training was the sole property of the master.

Nowadays, no one should treat the theory and principles as a deep secret. As long as you are willing to dig, you will be able to find the real meaning and theory of the Shii Soei Ching training. Once you have grasped the keys and understood the theory, the training process will become easy for you to follow.

In this chapter, I will summarize the training processes which have been recorded in the available Buddhist and Taoist documents, and I will add theoretical explanations when I can. Before you continue, you should understand that the theory and principles are the same in both the Buddhist and the Taoist versions of the training, even though their approaches to the training are somewhat different.

In the first part of this book we pointed out the main differences between the Buddhist and Taoist Yi Gin Ching and Shii Soei Ching training. We will not repeat them here. However, we would like to remind you of one thing, that generally Buddhist training is more conservative, gentle, gradual, slow, and focused more on the spiritual accomplishment than physical cultivation. The Taoist training is more open-minded, aggressive, fast, and looking for quick results. This is especially true in the Essence-Chi conversion process, where they use physical stimulation.

A large portion of the training discussed in this book is from Taoist documents, although they may have originally come from the Buddhists. When available, the original verse, poetry, or songs which are related to the training will be translated and commented upon. I hope that through this effort you will be able to understand and really feel the heart of the training. As mentioned before, Shii Soei Ching Chi Kung is a new field for me. Even though I feel that I have an understanding of most of the keys and principles, there is still one big void in this book. That is experience. Therefore, I hope that those few masters who are qualified and experienced in Shii Soei Ching will share their experience and fill up this void. Naturally, no single Chi Kung master is able to fill up this void alone. The art is a result of more than a thousand years of experimentation, and many, many qualified masters will be needed to explain it fully.

In the rest of this chapter, we will discuss who can accept the Shii Soei Ching training first. In order to build up a foundation for the further discussion of the training, two major documents from two different sources are translated and commented upon. Finally, the four main Shii Soei Ching training processes and techniques will be discussed in the following sections to complete this chapter.

8-2. Who is Qualified to Train?

In order to understand who is qualified to train Shii Soei Ching, let us first review the purposes of the training.

According to our previous discussion, it is clear that originally Shii Soei Ching Chi Kung was invented for monks who were interested in reaching enlightenment. In order to do this, a monk must first train Yi Gin Ching to increase the quantity and improve the quality of Chi. In addition, he must generate and refine the semen and convert it into Chi to fill up the Chi reservoirs (eight vessels) more fully. From the Chi vessels, the Chi will be able to spread into the Chi rivers (the 12 channels) and reach the limbs and internal organs. In addition, this abundant Chi can be used to wash the marrow. When one has accomplished this stage, he will have gained good health and be able to increase his longevity. However, for a priest to reach enlightenment, he must lead his Chi to the brain and Upper Dan Tien to nourish the brain and raise up the Shen.

In Shii Soei Ching practice, the Thrusting Vessel is considered the most important Chi reservoir, because it is the route by which Chi is led to the brain to nourish it. When the brain is filled up with Chi it is energized and it will begin to function more fully, using more than the usual 30-35% of the brain cells. This will increase the sensitivity of the brain, make your thinking more effective, and it will energize and raise up your spirit. Through training, the condensed energy will raise up the spirit and enable it to separate from the physical body and remain alive even after the death of the physical body. In order to reach this level, a monk must first let go of all the usual thoughts and emotions, including sexual ones, which tie him to the physical world.

Even though the Shii Soei Ching was designed for reaching enlightenment or Buddhahood, many Chi Kung practitioners have discovered that it is also the most effective way of maintaining health and increasing longevity. In addition, it has also been found that the training can significantly improve their sex life. Naturally, people who are aiming only for longevity or sexual ability will not have to reach the higher levels of spiritual cultivation.

You can see that the question of who can train Shii Soei Ching is relative. It depends on the person's goals. Also, when a person can accept the Shii Soei Ching has always been a controversial subject. In Henan province, where the Shaolin temple is, there are a number of records of teenage boys receiving this training, especially in Jwing Hsien, An Yang, and Wu An counties. It was common in rich families for the teenage sons to complete the first stage of Shii Soei Ching Chi Kung training to increase their sexual capability before marriage so that a good marriage could be arranged. It was common at that time for boys of sixteen to get married. The first stage of the Shii Soei Ching Chi Kung could speed the maturation process.

However, other documents say that one should not start Shii Soei Ching training before he is thirty-five. This is because it is hard for a person to understand Chi Kung theory and training to a deep level before this age. Therefore, these documents state that before one starts the Shii Soei Ching training, he must first understand and have completed some level of Yi Gin Chi Kung training. Other records tell of men in their sixties who start the training. They grow younger, their hair color changes from grey to black, their sexual activity resumes, and their bodies become healthy.

From this you can understand that if you are training in order to improve you sex life, you can practice the first stage of Shii Soei Chi Kung training. This will increase the amount of semen and sperm you produce, and also increase your sexual "staying power." For this purpose you may start at any age, from just after puberty to the retirement years.

However, if your goals are greater, and you desire good health and a long life, then you must convert the semen into Chi and lead it to fill the vessels, energize the brain, and lead this Chi to the entire body. In order to do this, you must know the complete theory and training methods of converting. In the beginning, you may not be able to convert much of the semen into Chi, but after you practice for a long time you will find yourself converting more and more effectively, either through the physical method or the meditative method.

If you want to reach this level, you must start watching your diet, managing your sexual thoughts and desires, and eliminating stress and distractions from your life as much as possible. You must eliminate your desire for such things as power, wealth, and sex. You must train yourself so that you do not have such feelings as anger, happiness, or worry. Then your thoughts will be neutral, and nothing will bother you.

Since such an extensive knowledge of and experience with Chi is required to do the Shii Soei Ching safely, it has proven extremely difficult for young children to do. Most people don't develop sufficient maturity and experience until at least their late twenties.

However, if you wish to train Shii Soei Chi Kung to reach enlightenment, then you will find that it is a long road which demands a great deal of patience. It is said that after ten months of converting Chi into Shen (spirit), you will need at least three years of meditation to protect the spirit baby and allow it to grow. Then you will need at least nine years of meditation (facing the wall) to reach the level of no feeling, then you will be able to separate your spirit and soul from your physical body. When you reach this level, you have reached the level of immortality, where death has no power over you.

8-3. Poetry

According to the available documents, there are two sources which claim to be the original Shii Soei Ching. Before we start discussing the techniques, I would like to first translate the portions of both documents which deal with training methods. As with the other documents, the original Chinese will be included for those who read Chinese and would like to have the feeling of the original verse.

Document 1

This document was published in the Chinese Book "The Real Meaning of Chinese Marrow/Brain Washing Kung Fu" (Jong Gwo Shii Soei Kung Fu Jy Jen Dih), by Chyau Charng-Horng:

Marrow/Brain Washing Spiritual Kung (Fu), in the beginning use instruments, (make) the Chi reach the four extremities: tongue, teeth, nails, and hair. Beat with a paddle to protect the bone marrow.

流髓神功，初用道具，氣串四捎，舌牙甲髮。搥打以杵，護其骨髓。

Since Marrow/Brain Washing is a Kung Fu which specializes in training the Spirit (Shen), it is called Spiritual Kung (Shen Kung). The single word "Kung" is commonly used by the Chinese to mean "Kung Fu," which refers to something which needs time and energy to train. In the beginning, since your Yi (mind) is still weak, you must rely on training equipment to lead the Chi to reach the four extremities - the tongue, teeth, nails, and hair. Later, after you have learned how to use your Yi to lead the Chi efficiently, you may dispense with the equipment. In addition, you will be able to lead the Chi to reach your head to energize the brain and raise up your spirit. When the spirit is raised, it can govern the Chi flow and make it reach throughout the entire body in a more efficient way. It is very common for Chinese doctors to diagnose your state of health from these four extremities. If you can make your Chi reach them, it will reach everywhere and you will have real health.

Also, in this beginning training you must use a rod or paddle to beat or slap the body along the Chi meridians. This was usually done with a "Chuu" a pestle-like rod commonly used to separate grain from chaff, or to beat clothing when washing. This body beating exercise will lead the Chi which circulates in the marrow to reach the surface of the skin, which serves two major purposes. The first is to open the millions of small Chi channels which move Chi out from the meridians and connect the marrow with the surface of the skin. The second is to lead the Chi to the surface of the skin and form a Chi shield (Wey Chi; Guardian Chi) which protects the body from negative external influences.

(If you) do not advance and cultivate thusly, there is no root to your Taoist learning. (When you) train to seven sevens (i.e., forty-nine days), the five Chis (of the heart, liver, spleen, lungs, and kidneys) return to (their) origins.

不此進修，學道無根。功至七七，五氣朝元。

In Shii Soei Ching Chi Kung, it is said that you will need at least 100 days to build the foundation. This foundation is the root of your entire training. If the root you have built is weak and unhealthy, you will have wasted your time and energy, for your training will not bear fruit. In the beginning of the 100 days of foundation training, you first train for forty-nine days to bring the Chis of the five major organs back to their origins.

During everyday life the Chi of the various organs tends to stray away from where it belongs, and the Chi level is either in excess or deficient. This means that the functioning of the organs is impaired. It is very important for the organ Chis to return to their proper level, so that normal function is restored. When these five Chis are mixed up and do not circulate where they are supposed to, you will be sick and the organs will degenerate faster. When these five organ Chis are circulating in the proper channels and at the correct levels, the organs will have their proper Chi supply and they will be healthy.

There is another explanation for the sentence about the five Chis returning to their origins. Some people say that the word "origin" refers to the Original Spirit (Yuan Shen) which resides in the Upper Dan Tien. When the Chi is led to the spiritual center (Upper Dan Tien), the spirit can be raised to a strong, energized state. Then this spirit will become the Chi headquarters and be able to govern the Chi effectively. This Chi includes the Managing Chi and Guardian Chi. The Managing Chi deals with the functioning of the organs. Therefore, when the five Chis return to their origins it means that the Shen is effectively controlling the functioning of the organs.

(When your) training reaches ten tens (100 days), three flowers reach the top.

功至十十，三花聚頂。

When you have trained for 100 days, you have built your foundation and will gradually be able to lead the three treasures or flowers to reach the top of your head. When Chinese people refer to the three treasures they mean Jieng (Essence/semen), Chi (energy), and Shen (spirit). When you reach this stage, you will be able to convert your Essence/semen into Chi and transport it to the brain to energize the brain and raise up your Shen (spirit). You have now planted the seed of the Baby Shen (Shen Ing) and the spiritual embryo is forming.

Transport (the Chi through) the marvelous meridians, get through the eight vessels, every part of the body will meet the (Chi) source. The more you refine your training, the more you will advance, (you will) enter the door to the large Tao.

行奇經，通八脈，遍軀達源。功愈醇而愈進，大道入門。

Once the three treasures can reach to the top of your head, they will be able to energize the brain to a higher, more concentrated state. You will be able to transport the Chi to the twelve meridians and the eight vessels. When this happens, your Chi will have reached every part of your body. The more you train, the more you will advance.

(Of) the methods of training this Kung (Fu), one is with the testicles (Ju Luen) and one is with the penis (Herng Mo).

行此功法，一在珠輪，一在橫磨．

The poetry uses euphemisms here, referring to the testicles as "Ju Luen," or "rotating pearls," and the penis as "Herng Mo," a "cylindrical grindstone." This sentence states that when you train Shii Soei Ching Kung Fu you must start with your testicles and penis.

Thread together into one, say Yi, say Shii.

一以貫之，曰易曰洗．

The Chinese in this sentence is very idiomatic and colloquial. The first part expresses the idea of putting Chinese coins on a string. (Since ancient times Chinese coins have been made with a hole in them so that they could be strung together.) The coins are then together, yet they are still separate, individual coins. When Chinese refer to a list of several items, they will sometimes use the word "say" before each item. Yi means the exercises of the Yi Gin Ching, and Shii means the exercises of the Shii Soei Ching. This sentence means that when you train, you should train both methods together, instead of only training one and ignoring the other. As explained in the first part, Yi Gin Ching is a Lii (Fire) training while Shii Soei Ching is a Kan (Water) training. Together they bring Yin and Yang into balance. This is the way of the Tao.

For the testicles, the secret training words are: say Slip Out (Jeng), say Massage (Rou), say File (Tsuo), say Hang (Juey), say Slap (Pai).

在珠輪行功字訣：曰掙、曰揉、曰搓、曰墜、曰拍
。

The word "Jeng" means to struggle to get free. For example, if someone has grabbed your wrist, if you break free with force it is called "Jeng Kai," which means "struggle to open." This means that when you train you hold your testicles with your hand and let them slip out of your grasp. Naturally, you only hold them lightly at the beginning so as not to injure them. "Rou" means to massage. When you Rou, your finger(s) stay in one place on the skin and circle around. Because the skin is loose, you can massage the area under the skin without rubbing your finger against the skin. "Tsuo" means to rub or to file. When you Tsuo you use your hands or fingers to rub the skin and generate heat. "Juey" means to hang something and let the object drop naturally. The last word, "Pai," means slap. That means you use your hand to slap the testicles gently. Except for Juey (hang), which is used to convert the semen into Chi, the other four words refer to common ways of stimulating the testicles. We will discuss all of these techniques in the following sections.

For the penis, the secret training words are: say Hold (Woh), say Bind (Shuh), say Nourish (Yeang), say Swallow (Ien), say Draw In/Absorb (Sher), say Hold Up (Tyi), say Close (Bi), say Swing (Shuai).

在橫磨行功字訣：曰握、曰束、曰養、曰咽、曰攝
、曰提、曰閉、曰摔。

"Woh" means to use your hand to hold something. "Shuh" means to bind or tie something up. "Yeang" means to nourish, to enhance, to make grow. "Ien" means to swallow. "Sher" has the meaning of draw in, absorb, or take. "Tyi" means to hold up or raise. "Bi" means to close, and "Shuai" means to swing from one side to the other. All of the above are ways of stimulating or training with the penis, although, in fact, not all of them apply directly to the penis.

In addition to these thirteen key words, there is another secret word Gan (Hard) throughout all of the training.

此十三字訣外，另有剛字訣總滙行功法。

The thirteen secret words refer to methods used to generate semen or convert the semen to Chi. However, during all of this training, the most important factor of success is not the procedures or the training methods. The most important factor for success is having a mind and a spirit which are as strong and hard as steel. The mind must be firm, concentrated, persevering, and yet relaxed. With a strong mind and raised spirit you will be able to move the Chi and complete the training successfully.

Except for Close, Swallow, Nourish, Hang, Draw In/Absorb, Bind, the other seven words use the hands to do the training. From light to heavy, from forceful to peaceful, complete the cycle and repeat, do not count the times. Little training, little achievement, great training, great achievement.

除閉、咽、養、墜、攝、束外，餘七字用手行功。
自輕而重，自勉而安，周而復始，不計遍數。小煉
小成。大煉大成。

Except for those six words (Close, Swallow, Nourish, Hang, Draw In/Absorb, Bind), you must use your hand for the other seven trainings. In the beginning you must force yourself to train. You start gently and gradually become heavier, until you feel easy and peaceful. The more you train, the more you will accomplish.

Hold Up means the point at the Magic Gate (Shyuan Guan). Close means slowing down aging and restoring the functioning (of the organs). Swallow is the breathing in the cavities (Shiuh). Hold is to hold up the kidneys (here meaning testicles) to the top, Nourish is to use the stove and vessel to warm and nourish, Bind is to use soft cotton to bind the root (penis), Hang is to refine the Chi and to sublimate it. Draw In/Absorb is to nourish the body (through) sitting and transporting (Chi).

提乃玄關一點、閉乃遲老還機、咽乃穴位呼吸、握
乃兜腎貫頂、養乃爐鼎溫養、來乃軟帛束根、墜乃
煉炁昇華、攝乃補體坐輸。

"Hold Up" is applied to one point, namely the "Magic Gate" (Shyuan Guan), or Huiyin cavity, which is located between the groin and anus. From the previous chapter you understand that the Huiyin cavity is the intersection of three major vessels: Conception, Governing, and Thrusting. This is the main gate which adjusts Kan and Lii and affects the body's Yin and Yang. This point is also the key place for converting the semen into Chi. Hold Up can be done either with a finger or purely by thinking.

"Close" is the key to slowing down the aging process and returning all of the degenerated organs back to normal functioning. Close is one of the Nei Dan trainings which stimulates the testicles and penis to increase semen production. "Swallow" refers to cavity breathing. The cavity here means "Huang Ting" (yellow yard), which is behind the navel and above the Lower Dan Tien. "Hold" means to hold both testicles. Chinese believe that the testicles and kidneys are directly related. Therefore, the testicles are sometimes called external kidneys. When doing Hold, hold the testicles with both hands and raise them up. "Nourish" is to wash and stimulate the penis to nourish it.

"Bind" is to use soft cotton rope to bind the root (penis). "Hang" is another key which is used to refine the Chi and sublimate it. Sublimation is a process during which, when a solid is heated, it turns into vapor directly without changing into liquid first (like ice sublimates into vapor). In Taoist Chi conversion, it means to convert the material (semen) into energy (Chi) and raise it up to heaven (the head). "Draw In/Absorb" is one of the most important processes. From it you learn how to keep your Chi in your body and also how to draw in or absorb Chi from nature or a partner to nourish your body.

The marvelous secret of these eight words, (can enable you to) sneakily take over (i.e., escape from) the creation and conversion (cycle) controlled by heaven and earth. Their (i.e., the eight words) achievement can wash the marrow/brain and conquer the hair. Weak person (becomes) strong, soft (becomes) hard, shrunken (becomes) longer, sick (becomes) healthy, great husband.

此八字妙訣，巧奪天地造化，功能洗髓伐毛。弱者
強，柔者剛，縮者長，病者康，偉丈夫也。

These eight secret words are marvelous because they can help you to escape from the destiny which heaven and earth (nature) have laid out for you. Your natural destiny is to be born, grow old, sicken, and finally die. If you train with these eight words you can keep your marrow clean and your brain fresh, and even make your Chi reach all the way out to your hair. Since marrow is the source of blood, you will be able to keep your blood fresh and healthy. This blood will then circulate in your body, keeping you healthy and slowing down the aging process. Training with these eight words can make a weak person strong, and can make what is soft become hard, and what is short become long. If you are sick you will become healthy, and your sexual abilities will increase.

Use this (trained body) for the technique of striking (fighting), wood stone iron hammer, how could I be afraid.

认之技擊、木石鐵槌，吾何惴哉。

Once I complete the above training, if I fight a battle I will not need to be afraid even if I am struck with various weapons (of wood, stone, or iron). A properly trained body will be impervious to injury.

Use this (trained body) to do the man's job (i.e., sex), a hundred battles without exhaustion.

认之人事，百戰不殆。

The Shii Soei Ching Chi Kung will also develop your sexual stamina.

(If I) follow (the natural path, I give) birth to human beings. The tiger deprived of the dragon's saliva; (if I go) against (nature, I) become immortal, the dragon swallows the tiger's marrow. The true secret is only (in deciding) between one way or the other. Withdraw or release depends on me, follow and give, I choose the person.

順生人，虎奪龍涎；逆成仙，龍吞虎髓，真訣只在中間顛倒顛，收放在我，順施擇人。

In China, sexual intercourse is commonly called "Long Hwu Jiau Gow," which means Dragon-Tiger intercourse. The Dragon who generates saliva (semen) is the man, and the tiger is the women. When a woman has a bad temper she is called Muu Lao Hwu, which means "mother tiger." If the tiger receives the dragon's saliva (the woman receives the man's semen) a child may be born. However, if the man goes against the natural way and retains his semen during intercourse, he can become immortal if he can convert the semen into Chi and energize his brain. The man can also absorb energy from deep within the woman's body, in fact, from her bone marrow. This is what is meant by the dragon swallowing the tiger's marrow. The secret of mortality or immortality lies in choosing between emitting and not emitting. Release or withdraw depends on me. I choose who I will give my semen and Chi to.

Use this to reach great achievement, then the hair will be like the halberd with a hook; the Chi and the blood are (like a) booming drum, (and) can be heard as martial bravery.

认之功業，則有毛髮如戟生鈎。氣血鼓盪能聞之武勇。

The halberd is a dangerous weapon. If a halberd is also equipped with a hook, it is even more powerful and dangerous. If you achieve great success with this Chi Kung training, then your Chi will be full and far-reaching, and be able to reach to the ends of your hair. A person who knows how to evaluate your state of health from the state of your hair will recognize your exceptional achievement. Energy vibrates, and higher energy vibrates at a greater frequency. Success in Shii Soei Ching will fill your blood and Chi with so much energy that they will be vibrant like a reverberating drum. People will sense that you have the power of a martial hero, and you will be able to accomplish whatever you wish.

Use this (training) to prevent aging, then (it is) possible to set up my life myself, with no extremes, like heaven. I do not know if there is any other herb better than this in heaven and earth. Is there anything in the human world more important than this?

以之防老，則可命自我立，與天無極。吾不知天地
間更有何藥復佳於是。人世間更有何事大於是。

As discussed in the last section, the Shii Soei Ching exercises were used by the Taoist monks in their striving for enlightenment. There are four stages of training. The first of these two stages can help the average person have a long and healthy life. This prepares him for the more spiritual third and fourth stages, where one gets beyond the polarity and extremes which ordinarily afflict us. Unfortunately, these later stages are not discussed. After all, there are not too many people who are really interested in setting themselves free from all human emotions and reaching the enlightenment of the Buddha. Almost all of the documents which have been passed down to us discuss the first two stages in detail, but virtually ignore the last two stages.

This category (of) training method is outside of the Taoist transmission; if (a person) doesn't have a predestined relationship, luck, and morality, don't teach. Try it, try it.

此門功法，乃道外別傳，非有宿緣福德之信受者不
傳。勉之勉之！

There are many different schools of Taoism, with a multitude of training methods. Shii Soei Ching is not in the regular course of study in any of them. This sentence states that it should only be taught to special people. Most Chinese people believe that we have lived previous lives. These previous lives often determine the events and relationships in this one. A "night relationship" (Suh Yuann) refers to a very close friendship which may have been predetermined by experiences in a previous life. This is the kind of friend you can stay up all night talking to without getting tired. The poetry says that you should only teach Shii Soei Ching to someone you feel this close to, and who has demonstrated good morality. The "luck" referred to here means that, in addition to everything else, a person has to be lucky to meet a person who is willing and able to teach him.

Document 2
This document was published in the Book "The Chinese Spiritual Kung, Vol. 1" (Jong Gwo Shen Kung, Vol. 1), by Gong Jiann Lao Ren.

(After) gathering Chi for more than three hundred days, the front and the back, Conception and Governing Vessels are completely full, then train the lower (body) Kung Fu. In the mother's womb, Conception and Governing, the two vessels, were connected. After birth, food in and out (causes) the separation of front and back. Their passage: the Governing Vessel starts at the "Shang Yin" (i.e., Yinjiao cavity), runs along the top and passes through the spine, descending to the Weilu (tailbone, Changqiang cavity). The Conception Vessel starts from the Chengjiang, runs along the chest and reaches down to the Huiyin. (The) two (vessels) are not threaded (connected). Now train the lower (body) Kung Fu, then the Chi reaches (the level where it) begins to connect and exchange.

積氣三百餘日，前後任督二脈悉皆充滿，乃行下部
功夫，令其通貫；蓋任督二脈，在母胎時，原自相
通，出胎以後，飲食出入，隔其前後。通行之道，
督脈自上齦，循頂行脊，下至尾閭，任脈自承漿，
循胸下至會陰，兩不相貫，今行下部工夫，則氣至
可以相接，而交旋矣。

This document says that after you have trained at least three hundred days of Yi Gin Chi Kung, you have cleared obstructions in the Conception and Governing Vessels and filled them with Chi. Now you can start the "lower body Kung Fu," meaning Shii Soei Ching Chi Kung, which begins with groin training.

It is believed by the Taoists that the Conception and Governing Vessels were originally connected when you were an embryo. This connection started to break down when you were born and started taking food by mouth. An embryo receives nutrition and oxygen from the mother through the navel, and it must move its abdomen (Dan Tien) in and out like a pump in order to help draw the food in. Because of this abdominal exercise the Huiyin cavity, which connects the Conception, Governing, and Thrusting Vessels, was open. Once the baby is born, it starts taking food in through the mouth and oxygen in through the nose. Since abdominal breathing is no longer essential, the child starts breathing higher in the chest. The Huiyin cavity becomes inactive, so it gradually becomes sealed, and the connection between the Conception and Governing Vessels weakens. Therefore, the first exercise the Buddhist and Taoist emphasize in meditation is to reopen this cavity through abdominal exercises. After this, you must continue the Shii Soei Ching training to keep your Chi full and keep the Huiyin cavity open.

When training this Kung Fu, its methods are on two places. It includes eleven items. Two places: one is the testicles, one is the jade stem (i.e., penis).

行此工夫，其法在兩處，其目有十一段；兩處者，
一在睪丸，一在玉莖。

This means that when you train Shii Soei Ching Chi Kung, there are eleven important training keys for two places: the testicles and the penis.

At the testicles, say Collect (Tzaan); say Slip Out (Jeng), say File (Tsuo), say Slap (Pai).

在睪丸者，曰攢、曰撐、曰搓、曰拍。

To hold things together is called "Tzaan." This word has the same meaning as Hold (Woh) in the last document. Tzaan means to use your hands to hold or collect the testicles. Jeng, Tsuo, and Pai are the same as in the last document. You can see that there are two words which are not included in this document: Rub (Rou) and Hang (Juey). However, Tzaan (collect) can be said to be a mixture of Hold and Rub. I consider the training keys to be the same in both documents, except for the word Hang (Juey). Since Hang is the major key to converting semen into Chi, I do not doubt that it was deleted from this document on purpose, and only passed down orally to protect the secret.

On the Jade Stem (i.e., penis), say Swallow (Ien), say Swing (Shuai) say Caress (Fuu), say Wash (Shii), say Bind (Shuh), say Nourish (Yeang), say File (Tsuo).

在玉莖者，曰咽、曰摔、曰撫、曰洗、曰束、曰養、曰搓。

This document contains three words which are not included in the last document: Caress (Fuu), Wash (Shii), and File (Tsuo). Caress is using the hands to lightly rub, touch, and massage. This is only to stimulate the penis and energize it. Wash here means to wash the penis with a special herb. There are many herbal prescriptions for this purpose found together with this document. However, this word was not even mentioned in the last document. File was included in the last document for use with the testicles, but not with the penis. Here it means you use both of your hands to rub your penis.

However, I would like to point out that there are four words - Hold (Woh), Draw In/Absorb (Sher), Hold Up (Tyi), and Close (Bi) - which are in the last document but not in this one. Again, these four words are the keys to refining, keeping, and converting the semen. I believe that they were deleted on purpose in order to keep the heart of the process secret.

The above eleven words, except for Swallow (Ien), Wash (Shii), Bind (Shuh), Nourish (Yeang), the other seven words use the hands to do the training. All from light to heavy, from loose to tight, from forceful to natural; (when the) cycle is completed repeat from the beginning, do no count the times, every day six sticks of incense, train three times (a day).

从上十一字，除咽、洗、束、養之外，其餘义字，用手行功，皆自輕至重，自鬆至緊，自勉至安，周而復始，不計遍數，日以六香，分行三次。

You can see that this sentence expresses ideas similar to those in the other document. In ancient China there were no clocks or watches, so time was measured by burning sticks of incense. Each stick lasts about 40 minutes. This means you should train three times a day, about one and one-half hours each time.

Hundred days, the training completed, then the Chi is full; (this Chi is) above the ten thousand objects.

百日成功，則其氣充，超越萬物矣。

Identical ideas are expressed in the other document. At least 100 days of training are needed to build your spiritual foundation, or Baby Shen. After 100 days of training, the Chi is full in your body. This Chi is more valuable than any material object you might possess.

For Collect, Slip Out, File, Slap, Swing, Caress six words, all use the hands to carry out (the training), gradually reach from light to heavy.

凡攢、挣、搓、拍、摔、撫六字，皆有手行之，漸至輕重。

This sentence repeats ideas expressed above.

For the Swallow word, at the beginning of the training, first inhale a mouthful of fresh air, use Yi to swallow it, silently send it to the chest. Then again inhale a mouthful of air, send it to the navel, again swallow a mouthful, and send it to the bottom to the training place.

若咽字着，初行功之時，先吸清氣一口，以意咽下，默送至胸，再吸氣一口，送至臍間；又咽一口，送至下部行功處。

While Swallow was discussed only briefly in the last document, this document tells you just how to do it. In the last document, Swallow implies cavity breathing, specifically the Huang Ting (yellow yard) cavity. However, this document implies that the cavity is the groin area, which includes the Huiyin cavity or "Magic Gate" (Shyuan Guan). This is the key to reopening this cavity.

Then carry out the Collect, Slip Out, etc. training.

然後乃行攢、挣等功。

This means that Swallow is the first practice you do.

For the Hold (Woh) training, always use Bow Chi to reach the top, and (train until it) becomes routine.

握字功，皆有弩氣至頂，乃為得力，日以為常。

Hold is another secret word which enables your Chi to reach the top of your head. This word was not mentioned before in this document, which seems to indicate that parts of the document have been deleted, perhaps on purpose. In the Hold training, your mind must be strong like a bow, and your will must be concentrated and directed. Bow Chi is equivalent to the idea of Hard used in the other document. It takes determination and concentration to bring the Chi to the top of your head. You must practice enough so that you can do it easily.

About Wash, use the herb water to wash twice every day. One (purpose) is the smooth circulation of blood and Chi, one is for (treating) the old skin.

洗者，汷藥水逐日燙洗二次也，一取通和血氣，一取蒼老皮膚。

Wash means to use an herbal solution to wash the penis twice a day. The herb helps the Chi and blood circulation, and also helps to prevent degeneration of the skin. This word was not mentioned at all in the last document.

About Bind (Shuh), after (the above) training, (after the) washing (is) completed, use soft cotton to make a rope, bind the stem and root, loose and tight just right, the purpose is so that it will be constantly extended and won't bend.

束者，功畢，洗畢，用軟帛作繩，束其莖根，鬆緊適宜，取其常伸不屈之義。

Shuh means to bind or tighten something up. Here it means that when the penis is erect you use a soft cotton rope to bind it along its entire length with the proper tightness, not too loose, not too tight. Then you use your Yi to expand it, and then relax it. This exercise will help keep your penis erect.

About Nourish, training completed and the object is big and strong, in every war (you will) defeat others, (this) is its original duty. But (if you're) afraid (it has become) lazy, or (you have) other worries, first use the old vessel, nourish it sometimes.

養者，功成物壯，靡戰勝人，是其本分，猶恐其懶，或至他虞，先用舊鼎，時戒養之。

This and the following sentences express an idea also mentioned in the other document, namely that you should always use warm and cold water (or an herbal solution) to stimulate the penis. This will keep it strong, big, and healthy. After you have finished the training you may find it useful or necessary to do the exercises every once in a while, so you will use the "old vessel" again to warm up some more herbs.

About Nourish, it means to use warmth (i.e., warm water or warm herbal solution) to nourish it peacefully. Do not loosen

and tighten suddenly. Must make (it) get used to the war, then (you) will not lose. (Do) this training for one hundred days, the longer the better. Weak (becomes) strong. Soft tough. Short long. Sick healthy. End up a strong husband. Even wood stone iron hammer, how could I be scared? Use this to face the battle, there is no stronger general in this world. Use it to pick and gain the magic pearl easily, use it to pass down the generation, then a hundred are all boys. I do not know if there is anything happier and greater than this in heaven and earth.

養者，謂安閒溫養，切勿馳驟，務令慣戰，然後能無失也。此功行滿百日，久久益佳，弱者強，柔者剛，縮者長，病者康，居然烈丈夫矣，雖木石鐵槌吾何惴哉，以此鏖戰，世間應更無勁將也，以之採取即得玄珠，以之延嗣，則百斯男，吾不知天地間，更有何樂孰大於是。

The same ideas are expressed in the last few sentences of the other document. After reading both documents you can see the following things:

1. The discussion of the training is very brief and unclear. That is why oral instruction was necessary in ancient times.

2. Both documents have the same information about 70% of the time. The second document is incomplete, with some of the key training deleted.

3. The second document includes the Wash technique, which was not included in the first document. Washing with herbs might have developed out of the Nourish practice. Both processes are identical except that Nourish uses water and Wash uses an herbal solution.

8-4. Refining the Essence and Converting It into Chi (Liann Jieng Huah Chi)

This is the first stage, that of 100 days of building the foundation. In this stage, you learn how to increase the production of Essence and convert it into Chi. Although you have built up a large store of Chi through the Yi Gin Ching training, it is still not enough for the Shii Soei Ching training. It was discovered that you could greatly increase the Essence-Chi conversion by stimulating the genitals and converting the semen Essence into Chi. This method is especially critical for those Shii Soei Ching practitioners who did not train the Yi Gin Ching and build up a large store of Chi through that training. If they do not generate enough Chi, their bodies will become too Yin and be damaged. Those who did not do the Yi Gin Ching training will also find that the Shii Soei Ching will only take them so far.

The most common way of increasing Essence (semen) production is through stimulation. This stimulation can be from Wai Dan or Nei Dan techniques. In Chinese Chi Kung society, Wai Dan stimulation is considered more effective and faster, and it has become more popular. Although Nei Dan training is slower and the result is not obvious in a short time, it is considered the better stimulation method because it does not disturb your peace and calmness and interfere with your mental cultivation. For this reason the Buddhists prefer the Nei Dan methods.

Theoretically, in order to generate more Chi for Shii Soei Ching training, you must first have more semen than you normally need. Although the available documents list many ways to stimulate the genitals, just about any way you may think of will work, as long as you do it for the purpose of semen production. This is especially true for the Wai Dan stimulation. The document has a song which talks about this stage of training:

In the Yinchiao vessel, Chi is misty. How many real originals are (hidden) inside; (if you can) pick (them up) and (lead them to) enter into the emptiness and refine into Chi, (even) Perng Lai ten thousand miles away, the road is open (to you).

陰蹻脈上氣濛濛，多少真元在此中；採入虛無煉成炁，蓬萊萬里路相通。

When you stimulate the groin and generate semen, the Chi first fills up the Yinchiao vessel. It is called misty because it is as heavy as a thick fog. This Chi is considered semen Chi, since it is converted from semen. Semen is considered part of the Original Essence. The originals here refers to Original Jieng (Yuan Jieng), Original Chi (Yuan Chi), and Original Shen (Yuan Shen). If you know how to pick up (use) and lead this Chi and to refine it into your Shen (spirit), you will be able to live forever like the immortals. Perng Lai is an island in ancient Chinese folk legends where the immortals were said to live.

As mentioned previously, after you have generated plenty of semen, you must convert it into Chi. If you do not convert it efficiently, the extra semen will stimulate your sexual desire to a high level. Therefore, after you have completed the groin stimulation process, you must continue with the conversion process. The trick of increasing the efficiency of the conversion is to lead the Chi from the four vessels in the legs upward to the Huang Ting and the head. This is especially important for the Yinchiao (Yin Heel) vessel. We will explain the reason in the Nei Dan training later. When the Chi in the four leg vessels is led upward, the semen-Chi conversion will increase to refill the four vessels.

In the next stage of the Shii Soei Ching training, leading the Chi upward to the Huang Ting and the brain is called "Liann Chi Sheng Hwa," which means "train the Chi and sublimate it." It is also called "Faan Jieng Buu Nao," which means "return the Essence to nourish the brain."

For your reference, we will discuss in this section some of the Wai Dan and Nei Dan methods for semen production. First we will discuss testicle stimulation, and then penis training.

Wai Dan Training:
1. Pearl-Wheel Kung (Ju Luen Shyng Kung)-Testicle Stimulation Training
Ju means pearl and Luen means wheel or turning. Shyng means to do or to execute, and Kung means Kung Fu or training. Testicle stimulation is a method of increasing semen production by working directly on the semen factory. The methods are effective and easy. You can easily train all of the following Wai Dan stimulation methods when you are taking a shower or bath. In the following techniques, whenever you have to use your hands you should first make sure your hands are

clean. Also, if your hands are cold you should rub them together until they are warm. When you train, you may start with about only twenty times for each exercise, and gradually increase the number and the force each training session.

The two documents discussed in the last section each refer to this training:

For the testicles, the secret training words are: say Slip Out (Jeng), say Massage (Rou), say File (Tsuo), say Hang (Juey), say Slap (Pai).

At the testicles, say Collect (Tzaan); say Slip Out (Jeng), say File (Tsuo), say Slap (Pai).

All of these techniques are used to increase semen production except Hang (Juey), which is used for the second stage of the Chi sublimation training. Hang will be discussed in the next section. We will now discuss the other techniques listed in these two documents.

A. Slip Out (Jeng)(to make an effort; to get free from; to slip out)

Jeng means to get free by making an effort. In this exercise, you simply use your fingers to gently grab or hold the testicles and let them slide out of your grip.

a. Dragon Pearl Finger Kung (Long Ju Jyi Kung)

Place both of your hands under the testicles with palms facing up. Use all five fingers to gently grab and press the testicles. Then use your thumb to circle the testicles for a few times, and then let them slide out (Figure 8-1).

b. Palm Slip Out Kung (Jaang Jeng Kung)

In this technique, use both hands to sandwich the testicles between the palms. Gently press the testicles and let them slip out (Figure 8-2).

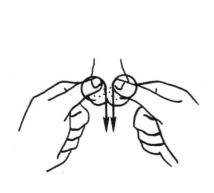

Figure 8-1. Dragon Pearl Finger Kung (Long Ju Jyi Kung)

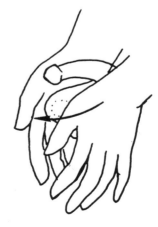

Figure 8-2. Palm Slip Out Kung (Jaang Jeng Kung)

B. Massage (Rou)

Rou means to massage. When you massage, your hands move together with the skin as they circle around. The hands and the skin should not rub against each other.

a. Dragon Pearl Palm Kung (Long Ju Jaang Kung)

This exercise is very similar to the Palm Slip Out technique. The main difference is that in this exercise you simply use both of your palms to rub the testicles with a circular motion. Hold your hands horizontally, palm to palm, with your testicles sandwiched in-between. Keep your penis on the side out of the way so that you can circle easily (Figure 8-3).

b. Dragon Tendon Extending Chi Kung (Long Gin Shen Chi Kung)

Use your thumb and the second finger to hold the vas deferens (the tube which carries sperm from the testes). Rub the two fingers against each other, moving down the tube away from the root of the penis down to the testicles (Figure 8-4). This will clear the tube of obstructions.

c. Dragon Tendon Develop Chi Kung (Long Gin Jaan Chi Kung)

Hold the vas deferens with your thumb and second finger and rub forward and backward while moving the two tubes apart (Figure 8-5). This stimulates the tubes instead of the testicles themselves, and will also clear the tubes of obstructions.

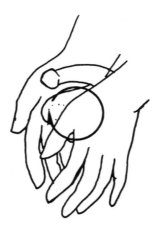

Figure 8-3. Dragon Pearl Palm Kung (Long Ju Jaang Kung)

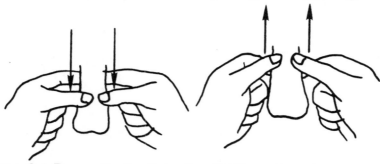

Figure 8-4. Dragon Tendon Extending Chi Kung (Long Gin Shen Chi Kung)

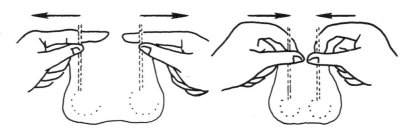

Figure 8-5. Dragon Tendon Develop Chi Kung (Long Gin Jaan Chi Kung)

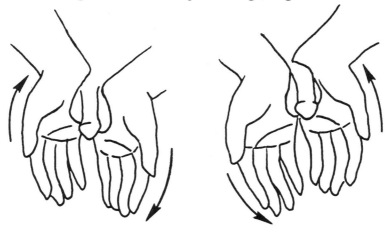

Figure 8-6. Hand Knife Kung (Shoou Dau Kung)

C. File (Tsuo)(to rub; to file)

Tsuo means to file or rub. In Tsuo, your hands rub against the skin until heat is generated. Tsuo is also used for the penis, which will be discussed later.

a. Hand Knife Kung (Shoou Dau Kung)

Use the edge of both hands to rub and file near the top of the scrotum (Figure 8-6). This exercise has two purposes. One is to stimulate and clear the vas deferens, the other is to toughen the skin in preparation for the hanging exercises, which will be discussed later.

D. Slap (Pai)(to pat; to slap)
a. Hand Pat Kung (Shoou Pai Kung)

Practice this in the morning, after you have gone to the toilet. When you practice, face the east, your eyes half closed, squat down into a horse stance. Hold the root of your penis with your left hand, and slap your scrotum with your right hand. Start hitting lightly, and gradually increase the force. At every slap, inhale, pull in the anus, open your eyes and stare at a distant point (Figure 8-7).

E. Collect (Tzaan)
a. Turning the Pearl Kung (Joan Ju Kung)

Tzaan means to collect or to hold something together. Hold both testicles in one hand and roll them around in a circle like you would two small balls, then do the same with your other hand for the same number of times. When you circle the testicles, do not press them. Simply move them around in a circle in your hand (Figure 8-8).

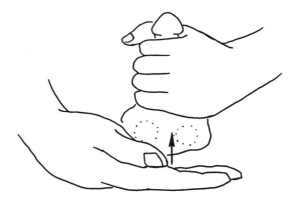

Figure 8-7.   Hand Pat Kung (Shoou Pai Kung)

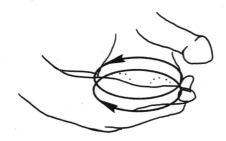

Figure 8-8.   Turning the Pearl Kung (Joan Ju Kung)

2. Jade Stem Training (Yuh Jing Kung) or Side Grindstone Training (Herng Mor Shyng Kung)-Penis Stimulation Training

Yu is jade and implies something precious, and Jen means stem, which implies the penis. Herng in Chinese means sideways, Mor means grindstone. When a cylindrical grindstone was used it was put sideways on a flat place to do the grinding. Herng Mo has also been commonly used by the Taoists to refer to the penis. Shyng Kung means to do the training.

The penis is a very sensitive organ. Stimulating it increases sexual desire and also the production of semen. This training will help you get used to the stimulation, and will increase your endurance during intercourse. In Shii Soei Ching Chi Kung training you must train yourself so that you can ejaculate or hold as you choose. This is what is meant by: "Withdraw or release depends on me, follow and give, I choose the person."

The documents discussed in the last chapter each has a paragraph listing the penis training:

For the penis, the secret training words are: say Hold (Woh), say Bind (Shuh), say Nourish (Yeang), say Swallow (Ien), say Draw In/Absorb (Sher), say Hold Up (Tyi), say Close (Bi), say Swing (Shuai).

On the Jade Stem (penis), say Swallow (Ien), say Swing (Shuai) say Caress (Fuu), say Wash (Shii), say Bind (Shuh), say Nourish (Yeang), say File (Tsuo).

All of these techniques are used to increase semen production, except Hold and Hold Up, which are used in the Chi sublimation training. Hold and Hold Up will be discussed in the next section. Among the others, Swallow, Draw/Absorb, and Close are considered Nei Dan trainings, while all the others are Wai Dan stimulation practices. First we will discuss the Wai Dan techniques, and then the Nei Dan ones.

A. Nourish (Yeang)(to nurture, to nourish); Wash (Shii)

Yeang means to raise, to nourish. Shii means to wash. I am placing these two words together because I believe that they refer to the same training. This training is mentioned in several places in the documents. One of the documents says:

Nourish is to use the stove and vessel to warm and nourish.

This means you should place your penis in a vessel with warm water or herbal liquid to warm and nourish it. The other document explains more about this training. It says:

About Wash, use the herb water to wash twice every day. One (purpose) is the smooth circulation of blood and Chi, one is for (treating) the old skin. About Nourish, training completed and the object is big and strong, in every war (you will) defeat others, (this) is its original duty. But (if you're) afraid (it has become) lazy, or (you have) other worries, first use the old vessel, nourish it sometimes. About Nourish, means use warmth (i.e., warm water or warm herbal solution) to nourish it peacefully. Do not loosen and tighten suddenly. Must make (it) get used to the war, then (you) will not lose.

You can see from these documents that in Wash and Nourish you place your penis into a vessel filled with an herbal solution or simply warm water. The prescription will be listed in Appendix A. The main purposes are to increase the circulation of the blood and Chi and also to increase the endurance of the penis to stimulation. Some other sources mention that to Wash and to Nourish means to place your penis alternately into warm and cold water to stimulate it. Other document claim that the vessel referred to is the woman's vagina, where you nourish yourself by absorbing Chi from her.

B. Bind (Shuh)(to bind, to tie up)

One of the documents says:

Bind is to use soft cotton to bind the root (penis).

The other one says:

About Bind (Shuh), after (the above) training, (after the) washing (is) completed, use soft cotton to make a rope, bind the stem and root, loose and tight just right, the purpose is so that it will be constantly extended and won't bend.

Shuh means to bind or to tie up. When you train this word, first stimulate your penis until it is stiff. Then tie a rope made of soft cloth around the root of the penis. Inhale and pull in your abdomen and anus, then exhale, expanding your abdomen and relaxing your anus. While your are exhaling, use your mind to expand the penis. This training is simply to increase your mind's control over the penis.

C. Swing (Shuai)(to swing; to cast away)

Shuai means to swing or to cast away. When you train this word, you squat down in a horse stance, then you use the first two fingers of one hand to grab the root of the penis and swing it from side to side. Swing fifty times and then repeat another fifty times with the other hand.

D. Caress (Fuu)

Fuu means to touch or rub lightly with the hand. To train this word, hold your penis tightly with one hand, with the head of the penis protruding. Use the palm and fingers of the other hand to caress and lightly rub the head of the penis with a circular motion. Repeat fifty times and then change hands and repeat another fifty times.

E. File (Tsuo)

Tsuo means to rub against each other. When you train this word, sandwich your penis between both palms and rub your hands forward and backward about fifty times.

Nei Dan Training:

The methods of increasing semen production through physical stimulation (Wai Dan) described above are easy and effective. However, they will also stimulate an increase in the production of hormones, which will increase your sexual desires. You must therefore also regulate your mind to stop thinking about sex. If you lapse and indulge in sex, all of your training will have been in vain.

Some practitioners believe that the production of semen can also be increased by the use of your imagination. The problem is that when you stimulate your semen production through imagination, the fantasizing usually also increases your sexual desire. This will disturb and scatter your mind, and affect your training. However, if you have a strong will and are able to handle your emotions, mental stimulation is one of the most effective ways. As for mental stimulation, everyone has his own fantasies and dreams, which are the best way for him to achieve the purpose.

Although mental stimulation is an effective way of producing semen, the Chinese Buddhists consider it to be an improper way to train. They believe that you should get rid of your emotions and set yourself free from the bondage of desire.

Although physical stimulation is sometimes mentioned in Buddhist Chi Kung documents, it is believed that most Buddhist Chi Kung practitioners prefer the production of semen through Nei Dan training. Theoretically, in the Nei Dan training you use your mind and different breathing techniques to lead the Chi to the groin and energize the penis and testicles at the same time. Naturally, these methods are more difficult than those used in Wai Dan, and you won't see results in a short time. However, after you train for a while and have grasped the trick of leading Chi to the groin, you may practice anywhere and anytime you want. Most important of all, your mind will be much calmer and more peaceful without the emotional disturbance. According to the available documents, there are three techniques which are commonly used in the Nei Dan practice: Swallow, Draw In/Absorb, and Close.

A. Swallow (Ien)

In order to understand the trick of this technique, we should first look at what the two documents say about it. The first one says:

Swallow is the breathing in the cavities (Shiuh).

The second document says:

For the Swallow word, at the beginning of the training, first inhale a mouthful of fresh air, use Yi (the mind) to swallow it, silently send it to the chest. Then again inhale a mouthful of air, send it to the navel, again swallow a mouthful, and send it to the bottom to the training place.

The first document tells you that the Swallow technique involves breathing in the cavities. The cavities here include the Huang Ting (yellow yard), the Lower Dan Tien, and the Huiyin. After you train for a while, you will be able to lead the Chi downward and mix the Fire Chi with the Water Chi at the Huang Ting. This Chi is then led to the Huiyin and the groin area to energize the penis and testicles. When you are leading the Chi to the Huiyin and groin through breathing techniques, all these cavities will also be expanding and withdrawing, and they will also seem to be breathing. This is why Swallow is also called cavity breathing.

The second document teaches you how to do this Swallow technique. You should squat down in a horse stance with both fists in front of your thighs, inhale and pay attention to the Fire Chi in your Middle Dan Tien (solar plexus), and then exhale smoothly. Inhale again, and use your mind to lead the Fire Chi to the Huang Ting at the same time that you lead the Water Chi from the Lower Dan Tien to Huang Ting. When you exhale, relax your mind and body and let the Fire and Water Chi mix (interact) together. Inhale once more and use your Yi to lead the Chi to the Huiyin and groin. When you exhale, expand your groin (Figure 8-9). When you train, you must continuously hold up your anus and Huiyin (Magic Gate). This will stop the Chi from reaching the tailbone and Magic Gate, and lead it to the groin. If you train every day you will find that in a short time you will be able to lead the Chi to the groin and energize it as you wish.

B. Draw In/Absorb (Sher)

Draw In/Absorb is a technique which allows you to absorb Chi from or exchange it with nature or a training partner. Strictly speaking, a Buddhist Chi Kung practitioner would prefer to absorb or exchange Chi from nature, while a Taoist would use both nature and a partner. The Taoists say: "Yin and Yang are not necessarily distinguished by male or female, Yin and Yang can be just the body's strength or weak-

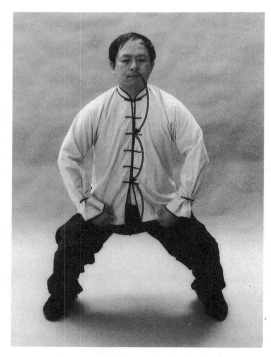

Figure 8-9.   The Posture for Swallow Training

ness."(*1) They also say: "Two men can graft and plant and a pair of women can adapt and nourish."(*2) This means that, in obtaining Chi nourishment from a partner, male or female is not important. For example, a teenage boy can be very strong and Yang, and an old man weak and Yin. Therefore, through mutual Chi transportation the Chi of both can be balanced to their mutual benefit. The Taoists also studied how men and women can transport Chi and nourish each other through sexual activity. Naturally, these techniques have never been adapted by the Buddhists. In the Buddhist Draw In/Absorb training, they train absorbing Chi from nature and also from a partner through still meditation. Next, we will discuss the methods of absorbing natural Chi, and then we will consider the non-sexual methods for exchanging Chi with a partner through still meditation.

a. Draw In/Absorb from Nature:
     The main sources of the energy you try to absorb are the sun, the moon, and the earth. The sun and the moon radiate electromagnetic energy onto the surface of the earth. If you know how to absorb and use this energy to nourish your body, you will find that it speeds up your training. In the wintertime, when your body is more Yin, you like to expose your body to the sun and absorb its radiation. However, it is important to understand the correct timing. For example, in the summertime both your body and the sun are very Yang, and so you should

---

(*1).陰陽不必分男女，體氣强弱即陰陽。
(*2).兩個男人可栽接，一對女人能採補。

not try to absorb the sun's Chi except in the early morning. However, when you practice this exercise, you don't just absorb the energy into your skin, you use Yi and breathing coordination to draw it deep into your body. Once you know how, you can use this natural energy to nourish almost anywhere in your body. For example, you can lead it to your groin to stimulate Essence production, or to the marrow to clean it, or you can lead it to nourish your brain. Naturally, you must know how to balance Yin and Yang, because too much of the energy can make your body too Yang and cause problems.

To absorb earth energy or Chi is to absorb the magnetic energy generated in the center of the earth. If you know how, you can use this magnetic Chi to smooth out your Chi circulation and find your mental balance. For example, if you are in the Northern Hemisphere, you should face south when you sleep or meditate. This lines you up with the earth's magnetic field and helps you to best absorb the magnetic Chi. This is discussed in detail in Chapter 4 of "The Root of Chinese Chi Kung."

Before we discuss further about how to absorb natural energy to stimulate your Essence production, we would like to translate a section of the document.

1. Absorb the (Nature) Essence Kung

採精華功

The Essence of extreme Yang, the refinement of extreme Yin, (when) the two Chis interact harmoniously, it derives into and gives birth to millions of living things. Ancient people who were good at picking up and swallowing (i.e., absorbing these Essences), (after) long long (absorbing) they all became fairies. Its methods were kept secret, people in the world did not know. Even when there were some who knew, they endured no perseverance and strong will, and further were without patience, so therefore it was worthless even when they knew, and there were few who achieved (success).

太陽之精，太陰之華，二氣交融，化生萬物。古人善採咽者，久久皆仙，其法祕密，世人莫知；即有知者，苦無堅志，且無恆心，是為虛員居諸，而成之者少也。

It has been mentioned several times in previous documents that the millions of living things are generated from the harmonious interaction of Yin and Yang. These methods of absorbing the natural Yin and Yang are able to make you "immortal," or a "fairy." Absorbing is commonly called Tsae Ien, or "picking up and swallowing." However, knowing about the methods is not enough, for without strong will, perseverance, and patience you will not succeed.

Whoever is training internal (Chi Kung), from the beginning of the training to his success, and finally his death, no matter (whether he is) at leisure or busy, he cannot discontinue. If the

training of picking up and swallowing is not discontinuous, then it is not hard to become a fairy or Buddha. The reason for picking up and swallowing is to take the Essence of Yin and Yang, (and use it) to benefit (i.e., nourish) my Shen and wisdom, enabling (me) to gradually remove the condensation and stagnation and (help) the clean spirit grow daily; millions of sicknesses will not be generated. It is of the greatest benefit.

凡行內煉者，自初功始，至於成功，以致終身，勿論門忙，不可間斷。若採咽之功無有間斷，則仙佛不難於成。其所以採咽，蓋取陰陽精華。益我神智，俾凝滯漸消，清靈日長，萬病不生，良有大益。

The Essence of Yin and Yang means the Essence of the sun and moon, two major natural Chi sources. This training is very important for those people who are training internal Kung. They should train without interruptions or stops. If you are able to train continuously, you will be able to use the natural Chi to nourish and raise your spirit, as well as to nourish your brain to increase your wisdom. Furthermore, this Chi Kung can remove condensed and stagnant Chi.

The method for the sun - choose the first day of the lunar month. It is said that at the beginning of the moon, its Chi is new and therefore it is good to pick up the sun Essence. For the moon (Essence), choose the fifteenth day of the moon (i.e., month). It is said the gold water is full and the Chi is abundant. It is good to absorb the Essence of the moon.

其法日取於朔，謂於月初之交，其氣方新，堪取日精。月取於望，謂金水盈滿，其氣正旺，堪取月華。

If you want to absorb the Essence of the sun, it is recommended that you train on the first day of the lunar month. The Chinese use the lunar month, and use the term "moon" for "month." Each month normally varies from twenty-eight to thirty days. It is believed that at the beginning of the month, the Chi emitted by the sun is fresh and gentle. The Chi from the sun is classified as Yang (Fire), while the Chi from the moon is classified as Yin (Water).

When you absorb the Essence of the moon you should practice around the fifteenth, or middle, of the month, when the moon is full and its Water Chi is full and abundant.

If it is gloomy or raining on the first and fifteenth, or because of business, then choose the second or the third, the sixteenth or seventeenth. You can still condense the Shen and absorb (the Essence). If it passes these six days, then the sun is weakening and the moon is softening, it is insufficient and should not be absorbed.

設朔望日遇有陰雨，或值不暇，則取初二、初三、

十六、十七，猶可凝神補取；若過此六日，則日昃
月虧，虛而不足取也。

You can delay the training a day or two because of rain or business obligations, but if you have to wait longer than this you shouldn't train, because the energy is no longer beneficial. When you train, to absorb effectively you must concentrate your mind and condense your Shen.

(When) absorbing the sun's Essence at the beginning of the moon (i.e., lunar month), should be 5 to 8 AM when (the sun) has just risen. Stay at a high place and face the sun quietly. Regulate your nose breathing uniformly, absorbing the light's Essence through inhaling, until it is a mouthful. Hold your breath and condense your Shen. Then swallow it very finely. Use the Yi to send it down to the center palace (i.e., Lower Dan Tien). This is one swallow. Like this for seven swallows, keep calm for a while, then move to take care of (your) daily affairs without disturbance.

朝取日精，宜寅卯初出時，高處默對，調勻鼻息，
道吸光華，令滿一口，閉息凝神，細細咽下，以意
送之，至於中宮，是為一咽；如此七咽，靜守片時
，然後起行，任從酬應，毫無妨礙。

The best time to absorb the sun's Essence is just when it has risen. At this time the sun is soft, fresh, and getting stronger and stronger. If you wait until the sun is already high, then the Essence will be too Yang and it can harm you to absorb it. When you train, you should sit or stand quietly facing the sun. Regulate your mind and breathing. You should chose a high location because the air is fresher there. When you inhale it seems as if you are taking in the sun's Essence and holding it in your mouth. Next, hold your breath and condense your spirit, swallow the Essence and lead it to the Lower Dan Tien. You should repeat the practice seven times. Then stand quietly for a while, then go calmly about your daily business.

(When) absorbing the moon's Essence on the fifteenth of the (lunar) month, also use the same method. Should be at 8 PM to 12 PM. Pick up and swallow seven times, this is the natural benefit of the heaven and the earth. Only he who has a persevering heart is able to enjoy it. It is only those who have confidence (who) will be able to take it. This is one of the great trainings among the methods, remember do not ignore it and miss it.

望取月華，亦準前法，於戌亥時，採吞七咽，此乃
天地自然之利；惟有恆心者，乃能享用之；亦惟有
信心，乃能取用之。此為法中之一部大功，切勿忽
誤也。

When you train to absorb the moon Essence, the method is the same as when you absorb the sun Essence, except the practice time is from 8

PM to midnight. At this time, the Water Chi from the moon is considered to be at its strongest.

You can see that the training methods are quite simple. Whether the training is successful or not depends on your will, patience, and perseverance. This document has given you a general idea of how to absorb natural energy. After you have practiced and experienced this for a while, you will realize that you may absorb almost any Chi which is around you. For example, if you feel your body is too Yang, you can put your arms around a tree and let it regulate your Chi and absorb the excess. You may use the air Chi near a stream to clean your lungs and freshen your mind. Remember that the key to success is knowing how to coordinate your Yi and breathing to lead the Chi deep into your body and to release the excess Chi out of your body to reach a balance of Yin and Yang.

Next we will discuss the Absorb methods which can be used to nourish the groin and to help build up the Chi in the Huang Ting. Only one of the sources discusses this technique. It says:

Draw In/Absorb is to nourish the body (through) sitting and transporting (Chi).

Face the sun or moon or other Chi source, sitting on a chair (Figure 8-10) or on the floor (Figure 8-11), and place your hands on your Lower Dan Tien. Pull your toes slightly upward, which will stop the Chi from leaking out from the Bubbling Well (Yongquan) gates on the bottom of your feet. Then inhale and imagine that you are absorbing the Chi from the source through the Baihui, face, and the skin. While you are

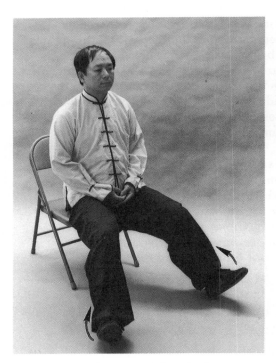

Figure 8-10. Draw In/Absorb the
Natural Chi while
Sitting on a Chair

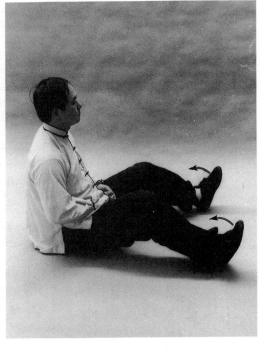

Figure 8-11. Draw In/Absorb the
Natural Chi while
Sitting on the Floor

doing this, you should hold up your Huiyin and anus slightly. Remember, **WHEN YOU HOLD UP YOUR HUIYIN AND ANUS, DO NOT TENSE THEM. SIMPLY HOLD THEM UP, USING MORE YI THAN PHYSICAL ACTION**. If you do not catch the trick of how to hold your Huiyin and anus, the Chi will stagnate there. Furthermore, the muscular tension there will also cause your stomach to tense, causing problems with your digestive system. The worst problem that a tense Huiyin and anus can cause is that the Chi will become stagnant and you won't be able to lead it to the Huang Ting smoothly. The Huiyin cavity is one of the gates which is called the "tricky gate" (Shyuan Guan), because whether or not you work with it correctly determines whether or not your training is successful.

When you inhale, use your Yi to lead the Chi to your Huang Ting; and when you exhale, lead the Chi in the Huang Ting to the groin and hold your breath for a couple of seconds. As you do this, imagine that the Chi is filling up the entire groin and energizing it. Naturally, the key to success is again the Huiyin and anus control. While you are doing this, you should hold up your Huiyin and anus during both the inhale and the exhale. If you do not do this, the Chi will pass the Huiyin and enter the Governing Vessel, and you won't achieve the goal.

b. Mutual Transportation with a Partner:

There are many ways of mutually transporting Chi with a partner. We will only discuss two of the common ways. The first one is used to nourish the groin, and the second one is to help each other to complete the Small Circulation.

Method 1:

Face each other, with your bodies touching as if you were hugging each other. Your minds should be calm and peaceful so that you can concentrate completely. Match your breathing so that when one inhales, the other exhales. After you have practiced for a while and are matching each other smoothly, you will feel that both of your Chi bodies have united into one. When this happens, you will feel that you are transparent and there is nothing separating you to interfere with the Chi circulation between you. Now, when you exhale use your Yi to lead the Chi from your body to the partner's body until it reaches the groin. Naturally, your partner should inhale and lead the Chi to his or her groin. After you have completed the process, then your partner exhales while you are inhaling, and you both lead the Chi to nourish your groin. Remember, the most important key to the training is that both of you should hold up your anus and Huiyin gently throughout the practice. The training can last as long as you wish.

This is only an example of the training that is possible. There are many other methods which can be used. As long as you know the theory, you should able to find many other ways of transporting Chi to nourish each other.

Method 2:

This mutual transportation training is commonly used to help each other complete or enhance the Chi circulation in the Conception and Governing Vessels (Small Circulation). It is only for those who understand the methods of Small Circulation practice. If you are unfamiliar with it, please refer to the book: "Chi Kung - Health and Martial Arts."

Sit with crossed legs, with your backs touching. Before you start to exchange the Chi, you should both first calm down your minds and regulate your breathing. The path which you would like to help each other with is from the tailbone (Changqiang, Gv-1) to the top part of your back. You can transport the Chi in this section of the back either when you are inhaling or exhaling; both ways are acceptable, but both of you must use the same method in order to help each other.

C. Close (Bi)

Close means to close or hold your breath and keep the Chi in the groin area. It is one of the more effective ways of stimulating the groin.

Close means slowing down aging and restoring the functioning (of the organs).

When you stimulate the groin, the production of Essence increases. This maintains your sexual activity and slows aging. The increased production of Essence increases the production of Chi and regenerates the internal organs.

To practice Close, inhale deeply and lead the Chi to the Huang Ting cavity. Then exhale and lead the Chi to the groin, and refrain from inhaling as long as you can. When you do this, it feels like you are inflating a balloon in the groin area. While training, continuously hold up your Huiyin and anus slightly.

Exhale any remaining air you have been holding in five short breaths. This allows you to hold air in your groin even longer. If saliva has accumulated in your mouth, swallow it and lead the Chi to the Lower Dan Tien. After your training, do not go to the toilet. If you do, all of the Chi accumulated in the groin will be lost. As a matter of fact, in all Chi Kung training, you should not go to toilet for at least an hour after practice.

8-5. Purifying Chi and Converting It into Shen (Liann Chi Huah Shen)

This stage is the ten months of pregnancy for the Spirit Embryo. You are now refining the Chi you have converted and leading it upward to the Huang Ting and to the head. This process is called "Liann Chi Sheng Hwa," or "to train and sublimate the Chi." In the documents, there is a song about this stage of training. It says:

Shen and Chi mutually interact and enter the dark and obscure. The Magic gate (Shyuan Guan) gold stamp one point through; five Chis moves toward their origins and come to surround it, conquer the hair and wash the marrow, rely on (this) real classic.

神氣交加入杳冥，玄關金印一點通；五氣朝元來環繞，伐毛洗髓賴真經。

When you lead the Chi to the top to meet your Original Spirit (Original Shen), this Chi and Original Shen will interact with each other. According to Chinese Chi Kung, the Upper Dan Tien is the residence of the Shen. This residence is dark and closed (obscure). You must lead the abundant Chi to this residence to interact with your Shen and open the gate. When this happens it is called "Kai Chiaw," which means "opening the tricky gate." In order to lead the Chi upward, you must learn how to use the golden stamp (the middle finger) to press the point which is called the "Magic Gate" (Shyuan Guan or Huiyin).

When the Chi is led to the Upper Dan Tien, the spirit can be raised. This raised spirit will be able to effectively govern and regulate the Chi circulation in the body. When you have done this, the Chi circulation for the five Yin organs (heart, liver, spleen, lung, and kidney) will return back to their original Chi level. Once you have reached this stage, you will also be able to lead the Chi into the marrow to clean it and to the surface of the skin to "conquer the hair." This means to stop aging, which is normally visible in the skin and hair.

This stage of training can again be divided into Wai Dan and Nei Dan. It does not matter which method is used, the main purpose is to sublimate the Chi upward to the brain to nourish it and raise up the spirit.

Wai Dan Chi Sublimation:
A. Hang (Juey)(to fall; to drop; to hang)
The document says:

Hang is to refine the Chi and to sublimate it.

Hanging something from a rope is call Juey. Juey is one of the most important processes in Taoist Shii Soei Ching Chi Kung training. It is the hanging which enables you to lead the Chi upward from the vessels in the legs and consequently to increase the efficiency of the Jieng-Chi conversion. This process has been used mostly by the Taoists. The Buddhists usually use the Yi and some minor body controls to do the converting. That is considered a Nei Dan conversion process and will be discussed later. Generally speaking, the hanging training is a quicker and more effective way for people whose level of meditation is still shallow. Converting with the Yi is difficult, and requires a lot of experience and a deep knowledge of meditation.

Basically, to train this process you hang a weight from your genitals and swing it back and forth. As the weight pulls down on your genitals, you must have the Yi (intention) of holding upward. This intention of lifting generates the Chi to carry out the lifting, and so the two forces of pulling down and pulling up are balanced. When you use your mind to coordinate this exercise, you will lead the Chi up to the Huang Ting, and also through the Thrusting Vessel to the brain. This process is called "Faan Jieng Buu Nao" (Returning the Semen and Nourishing the Brain).

Before you start the hanging and swinging training, you must first train two things to strengthen the groin.

Preparation:
a. Shoou Dau Kung (Hand Knife Kung):
This training has been discussed in the first stage of training. Simply use the edges of both hands to rub the root of the genitals. This strengthens the area which supports the weight.

b. Dragon Tendon Strengthening Kung (Long Gin Renn Kung):

Form a ring with your thumb and index finger, and hold the top part of the genitals which is closest to the abdomen (Figure 8-12). Pull down about 80 times, then switch hands and pull another 80 times. This also strengthens the area which holds the weight.

Materials Needed for Hanging:

a. A piece of silk or satin cloth measuring about four and a half feet by one foot. The edge of the cloth should be sewn to prevent fraying. The cloth is rolled into a rope when used. Satin cloth is used because it is soft and will not cause friction burns during the training. You will also find that with satin it is also easier to untie the knot than with other materials such as cotton.

b. Weights. You can buy barbell weights in many sporting goods stores. They have a hole in them that you can slip the cloth through, and they are flat, so they will easily pass between your legs. They are also marked with their weight, so you can know exactly how much you are lifting.

Training Procedure:

a. Remove your pants and underpants. You can either sit on the floor, or stand in front of a chair with the weights on it. Tie the satin rope around the top of the genitals close to the abdomen.

b. Pass the satin rope through the center hole of the weight and tie the ends. Check that the length is short enough so that the weight will clear the floor when you stand up (Figure 8-13).

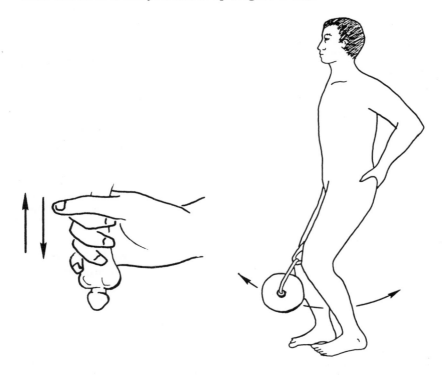

Figure 8-12. Dragon Tendon
Strengthening Kung
(Long Gin Renn Kung)

Figure 8-13. Hanging Training

c. Stand up into Ma Bu (horse stance) with your feet shoulder distance apart.

d. Swing the weight forward and backward until it becomes uncomfortable. Start with the lightest weight, and slowly increase the number of swings and the weight.

Training Keys:
1. Close the mouth.
2. The tip of the tongue touches the roof of the mouth.
3. Clench your teeth.
4. Clasp your hands behind you.
5. Hold up your anus and withdraw your penis.
6. Breath normally and uniformly.
7. The body is upright.
8. Upper body stays relaxed.
9. The eyes stare straight ahead.
10. Keep your Yi on your Huang Ting or Lower Dan Tien.
11. Hold up the Huiyin cavity (Magic Gate).

Diet During Training:
1. Keep away from ice cold food and drink. They keep your Chi in your lower digestive system and prevent it from moving upward.
2. Do not drink alcohol, it can affect your concentration, judgement, and sensitivity.
3. Keep away from strong tastes such as sour, spicy, hot food, and coffee. These foods will usually generate a heavy Chi disturbance in your digesting system. This will also interfere with your leading the Chi upward.

Times to Train:
Past experience indicates that the best time for hanging training is right after midnight. This time is called "Hwo Tzyy Shyr," or "alive midnight time." This is because right after midnight the Chi is normally gathered in the groin, where it stimulates semen production. It is believed that if you train at this time to lead the Chi upward from the vessels in the legs, you can increase the efficiency of the semen-Chi conversion. The Taoists call leading the Chi upward to the Huang Ting and the brain "Tsae Yaw," or "picking up the elixir." When you know how to pick up this elixir at midnight, it is called "Dang Ling." This means "seasonable" or "fashionable," and implies that it is the "right time."

Of Special Importance:
1. No sex for one hundred days. When you start to train Shii Soei Ching, you should not have sex for the first 100 days. The reason is very simple. In the first 100 days you are building up the Chi in your Huang Ting to an abundant level. If you have sex before you have built up your Chi to a suitable level, you will lose what you have built up. Each time you ejaculate you lose a great amount of semen and Chi.
2. Hold up your penis, anus, and Huiyin (Magic Gate) from the beginning to the end of your hanging training. This is the only way you can keep the rising Chi from going up the Governing Vessel (Du Mei) and entering the Fire path. When you hold up your penis, anus, and Huiyin the Chi will be led to the Water path and enter

the Thrusting Vessel (Chong Mei), which connects to the Huang Ting and the brain.

3. After you finish your training, you should not use the toilet for at least one hour. Chi will continue to move upward for a while after you finish training. If you go to the toilet, you will lead the Chi downward and it will pass out of your body. It is therefore a good idea to use the toilet before you start training.

4. The amount of weight you use is not important. You do not need a heavy weight to sublimate the Chi upward successfully. You may find that swinging a lighter weight more times is more effective than swinging a greater weight a few times.

5. After hanging you should do the beating practice to complete the Chi circle. This leads the Chi into the marrow and to the surface of your body. This stimulation will fill up your entire body with Chi.

6. When your penis is erect, do not hang. Many practitioners suggest that you should not hang when your penis is erect lest you injure yourself. However, it depends on how much weight are you hanging and how careful you are.

7. Do not hang when ill or recuperating. If you are sick, you should stop your training, and not resume until you have recovered completely. When you are sick your Chi is weakened or disturbed, and the hanging will bring more harm to your body than benefit.

8. If your skin is injured by the hanging, stop hanging until it is healed.

B. Hold (Woh)

There are two sentences in the documents which talk about this key word:

Hold is to hold up the kidneys (here meaning testicles) to the top.

For the Hold (Woh) training, always use Bow Chi to reach the top, and (train until it) becomes routine.

Woh means to hold with the hand. There are two ways of training Woh. In the first one you sit on the edge of a chair so that your genitals hang loose. Rub your hands together until they are warm. Breathe regularly and smoothly. Use one hand to hold the penis with the palm facing down. Then inhale while drawing your abdomen in, and at the same hold your penis tighter and tighter. While you are inhaling, pull in your penis and hold up your Huiyin and anus. This is called "Withdrawing the Sword Kung" (Shou Jen Kung) or "Withdrawing the Turtle Kung" (Shou Guei Kung). After inhaling as much as you can, exhale slowly, and at the same time gradually loosen your grip until it is completely loose; at the same time release your anus. Repeat at least ten times, then repeat the exercise the same number of times with your other hand.

The second way to Woh is to use both hands to hold the testicles and penis, palms up. When you train, you should stand with your feet shoulder-width apart. Calm and center your mind, then sit down. Keep both knees bent, your heels on the floor, and lift up the front of your feet. Rub both hands until they are warm. Finally, use both hands to hold up the testicles and use the thumbs to press and rub them (Figure 8-14). When you are doing this, you must hold up your

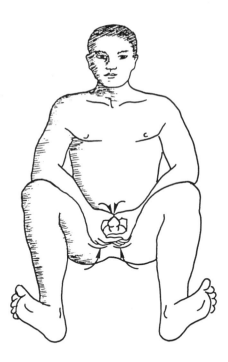

Figure 8-14. Hold Training

Magic Gate cavity (Huiyin) in the perineum, and hold in your penis and anus. Keep your mind calm, and breath deeply and regularly.

Now that you have some idea of the training, I would like to use an ancient poem to explain this key word:

Hands hold the pearl wheel, lift up to Kuen Luen (a famous mountain); descend, contain, absorb in, and press heavily; Jieng, Chi, and Shen condensed. Chi (is able to) reach four extremities, tongue, teeth, nails, (and) hair; man and heaven united into one, no death, no aging. One holds one rubs, left and right change hands; nine nine the number (i.e., 81 times), the real Yang (Chi) will not walk (away). Large Tao's training, (its) achievement involves creation and variation; sit, meditate into the depths, return the aged to childhood.

手捧珠輪，提上崑崙；降持攝擩，精氣神凝。
氣貫四稍，舌牙甲髮；人天合一，不死不老。
一兜一搓，左右換手；九九之數，真陽不走。
大道之行，功參造化；坐息冥冥，返老還童。

When you practice the secret Hold technique, hold your testicles with both hands and lift them up as far as they will go. Kuen Luen is one of the highest mountains in China. Chinese people commonly used this mountain to express great height. Here it conveys the idea that you are not only holding your testicles high, but that you are also raising your mind to the top of your head. When you train, it does not matter if you lift, descend, contain, or use the palm to press and rub, in any case your Jieng, Chi, Shen will be condensed.

Eventually your Chi will be able to reach the four extremities: tongue, teeth, nails, and hair, and your Chi will be able to combine with the energy in nature (heaven), and you will not age.

When you train, use one hand to hold up the testicles, and use the other to press and rub. After 81 times, change your hands and repeat the process. This procedure is also a method for converting semen to Chi, which will keep the Yang Chi you are generating from being lost.

Once you achieve this large Tao you will be able to improve your life and health. When you train, your mind must be calm and meditating deeply, then you will be able to convert the semen (hormone) into Chi and reach the goal of returning to youth.

C. Pointing (Dien)

The document contains a song believed to be an oral secret which talks about this key word. It says:

Hand lifts the golden stamp to reverse (the situation), (press) one point (on the) Yellow River, the water reverses its flow. (If you are) able to use this method to turn around the Water (Kan) and Fire (Lii), (your Chi will be able to) reach the top of Kuen Luen Mountain and abide there.

手提金印倒轉紐，一指黃河水逆流，能用坎離顛倒法，直至崑崙頂上遊。

The "golden stamp" means the middle finger. When you use this finger to point or press, it is like using a stamp such as the Chinese use for stamping their signatures. This technique is so valuable that it is called the "golden" stamp. The Yellow River is one of the largest rivers in China. Here it means the Chi flow in the vessels. If you know how to use finger pressure on one point, you will be able to reverse the Chi flow from the Fire path to the Water path. The Fire path is the Chi circulation in the Conception and Governing Vessels, and the Water path is from the Conception Vessel through the Thrusting Vessel to the brain. Kuen Luen mountain is one of the highest mountain in China. Here it refers to the brain.

This secret oral poetry clearly points out that if you wish to control the Kan and Lii effectively, you must first learn how to use one finger to change the Chi flow from the Fire path to the Water path. You apply pressure with one finger to the Huiyin cavity (Magic Gate). This causes the gate to tense up slightly and thus seal the way to the Fire path.

Pointing is used by the beginner who cannot easily use his Yi to control the Magic Gate. Once you are familiar with the feeling, you may use your Yi to gently hold up the area and achieve the same end. This is called Tyi (Hold Up), which we will discuss in the next section.

You usually do not start Pointing training until after 20 days of hanging. By that time you are beginning to understand how to lead the Chi from the vessels in the legs upward to the lower abdomen. You can now add this technique to prevent the Chi from flowing to the back of your body and entering the Governing Vessel.

When you train Pointing, you may stand, sit, or even lie down. Hold up your anus and place the tip of your tongue on the roof of your mouth. Then press the Huiyin lightly with your middle finger, and at the same time inhale and use your mind to lead the Chi upward to the Huang Ting and then to the head. Train several times a day, and try to become familiar with the inner feeling of this practice.

Nei Dan Chi Sublimation:
Although Nei Dan Chi sublimation training uses a slight tensing of the body in some places, the coordination of the Yi and the breathing is the main key to success. There is only one key technique which is known.

A. Hold Up (Tyi)(to raise; to pick up)
The document says:

Hold Up means the point at the Magic Gate (Shyuan Guan).

One of the Taoist classics states:

The Magic Gate (Huiyin) is one point, (where) the Original Chi reverses flow. Change Yang Jieng into shapeless pre-birth real Chi. Return the light shining on you seven times, that means pick up the herb. This also means the dual cultivation of Shing (personality) and Ming (body, life), this is the achievement of the Golden Elixir and Large Tao.

玄關一點，元炁逆流，化陽精為無形的先天真炁，回光返照之返，是謂採藥，亦即性命雙修金丹大道之能事也。

The Magic Gate refers to only one point, the Huiyin cavity. As explained before, the Huiyin cavity is the place where the three main Chi vessels, the Conception, Governing, and Thrusting Vessels, connect and communicate with each other. This spot is a gate which can regulate the Chi level in the three vessels. Semen (and sperm) is considered a Yang Essence which is able to generate life. Chi can be generated from this Essence. According to Chinese medicine, there are two places which store Original Essence and thus can generate Original Chi or Pre-birth Chi. One is on the Kidneys (called the internal Kidneys) and the other is the testicles (called the external Kidneys).

In Chinese Chi Kung it is believed that when the excess Chi is led to your brain you will feel and sense an internal enlightenment like lightning in your brain. Scientifically, we can say that when the excess electricity is led to the brain to activate the brain cells, the energization is perceived as a kind of lightning or visual flash in the brain. According to Chinese Chi Kung, you should practice until your feel the lightning in your brain seven times. When you have reached this stage, it is said that you have picked up the herb (golden elixir). Your spirit can be raised to a higher level to understand yourself and nature (Shing) more clearly. This raised spirit is also able to govern the Chi circulation more effectively and therefore gain you physical health (Ming). This is what is referred to as "dual cultivation" because you develop both your spirit and your physical body.

These two documents make it clear that the Magic Gate is the main key to leading the Chi upward and consequently increasing the semen-Chi conversion. It is also believed that Tyi in the Magic Gate is able to make the three flowers (Jieng, Chi, and Shen) reach the top (San Huea Jiuh Diing), and the Five Chis (heart, liver, spleen, lung, and kidney Chi) move toward their original levels (Wuu Chi Chaur Yuan).

Theoretically, you may practice Tyi any place and any time you want. Posture is not strictly important. However, you should understand that your body must be very relaxed, especially the lower part of your body. Only when you are in a relaxed state may you use your Yi to lift the Magic Gate effectively. According to my personal experience, the best posture to feel and sense the Chi's sublimation is sitting on a couch leaning slightly backward. Have your feet on the floor, and pull the front of your feet up slightly (Figure 8-15). Close your eyes and use your Yi to hold up the Huiyin and anus for the duration of the practice. Breathe deeply, and every time you inhale use your Yi to lead the Chi upward through the Thrusting Vessel, and at the same time concentrate on your Upper Dan Tien (the third eye). This will lead the Chi to nourish your spirit. You may also lead the Chi upward to the Baihui (Gv-20) and use the Chi to nourish your brain.

Some Chi Kung practitioners claim the best posture is the embryo posture (Figure 8-16). According to this theory, when the embryo is formed and growing, its posture enables it to hold the Chi inward to aid its growth. This may be related to the tendency, when you feel cold, to pull your arms and legs inward to your body to conserve energy.

You may very likely find other postures which suit you better. When you are doing it right, you will have a sensational feeling in your ankles and the Huiyin area. You will feel like you are very light and

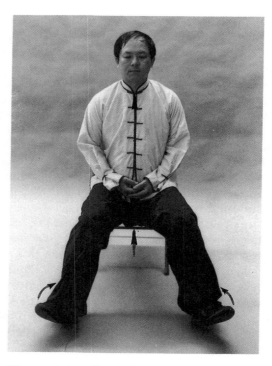

Figure 8-15. Chi Sublimation Training

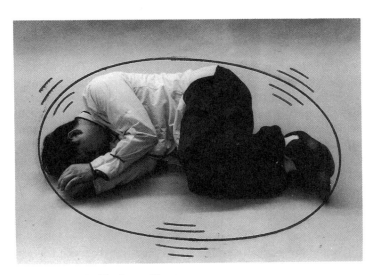

Figure 8-16. Embryo Posture

your body is floating, and at the same time you will feel the Chi growing in your head. When you lead the Chi upward to the brain through the Thrusting Vessel, it moves very rapidly because it is passing through the spine where there are no muscles to tense and slow it down. This feeling you get when you circulate Chi through the Water path is quite different from what you experience when you circulate Chi through the Fire path.

8-6. Washing the Marrow and Conquering the Hair (Shii Soei Fa Mau)

Many laymen are interested in Shii Soei Ching training only until the second stage of Shen and brain nourishment. The third and fourth stages of spiritual enlightenment and becoming a Buddha are usually trained only by monks who are willing to separate themselves from human society. Laymen who complete the second stage can increase their health and longevity significantly. This requires that they learn how to lead Chi to the marrow to revitalize it and to the skin to maintain its health and youthfulness. The document says:

Marrow/Brain Washing Spiritual Kung (Fu), in the beginning use instruments, (make) the Chi reach the four extremities: tongue, teeth, nails, and hair. Beat with a paddle to protect the bone marrow.

You can see from this that, in order to lead Chi to the marrow and to the surface of the skin, you must use the beating exercise. In fact, however, beating training is only the Wai Dan way to do this. It is an easier and much more effective approach for the practitioner who has not reached a high level of Nei Dan training.

If you have mastered Nei Dan Chi Kung, you may instead use your Yi in coordination with your breathing to accomplish the same goal. In this section we will only discuss the beating exercise briefly, since we have already discussed it thoroughly in Part Two. However, we will go into bone breathing more deeply, since it is the key method for Nei Dan marrow washing in the Shii Soei Ching.

Wai Dan Marrow Washing:
A. Beating Exercises:

The theory of the training is very simple - the beating stimulates the muscles, which leads Chi to the surface of the skin. This also increases the lateral movement of Chi, generating Chi circulation throughout the whole of each bone (Figure 8-17). The end of a bone is its weakest part, but it is also the gate whereby the Chi in the marrow communicates with the tendons around the joints. Beating increases the circulation of Chi, which cleans the marrow and leads Chi to the surface of the skin. Many practitioners also emphasize beating on the joints, claiming that it increases the Chi communication through the gates at the ends of the bones. Naturally, you should be careful not to injure the joints.

For more detailed information on beating, please check Part Two.

B. Biting Exercise:

In the biting exercise, your training partner lightly bites the joints and the bones which are near the surface. This stimulates the Chi to a higher stage, and increases the Chi circulation in the marrow. Naturally, you may also find or design an implement to do the same job. When you stimulate the joints like this you normally have a cold but marvelous feeling deep in the bones. Obvious places to do this are the knees and ankles.

According to the science of bioelectricity, stimulating the bones near the skin increases the bioelectric current there, and also increases the Chi circulation from the bones. The obvious places for this stimulation are the shin and the hip bones.

When you do this practice, be careful not to injure the skin or muscles. Also, do not repeat this practice too often. It will make your body too Yin and also affect your nervous system. Once or twice a week should be enough to stimulate the Chi exchange in the marrow.

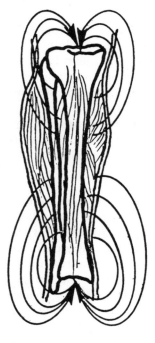

Figure 8-17. Bone Breathing Through Beating Stimulation

Nei Dan Marrow/Brain Washing:

In the discussion of Kan and Lii in Part One we mentioned that breathing is the strategy in Chi Kung training. During inhalation you may condense the Chi from the primary Chi Channels inward, and during exhalation you may expand the Chi from the primary Chi Channels outward to the surface of the skin. Through breathing you can adjust the Kan and Lii and make your body more Yin or Yang. When you have reached this level, you feel like your entire Chi body is breathing when you breathe. The more you train, the better and more efficiently you are able to lead the Chi inward and outward.

In the Nei Dan Marrow/Brain Washing, the Yi, breathing, and Huiyin are the keys to success. When you practice, you may sit on a couch with your feet resting gently on the floor, and the front of your feet lifted slightly. Concentrate your mind and regulate your breathing. According to my personal experience, the Taoist reverse breathing is more effective than the Buddhist breathing.

Once you have calmed down and regulated your breathing, you may start the bone breathing practice. Use your Yi to hold up the Huiyin and anus when you inhale, and relax them when you exhale. Remember: **THE YI IS MORE IMPORTANT THAN THE ACTUAL MOVEMENTS OF THE HUIYIN AND ANUS**. Although they are held up lightly, they remain very relaxed. As you inhale, draw Chi into the ends of the bones, and as you exhale, circulate the Chi out the sides of the bones and out to the surface of the skin.

In the Nei Dan technique of leading Chi to the brain, the keys to the practice are exactly the same as in the bone breathing, except that you should hold up your Huiyin and anus all during the training. When you inhale, your Yi should be either on the top of your head (Baihui) or your Upper Dan Tien. When you exhale, relax your mind, and the Chi will circulate smoothly by itself. After a while, you will gradually begin to understand the practice, and you will start to feel the Chi sublimating to the head. Practice thirty minutes a day. In no time, you will find that you can lead Chi to the brain more and more easily.

8-7. Refining Shen and Returning it to Nothingness (Liann Shen Faan Shiu)

This is the stage of three years of nursing. It is for those practitioners who wish to reach enlightenment or Buddhahood. In this stage you use the Chi to open the gate of the Shen residence, giving birth to the Shen baby. This spirit baby now needs three years of nourishment to grow stronger. You must regulate your mind and get rid of your human emotions and desires. Since all of these human emotions and desires end up as nothingness and have no meaning after you die, they are called "nothingness." Only when your mind is able to reach the stage of nothingness can the spirit baby grow stronger and gradually separate from your physical body. In Chinese religious society, this process is also called "Liann Shen Leau Shing," or "train your spirit and end human nature."

The document contains a song which talks about this training process. It says:

Every morning transport your Chi to Ni Wan, moistening the sweet saliva on the tip of your tongue; watering three fields and

and generating hundreds of vessels, to disembody and become immortal come from this.

朝朝運炁上泥丸，浸浸甘津長舌端：灌溉三田生百脈，脫胎換骨此中求。

The best time for Shii Soei Ching brain nourishment training is from one to six o'clock in the morning. Ni Wan is a Chi Kung term meaning the top of the head where the Tian Ling Gay (Heavenly Cover, or Baihui) is. You have to learn how to generate sweet saliva. When you are very calm and your breathing is uniform, your mouth will secrete a saliva which is sweeter than usual, not the Yang, slightly bitter taste. This is a Kan technique which will water your three Dan Tiens (the "three fields") and prevent them from becoming too Yang. When the Chi in a Dan Tien is too Yang it can burn you out and make your body deteriorate faster than normal. The moisture or saliva which is generated from meditation is the key to bringing the Fire in the three Dan Tiens down. When the three Dan Tiens are watered, Yin and Yang will be balanced. This Chi will be able to run through all of the Chi vessels in your body.

The Chi channels or vessels are called Chi Mei. In addition to the twelve primary channels and eight vessels, there are thousands of small Chi channels which connect deep into your bone marrow and also to the surface of the skin. Many of these channels are sealed or narrowed, and the Chi circulation is stopped or stagnant. After you train Chi Kung, you will be able to reopen and regrow all of them. Once you can do this, your Chi will be able to reach everywhere in your body, including the extremities such as the hair, teeth, tongue, and nails. This also enables you to change your body from weak into strong.

If you ponder this poetry deeply, you can see that it was written by a Taoist who was seeking only a long life and a healthy body. There is no mention of becoming a Buddha.

The available documents have very little information about this stage of the training. According to my personal understanding of the different sources and also from my personal pondering, I have come to the following conclusions about this stage of training.

Theoretically, in this stage you would like to open the gate. In order to reach this goal, you must first build up an abundant supply of Chi to activate the brain and pass through the blockage on your Upper Dan Tien. Therefore, Chi must be built up continuously to a high level, and at the same time you must learn how to lead the Chi to the Upper Dan Tien. When you focus all of this Chi into a tiny spot, the power is very strong. The smaller the spot in which you can focus it, the stronger the power will be. It is just like using a lens to focus the sun. One day you will find the Chi will be strong enough to activate the bone cells and open the path to communicate with the outside world. This is considered the birth of the baby. After the baby is born, you must keep nourishing it so that it grows stronger and stronger.

From my personal understanding, it is almost impossible to use only Wai Dan to open the gate. Opening the gate must be done internally. However, there are some Wai Dan techniques which might help the internal concentration and focusing. Therefore, you should know that even though we discuss Wai Dan and Nei Dan separately, both should be used together.

Wai Dan Gate Opening Practice:

A. Beating the heavenly drum to clear the mind and increase the concentration. Beating the heavenly drum will also open up the tiny Chi channels which connect the brain to the outside of the head. There are two common methods of doing this practice. The first technique is simply using the fingertips to tap the entire head lightly (Figure 8-18). The second way is covering both ears with the palms and placing the index fingers on the middle fingers and snapping the index fingers down to hit the head (Figure 8-19).

B. Massaging or tapping the Upper Dan Tien. This makes it easier to concentrate your attention, and strengthens the focus of power there. After you train for a while, you will find that you can focus your mind there much more easily.

Nei Dan Gate Opening Practice:

In the last section, we discussed how to lead Chi to the brain. We would now like to point out a few related keys to the training:

A. Shen Breathing. Shen breathing combines your spirit with your breathing. Once they combine, the Chi can be led more efficiently to the Shen to nourish it before and after the spirit baby is born. Only after the baby is born can it have its own spirit and become independent.

B. Shen focusing training. In this stage, you must nourish your spirit and make it grow. In addition, you must also learn to focus the

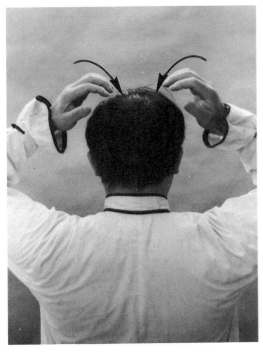

Figure 8-18. Tapping the Head to Beat the Heavenly Drum

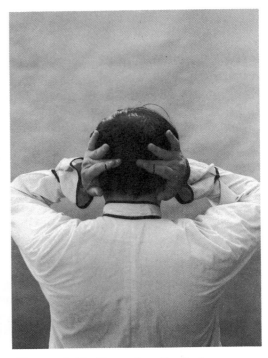

Figure 8-19. Snapping the Index Fingers to Beat the Heavenly Drum

spirit into a tiny point to make it strong until the "gate" is opened. Naturally, mind regulation is a vital key to success.

C. Separate the spirit and the physical body training. Once the gate is opened, you lead the spirit away from your physical body. However, this baby spirit cannot go too far from your physical body.

The document has only two key words which might concern the third stage of training:

A. Hard (Gan)
The document says:

In addition to these thirteen key words, there is another secret word Gan (Hard) throughout all of the training.

Hard here means mental strength. It is the key to strengthening your will power, raising the spirit to a higher level, and focusing the spirit power to a tiny point. If you are able to be strong internally, you will be able to reach all of the goals you plan more effectively.

B. Calm (Jing)
Calm is the second key word which can be found in the document. Since it was not discussed in the first two stages of training, I believe that it refers to the calmness which must be reached in Nei Dan still meditation. It looks very simple, but it is in fact very difficult. It is the calmness of the physical and mental bodies. In order to achieve it, you must regulate your body into a relaxed state, then you must regulate your breathing until it is smooth and calm. Then, you must learn to regulate your mind. Only if your have regulated these three have you grasped the key of calmness.

8-8. Crushing the Nothingness (Feen Suory Shiu Kong)
In the last stage of Shii Soei Ching training you must use your Yi to regulate your mind until your mind can be free from all emotional bondage. In this stage, you do not need your Yi to regulate your mind anymore. Remember **THE REAL REGULATING IS NO REGULAT-ING**. If you still need to regulate what you should regulate, then it is not the real regulating. It is just like when you start to learn how to drive, your mind is on how to drive. After you have mastered the skill of driving, your mind will not have to be on driving. Only then is the emptiness of emotions and desires the real emptiness. Therefore, "Crushing the Nothingness" means there is no difference whether you are in emptiness or not in emptiness. This implies that emptiness does not mean anything to you. We use the word "nothingness" here because it even goes beyond the idea of "emptiness," which implies the lack of something, or that something was once there. Only when you have cultivated your mind to this stage will your spirit be able to move far away from your body and travel anywhere it likes.

In order to reach this level, you should face the wall to meditate for nine years. When you face the wall, you see only wall, think only wall, the mind will gradually enter the domain of nothingness. This enables you to neutralize your emotional thoughts. In this stage of training, the spirit baby will grow up until it can be independent.

You can see that when you have reached this stage, it is all Nei Dan mind regulation training. When your mind is neutral, your spirit will be able to become part of the natural Chi and spirit world. When this happens, your spirit will not die even when your physical body dies. In this case, you have become a Buddha and your spirit will leave the cycle of reincarnation.

There is almost no information in the documents about how to train in this stage. However, I believe that when you have accomplished the third stage, you will know what to do for this stage, and how to do it. This is simply because, when you have reached the third stage, you will be able to see and feel more clearly than before, and know things you could not know before.

According to the limited information that is available, in order for your spirit to leave your body and travel around for a long time, you must learn hibernation breathing training. You need to be able to meditate very deeply, slow your heart beat down, and reduce your oxygen usage to the minimum. Only when your physical body has reached this very Yin stage will your spirit be able to leave. Hibernation breathing also serves to maintain your physical body while your spirit is away. It is said that, once you have reached this level, your spirit is able to leave your body for several months at a time.

PART FOUR

QUESTIONS AND CONCLUSION

Chapter 9

Questions

Because many of the Chi Kung practices have been kept secret in the past, the theories and methods have been passed down randomly. Only in the last twenty years have most of these secrets been revealed to the general public. Finally, interested practitioners have the opportunity to learn the secrets of other styles. Even so, because of the long years of secrecy, many of the documents that are available to us remain incomplete or unconfirmed. To compile all of these documents and finalize a systematic summary of theoretical explanations is very difficult. During the course of my study and research, many questions and answers have arisen. Some answers seem accurate but need further verification through modern technology. Some of the questions are beyond any test which can be done with modern scientific equipment.

Some questions may be due to my limited understanding of Chi Kung training, while others are generated from advances in modern science. I believe that during the course of my continuing research over the rest of my life, many of these questions will be answered. I also hope that I will obtain some of the answers from other experienced Chi Kung masters. Many of the questions need to be investigated through experimentation involving modern equipment. Some of the questions may remain mysteries, since I firmly believe that nobody is able to reach the level of Chi Kung practice attained by earlier masters.

The following are some of the questions I have had which relate to the Yi Gin Ching and Shii Soei Ching. There are many other questions concerning the general Chi Kung practices which have already been listed in the first volume of this series: "The Root of Chinese Chi Kung." We will not repeat these questions here. I hope that you will keep these questions or any question you might have in your mind during the course of your study, so that one day you will come to realize that you know much more than anybody else.

About Essence:

1. Can the stimulation of semen production be done in a modern way? For example, through minor electrical stimulation? Will this cause problems, since the person stimulated does not need to have regulated his mind?

2. Can the stimulation of semen production through modern technology achieve the same purpose of longevity? Can this be done to an old man without causing problems, for example, causing a heart attack?

3. Is there any way of increasing the efficiency of Essence-Chi conversion through modern technology? Such as using an electric or magnetic field to lead the Chi in the vessels upward to the Huang Ting and the brain?

4. Can artificial hormones benefit the body like the Essence generated inside of the body? Are there any side-effects?

5. What exactly is the biochemical reaction which occurs in the Essence-Chi conversion? If we know this process clearly, we may be able to figure out a way to increase the efficiency with modern technology.

6. Can we use modern technology to transport Essence from one person to another, like a blood transfusion?

7. How can we improve the quality and quantity of Essence?

About Chi:

1. Is there any modern way we can use to more rapidly stimulate and raise fasciae for Chi storage? Will this cause problems, since we may not be able to generate enough Chi to keep them active and full?

2. Is there any modern way which can help to build up the Chi internally? Will this cause any problems?

3. Since Chi and the brain are closely related, can we adjust the Chi nourishment of the brain and cure mental illness?

About Spirit (Shen):

1. How do we define spirit? Is it a form of energy? How can a spirit have its own thoughts?

2. Is it true that there is another dimension or world which is not known to science, yet can be reached by the spirit or soul? There are many stories of people dying and then coming back. They often say that they were outside of their physical bodies, and could see them. The Chinese believe that the world we are living in now is the "Yang World" (Yang Jian), and when a person dies, his spirit will enter the "Yin World" (Yin Jian). According to Yin-Yang theory, Yang must be balanced by Yin. Can this Yin world only be reached by energy or spirit?

3. Can we use modern technology to increase the flow of bioelectricity to the brain to activate more brain cells? Are there any side effects? Nowadays, many body builders use electricity to speed up the growth of their muscles to develop a super-looking body in a short time. Later they discover that because the inner body cannot produce enough bioelectricity to support the muscles, the muscles degenerate faster than normal. Will we encounter the same problem if we activate the brain cells the same way?

4. Can we open the gate on the Upper Dan Tien through external electrical stimulation? What will happen if we open the gate quickly, if we do not have enough Chi internally to support this wandering spirit? Will we go crazy?

5. When we reach a higher level of spiritual enlightenment, can we then communicate with aliens from outer space? If they are a thousand years ahead of us in science, they should have reached a high spiritual level and we should be able to contact them somehow.

6. Is the spiritual dimension a new dimension to human beings in which we can travel much faster than the speed of light? Is that how UFOs travel to the earth?

7. How important a role will the human spirit play in human history when science leaves its present stage of infancy and enters the stage of its youth?

8. What is the scientific explanation for the halo around the head, or the glow around the body, of a meditator? Though I try to explain these phenomena as air de-ionization generated by the body's electrical charge, an experiment needs to be conducted to determine whether this is true.

9. How do clouds and fog affect spiritual training? We know that low clouds are able to generate an electric field which affects the human energy field. Does fog do this as well? When you are in fog, do the charges surround you uniformly? Can this affect your spiritual cultivation?

10. How is spirit generated in a newly born baby? Where does spirit originate? Does it start when the baby begins to think? Does it exist only in humans?

11. What are the differences between the spirit and the soul? Since there is no exact translation from Chinese into English, I would like the exact difference and definition of these words.

12. How do we generate a "spiritual baby" in Chi Kung training? In the Chi Kung tradition, in order to reach the final goal of enlightenment you must train yourself until you have given birth to a spiritual baby. Only when this baby has grown to be independent will your spirit not die, but live forever. Is this true? Scientifically, how can this happen? Can we use modern science to explain this, or is it still beyond what today's science can grasp? If we believe that a highly cultivated mind is able to speed up the process of evolution, then this mind may be able to reach many other things which are still beyond human understanding.

13. Does a spirit make its own decisions or is it affected by natural Chi? Can a spirit think? How can it help a person who is alive? Through brainwave communication? Or is a spirit only some human energy residue roaming around in the energy world and being affected by surrounding energy forces?

14. Can a highly concentrated mind make an object move without touching it? What is the principle behind this phenomenon? If this is true, then how can brainwave energy become so strong that it can do this? Are miracles done with brainwaves or through the spiritual dimension?

15. Can the spirit really leave a living body and travel, or is it only that the brainwaves sense something and match its frequency so that you can be aware of it? Also, we have heard that when someone is hypnotized, he is able to sense many things which are beyond his capability while he is in a normal state of consciousness. Is this similar to what happens when a person seems to leave his body during meditation?

16. Can one person affect another person's thinking through brainwave correspondence?

17. Can modern technology create an electromagnetic wave whose wavelength is close to or equivalent to the human brainwave? Our technology seems to have already progressed that far. If this is so, will a brainwave machine be able to generate a wave which will thinking and judgement? This would truly be "brainwashing." Can we create a machine to generate brainwave "white noise" to act as a shield against such a weapon? Will the wars of the future be wars of brainwave machines?

18. If it is possible to make a brainwave machine, can we determine what frequencies are associated with crime and then somehow block those frequencies? Is it possible to really brainwash criminals? Of course, if such a machine fell into the hands of criminals, they would have a powerful tool for evil. Can we accept the moral responsibility for changing an individual's brainwaves?

19. Can a good Chi Kung meditator avoid being controlled and affected by a brainwave machine? Personally, I believe that a Chi Kung practitioner who has reached the stage of regulating his mind effectively would be able to avoid the effects of a brainwave machine. However, how long would he be able to do this?

20. What is the width of the brainwave band? What existing materials can shield them out? Metal is usually a good insulator against radiowaves, but can it also keep out brainwaves? If not, is there any material which can be used to shield against brainwaves?

21. What is the relationship between spirit (Shen) and brainwaves? I personally believe that when your Shen is high, your brainwaves will be stronger and, probably, more focused and sensitive in different wavelengths. Is this true?

22. Since our spirit is so closely related to Chi or the energy field, how much has our spirit been affected by energy pollution such as radio waves?

23. The Su Wen states that our lives run in cycles of 7 years for women and 8 years for men. When the book was written, boys reached puberty around the age of 16, and girls around 14. Now that puberty comes 2 to 4 years earlier, are the cycles changed? Do the cycles have objective reality, or were they more philosophical ideas?

Chapter 10

Conclusion

In conclusion, I would first like to remind you that this book is constructed of pieces of a puzzle. Although it has given you a general picture of the training, many unclear details and mysteries still remain. Therefore, when you study this book, you must use a neutral mind to judge the training theory and methods. You should always ask "Does it make sense?" and "Could it happen that way?" You have grasped the real meaning of the training only when you are able to **FEEL** that it is right. Only then are you qualified to start the training.

It has been my wish that this book open a general discussion of Chi Kung, and hopefully stimulate scientists to get involved in this study. This would make it possible to finally start using both the ancient practices and modern technologies to help mankind reach the goal of health and longevity. I deeply hope that this study will also help to improve the quality of people's lives. This can only be achieved through spiritual cultivation.

Finally, I would like to remind you that it is not possible for me alone to explain the entire Yi Gin Ching and Shii Soei Ching in a single book. These two arts are considered the highest levels of Chinese Chi Kung. You should also remember that this book is not an authority. It is only one of the reference books available for you to ponder, which I hope will guide you to the right path for spiritual training.

Appendix A

Herbal Prescriptions for Yi Gin Ching and Shii Soei Ching Training

Traditionally, Chinese herbs can be divided into two main categories. One is for external use and the other is for internal use. The general purposes of the external herbs are to help the Chi circulation, reduce swelling, dissolve bruises, assist in healing, and adjust Yin and Yang in the treated area.

Most of the external herbs cannot be taken internally. There are four different ways to apply external herbs. The first way is to place the herbs in a bottle with alcohol and let them sit for a long time. Later the liquid is used to rub and massage injured areas. The second way is to cook the herbs with either water or wine and then use the liquid to wash or rub the areas. The third way is to grind the herbs into powder, which is mixed with alcohol and applied to the injured area. The last way is to make an ointment out of the herbs.

Herbs that are taken internally are generally used to adjust the Yin and Yang of the body, remove internal bruises, and speed healing.

There are three common ways to take herbs internally. The first way is to cook the herbs with water or wine and drink the juice. The second way is to grind the herbs into powder and then mix them with honey to make pills. A number of the pills are taken with water or wine. The third way is to grind the herbs into powder. The correct dosage is then taken with water or wine.

Many herbal prescriptions are listed in the Yi Gin Ching and Shii Soei Ching documents. Generally, these prescriptions can be divided into four groups according to their purpose. 1. For the massage period of the Yi Gin Ching training (the first 200 days) to increase the Chi level internally. 2. For Yi Gin Ching training from the 200th day to the 300th day. 3. For the Yi Gin Ching training after 300 days. 4. For Shii Soei Ching groin washing. We will list and briefly discuss these prescriptions according to these four groups. In order to avoid confusion, the herbs will be listed in Chinese. Simply make a copy and show it to a Chinese pharmacist, and he will prepare it for you.

A word of caution. These prescriptions can be very potent. Except where specifically noted, **DO NOT TAKE TWO DIFFERENT PRE-SCRIPTIONS AT THE SAME TIME**. For example, if the two sources both have an internal prescription for a certain stage of training, only take one. However, after a month or so you can switch to the other one. Of course, you can take an internal and external prescription at the same time.

1. Prescriptions for Yi Gin Ching Massage (First 200 Days):
There are two main sources for the prescriptions used in this period.

Source #1:
A.

Almost every ingredient in this prescription must be prepared in a special way. You can either do the preparation yourself, or else ask the pharmacist to do it for you. For the first 100 days, take one pill with either water or wine before each massage session. This prescription has a main part and several secondary parts. The main prescription is:

Ten Brocade Pill (Shyr Gin Wan):

十錦丸方 (內服)

（Chinese prescription text）

The following extra ingredients should be added to the pill when the area indicated is being massaged:

1. When training the front of the body:

（Chinese prescription text）

2. When training the back of the body:

（Chinese prescription text）

3. This is used mainly during Nei Juang training to harmonize and concentrate the Chi:

如用過力量三次一一中午時服藥氛的之法方：：餘家服服十四過沉水粉四兩。

If your body is too Yang or too Yin you should take one of the following prescriptions before you take the Ten Brocade Pill. For the first 40 days of massage training, take one pill in the morning and one in the evening before you take a Ten Brocade Pill.

B. If you are deficient in Yang:

如陽虛者，先習功。先服五生丸十，令陽氣壯先持四十日，服四十丸。再服十錦丸。

Five Growing Pill (Wuu Sheng Wan)

丸其如彈子大。約重三錢，每日早晚各服二丸。白朮（炒）、戌黃「十」等分為末。然後白蜜十錦為。

五生丸方

C. If you are deficient in Yin:

如人陰虛者，先習功。先服五成丸十，令陽氣壯持至三十日，服四十丸。後再服十錦。

Five Achieving Pill (Wuu Cherng Wan)

用車前當歸二兩，每日二次，大熟地。白朮火上製過就熟藥、釐，為為末。

五成丸方

D. However, if you are having nocturnal emissions you should take a Ten Completeness Pill for the first 40 days each time before training. During this period, train holding up your Huiyin and anus and concentrating your mind on your Upper Dan Tien. When the emissions cease after 40 days you may start taking the Ten Brocade Pills. There are five different prescriptions called Ten Completeness Pill. Depending on the individual, one may be more effective than the others. Remember: only take one of these prescriptions at a time.

如遺精者有夢無夢小通有。先習功。河車大熟地。當歸十全大補丸。每日服十。人正人可用。全鹿丸。上中下用之法。每日服四十再加氣血持四十日。后不性時用大稽桂枝附桂方極好道。

Ten Completeness Pill (Shyr Chuan Wan) - #1

十全丸方一一

海石蜊(火煅)、牡蠣、龍骨、白粉(俱全上)、白礬石、韭子(炒)、金櫻
子、大赤金(五十張)、硃砂(飛五錢)、蓮肉(炒一兩)。
共為末，用銀杏肉十兩，煮熟，取出，入臼內搗成泥，加前藥，
打丸，梧子大，每服五錢，空心青鹽湯下，午用酒下，夕用炒杏仁
湯下。一日三服，接續三次，方見其效。

Ten Completeness Pill (Shyr Chuan Wan) - #2

十全丸方一二

白茯苓(鹽水炒十兩)、黃精(九蒸九晒十兩)、仙茅(人乳蒸十兩)，
為末，煉蜜丸，重三錢，日服三丸，湯酒任下，以前藥。

Ten Completeness Pill (Shyr Chuan Wan) - #3

十全丸方一三

硃砂(水飛)、雄黃(水飛)、木香(各十兩)，生蜜為丸，黃豆大。日服
三丸，三次用下。

Ten Completeness Pill (Shyr Chuan Wan) - #4

十全丸方一四

白茯苓(人乳浸蒸)、白朮(米泔浸土炒)等分為末，蜜丸，重三錢，
湯酒任下。

Ten Completeness Pill (Shyr Chuan Wan) - #5

十全丸方一五

建蓮肉(去心)、白茯苓(蜜浸)等分，為末，煉蜜丸，每服三錢，白
開水下。

Source #2:

The following prescriptions can also be used to strengthen the Nei Juang during massage training.

Internal Use:

Internal Strength Prescription (Nei Juang Yaw)

野荳蔻（酒製）、墨旱蓮（酒製）、當歸（酒製）、甘草（炒）（各二錢）。以上共為細末，煉蜜為丸，每丸重二錢。

Take one pill with water or wine right before the massage for the first 200 days of training.

External Use:

Internal Strength Washing Prescription
(Nei Juang Tang Shii Fang)

Cook the herbs with the same amount of salt in an appropriate quantity of water, and use the warm liquid to wash the area being trained. This will harmonize the blood and Chi and increase the circulation.

2. Prescriptions for Yi Gin Ching Massage (After 200 Days):

After two hundred days of massage, slapping, pounding, beating, and striking, the Chi is getting full in the body. The following prescriptions are recommended for when you are training the arms.

Internal Use:

Sideway Opening Internal Prescription (Hen Kai Fwu Fang)

Take two pills a day with water. Train twice a day, 90 minutes each time.

External Use:

Sideway Opening External Washing Prescriptions
(Hen Kai Shii Fang)

開洗方
草烏・丹參・附子各一兩・仙人杖二兩・自然銅・何首烏・紫丁香・花粉・甘草等分共末・水一日洗浴二次。

Place the herbs in a cloth bag and boil in water. Use the water to wash twice a day the areas being trained.

3. Prescriptions for Yi Gin Ching Massage (After 300 Days):

After three hundred days of massage, slapping, pounding, beating, and striking, the Chi is full in the body and you have started the Grand Circulation training. The following prescriptions are recommended for this period.

Internal Use:

Arising Internal Prescriptions (Pyng Chii Fwu Fang)

平氣服方
拜三日之後用此服方用甘草（一兩）・地骨皮（一兩）・紫丁香（一兩）・沉香（一兩）・紫尖（一兩）・土鱉（一兩）・乳香（一兩）・蛇蛻皮（一兩）・真血竭（八兩）・鐵砂・紅花自然銅（二錢半四個）・共細末・將飛過紅鉛和入煉蜜為丸。每服一錢・日服三丸・水下・不可將此方行功三百煉。

Take two pills a day with water. Train twice a day, 90 minutes each time.

External Use:

Arising Washing Prescriptions (Pin Chii Shii Fang)

平氣洗方
地骨皮各一兩・丹參・羌活・川烏防風依撞鹽・甲柏桃各依撞・馬蹄・肥皂之草共末・水一日洗三次。

Place the herbs in a cloth bag and boil in water. Use the water to wash the body twice a day.

4. Prescriptions for Shii Soei Ching Groin Training (After One Year of Yi Gin Ching):

After one year of Yi Gin Ching training, you should also start the Shii Soei Ching training. There are several prescriptions recommended for this period. Again, there are two sources which list prescriptions.

Source #1:

Internal Use:

-269-

Advancing Downward Internal Prescription
(Shiah Jinn Fwu Fang)

（下進服方）

Take two pills a day with water.

External Use:

Advancing Downward Washing Prescription
(Shiah Jinn Shii Fang)

（下進洗方）

Place the herbs in a cloth bag and boil in water. Use the liquid to wash the groin. Every prescription can be used about six times.

Source #2:

External Use:

Lower Portion Herb Washing Prescription
(Shiah Buh Yaw Shii Fang)

（下部洗方）

Cook the herbs in water, and wash the area being trained two or three times a day.

* * * * * * * * * * * *

There are four additional prescriptions found in the documents. They are not clearly classified into any of the four categories. We list them here for your reference.

A. Strike Tiger Strength Origin Elixir
(Daa Hwu Juang Yuan Dan) - #1

打虎壯元丹 - 一

人參(三兩)·鹿茸(一對)·黄芪(四兩)·附子(三兩)·茯苓(四兩)·遠志(八兩)·牛膝(四兩)·大茴(四兩)·白茯苓(四兩)·蛇床子(四兩)·肉蓗蓉(四兩)·巴戟(四兩)·山藥(四兩)·白茯苓(四兩)·木香(二兩)·杜仲(四兩)·當歸(四兩)·棗仁(四兩)·人參(四兩)。 共為細末，煉蜜為丸，每服一錢。

This prescription can be used to strengthen the internal Chi and build up Nei Juang. Take one pill in the morning and one in the evening before training.

B. Strike Tiger Strength Origin Elixir (Daa Hwu Juang Yuan Dan) - #2

打虎壯元丹 - 二

硃砂·當歸(各一兩)·白茯苓(四兩)·陳皮(四兩)·甘草(三錢)·人參(五錢)·肉桂(五錢)·川貝母(一兩)·茯苓(四錢)·澤瀉(泡淡鹽水炒)·夏用二錢·大附子(一錢)·連翹(三錢)·桃仁(少許)·夏加茯苓三錢·上行加一錢·中行加杜仲己一錢·夏加肉桂五錢·夏加膝行加牛膝·一錢·脚行加防己一錢。 蘇子夏加五錢·人參加一錢·

共為細末，煉蜜為丸，白水下。

This prescription is for the same purpose as the last one. The method of preparation and the dosage is the same. Remember, **DO NOT TAKE TWO DIFFERENT PRESCRIPTIONS AT THE SAME TIME!** You may overdose and have a severe reaction! Whenever you are taking one prescription, do not take another one during the training period, except as indicated above. However, you may change from one to another after a period of time.

C. Great Power Pill (Dah Li Wan)

大力丸

土茯苓(炒手斤)·全當歸(酒炒四兩)·牛膝(酒炒四兩)·枸杞(四兩)·廣膠(四兩)·續斷(四兩)·補骨脂(鹽水炒四兩)·菟絲餅(四兩)·虎脛骨(四兩)·酥炙梁前腿骨(酥炙蜜炒手斤)。 共為細末·

煉蜜為丸，每丸一錢，酒下。

This prescription can be used for strengthening the power of the limbs. I believe that it is used for the second and third years of Grand Circulation training.

D. Wash Hand Fairy Prescription (Shii Shoou Shian Fang)
(External Use)

"Fairy prescription" implies that this prescription is passed down from an immortal. It can be used externally right after rubbing and massage training to increase the Chi and blood circulation. When you prepare this prescription, use five cups of vinegar and five of water, and cook until only seven cups remain. Wash the area every day. Each prescription can be used only three times.

Appendix B

Glossary of Chinese Terms

Ann Mo: 按摩

Literally: press rub. Together they mean massage.

Ba Duann Gin: 八段錦

Eight Pieces of Brocade. A Wai Dan Chi Kung practice which is said to have been created by Marshal Yeuh Fei during the Song dynasty.

Ba Kua: 八卦

Literally: Eight Divinations. Also called the Eight Trigrams. In Chinese philosophy, the eight basic variations; shown in the I Ching as groups of single and broken lines.

Ba Kua Chang: 八卦掌

Eight Trigrams Palm. One of the internal martial styles, believed to have been created by Doong Hae-Chuan between 1866 and 1880 A.D.

Bae Ryh Jwu Ji: 百日築基

One Hundred Days to Build the Foundation. In Yi Gin Ching and Shii Soei Ching, the training of the first hundred days is the most important because you lay the foundation for further progress.

Bih Gang: 閉肛

Close the anus.

Charn: 禪

A Chinese school of Mahayana Buddhism which asserts that enlightenment can be attained through meditation, self-contemplation, and intuition. Charn is called Zen in Japan.

Charn Tzong Chii Tzuu: 禪宗七祖

The seven ancestors of the Charn (Zen) style. During the Tarng dynasty of Kai Yuan (713-742 A.D.), Shen Huey was added to the Six Ancestors of the Charn Style and became the seventh ancestor.

Charn Tzong Liow Tzuu: 禪宗六祖

The six ancestors of the Charn (Zen) style: Da Mo, Huoy Kee, Seng Tsann, Tao Shinn, Horng Zen, and Huoy Neng.

Chi: 氣

The general definition of Chi is: universal energy, including heat, light, and electromagnetic energy. A narrower definition of Chi refers to the energy circulating in human or animal bodies.

Chi Kung: 氣功
Kung means Kung Fu (lit. energy-time). Therefore, Chi Kung means the study, research, and/or practices related to Chi.

Chi Shuu: 氣數
Literally: Chi number. When Chi can be numbered, it means that it is limited, and therefore that that person's life is almost over.

Chii Ching Liow Yuh: 七情六怒
Seven emotions and six desires. The seven emotions are happiness, anger, sorrow, joy, love, hate, and desire. The six desires are the sensory pleasures associated with the eyes, ears, nose, tongue, body, and mind.

Chii Huoo: 起火
To start the fire. When you start to build up Chi at the Dan Tien.

Ching: 經
Channel. Sometimes translated meridian. Refers to the twelve organ-related "rivers" which circulate Chi throughout the body.

Ching Shiou Pay: 清修派
Peaceful Cultivation Division. A branch of Taoist Chi Kung.

Chong Mei: 衝脈
Thrusting Vessel. One of the eight extraordinary vessels.

Chow Pyi Nang: 臭皮囊
Notorious skin bag. A scornful Buddhist expression for the physical body. They believe that the physical body is of only temporary use as an aid to spiritual cultivation.

Chuu: 杵
A wooden bar which was used to remove the chaff from grain.

Chyi Ching Ba Mei: 奇經八脈
Literally: strange channels eight vessels. Commonly translated as "extraordinary vessels" or "odd meridians." The eight vessels which store Chi and regulate the Chi in the primary channels.

Da Chyau: 搭橋
To build a bridge. Refers to the Chi Kung practice of touching the roof of the mouth with the tip of the tongue to form a bridge or link between the Governing and Conception Vessels.

Da Jou Tian: 大週天
Literally: Grand Cycle Heaven. Usually translated Grand Circulation. After a Nei Dan Chi Kung practitioner completes his Small Circulation, he will circulate his Chi through the entire body. He is then said to have completed his Grand Circulation.

Da Mo: 達摩
The Indian Buddhist monk who is credited with creating the Yi Gin Ching and Shii Soei Ching while at the Shaolin monastery. His last name was Sardili, and he was also known as Bodhidarma. He was once the prince of a small tribe in southern India.

Da Mo Juang Chi Kung: 達摩壯氣功
A set of Wai Dan Chi Kung practices. Based on the theory of Da Mo's Wai Dan Chi Kung training.

Dai Mei: 帶脈
Girdle Vessel. One of the eight extraordinary vessels.

Dan Diing Tao Kung: 丹鼎道功
The Elixir Cauldron Way of Chi Kung. The Taoists' Chi Kung training.

Dan Tien: 丹田
Literally: Field of Elixir. Locations in the body which are able to store and generate Chi (elixir) in the body. The Upper, Middle, and

Lower Dan Tiens are located respectively between the eyebrows, at the solar plexus, and a few inches below the navel.

Dien Shiuh: 點穴

Dien means "to point and exert pressure" and Shiuh means "cavities." Chin Na techniques which specialize in attacking acupuncture cavities to immobilize or kill an opponent.

Du Mei: 督脈

Usually translated Governing Vessel. One of the eight Chi vessels.

Ermei Mountain: 峨嵋山

A mountain in Szechuan province where many martial styles originated.

Faan Hu Shi: 反呼吸

Reverse Breathing. Also commonly called Taoist Breathing.

Faan Jieng Buu Nao: 還精補腦

Literally: to return the Essence to nourish the brain. A Taoist Chi Kung training process wherein Chi which has been converted from Essence is lead to the brain to nourish it.

Feen Suory Shiu Kong: 粉碎虛空

To crush the nothingness. One of the Taoist training processes for enlightenment wherein the illusion which connects the physical world and the spiritual plane is destroyed.

Fu Shyi: 膚息

Skin breathing. One of the Nei Dan Chi breathing practices.

Fwu Chi: 伏氣

To tame the Chi. Tame means to control and to govern.

Gin Dan Dah Tao: 金丹大道

Golden Elixir Large Way. Major Taoist Chi Kung training in which the elixir is produced in the body through training, and later used to extend life.

Gin Jong Jaw: 金鐘罩

Golden Bell Cover. An Iron Shirt training.

Guu Shen: 谷神

Valley Spirit. The Baihui cavity on the top of the head, believed to be the place or gate where the body's Chi communicates with the heaven Chi.

Guu Soei: 骨髓

Bone marrow.

Harn Fen Lou: 涵芬摟

The Tower of Fragrance. Believed to be the name of a Taoist organization.

Herng Mo: 橫磨

Grindstone. A Shii Soei Ching term for the penis.

Hou Tian Faa: 後天法

Post Heaven Techniques. An internal style of martial Chi Kung which is believed to have been created around the sixth century.

Hsin: 心

Literally: Heart. Refers to the emotional mind.

Hsing Yi or Hsing Yi Chuan: 形意、形意拳

Literally: Shape-mind Fist. An internal style of Kung Fu in which the mind or thinking determines the shape or movement of the body. Creation of the style is attributed to Marshal Yeuh Fei.

Huang Ting: 黃庭

Yellow yard. In Taoist Chi Kung, the place in the center of the body where Fire Chi and Water Chi are mixed to generate a spiritual embryo.

Jeng Hu Shi: 正呼吸

Formal Breathing. More commonly called Buddhist Breathing.

Jeou Nian Miann Bih: 九年面壁

Nine year of facing the wall. The last stage of the Shii Soei Ching training for enlightenment or Buddhahood.

Jieng: 精

Essence. The most refined part of anything.

Jieng Chi: 精氣

Essence Chi. The Chi which has been converted from Original Essence.

Jieng-Shen: 精神

Essence-Spirit. Often translated as the "spirit of vitality." Raised spirit (raised by the Chi which is converted from Essence) which is restrained by the Yi.

Jing: 勁

A power in Chinese martial arts which is derived from muscles which have been energized by Chi to their maximum potential.

Ju Luen: 珠輪

Pearl wheels. The testicles.

Kai Chiaw: 開竅

Opening the tricky gate. In Chi Kung, opening the gate of the Upper Dan Tien.

Kan: 坎

A phase of the eight trigrams representing Water.

Lao Tzyy: 老子

The creator of Taoism, also called Li Erh.

Li: 力

The power which is generated from muscular strength.

Li Erh: 李耳

Lao Tzyy, the creator of Taoism.

Liann Chi: 練氣

Liann means to train, to strengthen, and to refine. A Taoist training process through which your Chi grows stronger and more abundant.

Liann Chi Huah Shen: 練氣化神

To refine the Chi to nourish the spirit. Leading Chi to the head to nourish the brain and spirit.

Liann Chi Sheng Hwa: 練氣昇華

To train the Chi and sublimate. A Shii Soei Ching training process by which the Chi is led to the Huang Ting or the brain.

Liann Jieng: 練精

Liann here means to conserve, to train, and to refine. A Chi Kung training process for protecting and refining the Essence.

Liann Jieng Huah Chi: 練精化氣

To refine the Essence and convert it into Chi.

Liann Shen: 練神

To train the spirit. To refine, strengthen, and focus the Shen.

Liann Shen Faan Shiu: 練神還虛

To train the spirit to return to nothingness. An advanced stage of enlightenment and Buddhahood training in which the practitioner learns how to lead his spirit to separate from his physical body.

Liann Shen Leau Shing: 練神了性

To refine the spirit and end human nature. The final stage of enlightenment training where you learn to keep your emotions neutral and try to be undisturbed by human nature.

Liann Shenn: 練身

　　Train the body.

Lii: 離

　　A phase of the eight trigrams representing Fire.

Ling Tai: 靈胎

　　Spiritual embryo.

Lingtai: 靈台

　　Spiritual station. In acupuncture, a cavity on the back. In Chi Kung, it refers to the Upper Dan Tien.

Lou: 絡

　　The small Chi channels which branch out from the primary Chi channels and are connected to the skin and to the bone marrow.

Mei: 脈

　　Chi vessels. The eight vessels involved with transporting, storing, and regulating Chi.

Mi Leh For: 彌勒佛

　　Happy Buddha. Chinese name of Pao Jaco, the first Indian priest to come to China to preach.

Mih Tzong Shen Kung: 宓宗神功

　　Secret Style of Spiritual Kung Fu. Tibetan Chi Kung and martial arts.

Ming Tian Guu: 鳴天鼓

　　Beat the heavenly drum. A Chi Kung practice for waking up and clearing the mind in which the back of the head is tapped with the fingers.

Nao Soei: 腦髓

　　The brain.

Nei Dan: 內丹

　　Internal elixir. A form of Chi Kung in which Chi (the elixir) is built up in the body and spread out to the limbs.

Nei Juang: 內壯

　　Internal strength. The strength of the Chi body which supports the external, or physical body.

Nei Kung: 內功

　　Literally: internal Kung Fu. Usually, martial Chi Kung.

Ni Wan or Ni Wan Gong: 泥丸、泥丸宮

　　Dust pill, or dust pill palace. Chi Kung terminology for the brain.

Ning Shen: 凝神

　　To condense or focus the spirit.

Pao Jaco: 跋陀

　　An Indian priest, called Mi Leh For (Happy Buddha) by the Chinese, who was the first Indian priest to come to China to preach.

Perng Lai: 蓬萊

　　A mythical island where the immortals reside.

Ren Mei: 任脈

　　Usually translated "Conception Vessel."

San Guan: 三關

　　Three gates. In Small Circulation training, the three cavities on the Governing Vessel which are usually obstructed and must be opened.

San Huea Jiuh Diing: 三花聚頂

　　Three flowers reach the top. One of the final goals of Chi Kung whereby the three treasures (Essence, Chi, and Shen) are led to the top of the body to nourish the brain and spirit center (Upper Dan Tien).

San Nian Yeou Cherng: 三年有成

　　Three years of achievement. The three years of Yi Gin Ching training.

San Tsair: 三才

The three powers. Heaven, Earth, and Man.

Sann Kung: 散功

Energy dispersion. Premature degeneration of the muscles when the Chi cannot effectively energize them. Caused by earlier overtraining.

Seng Bing: 僧兵

Priest soldiers. In the Tarng dynasty, the Shaolin temple was the only one the emperor permitted to have its own complete martial arts system.

Shaolin: 少林

A Buddhist temple in Henan province, famous for its martial arts.

Sheau Jeau Tian: 小九天

Small nine heaven. A Chi Kung style created in the sixth century.

Sheau Jou Tian: 小週天

Small heavenly cycle. Also called Small Circulation. The completed Chi circuit through the Conception and Governing Vessels.

Shen: 神

Spirit. Said to reside in the Upper Dan Tien (the third eye).

Shen Chi Shiang Her: 神氣相合

The Shen and the Chi combine together. The final stage of regulating the Shen.

Shen Guu: 神谷

Spirit valley. Formed by the two lobes of the brain, with the Upper Dan Tien at the exit.

Shen Ing: 神嬰

Spiritual baby.

Shen Jiau: 神交

Spiritual communication.

Shen Shyi Shiang Yi: 神息相依

The Shen and breathing mutually rely on each other.

Shen Tai: 神胎

Spiritual embryo. It is also called "Ling Tai."

Sheng Tai: 聖胎

Holy embryo. Another name for the spiritual embryo.

Sher Jieng: 攝精

Absorbing the Essence. Absorbing natural Essences, such as from the sun, moon, food, and air.

Shii Soei Ching: 洗髓經

Washing Marrow/Brain Classic, usually translated Marrow/Brain Washing Classic. Chi Kung training specializing in leading Chi to the marrow to cleanse it.

Shii Soei Fa Mau: 洗髓伐毛

Washing the marrow and conquering the hair.

Shing Ming Shuang Shiou: 性命雙修

Human nature life double cultivation. Originally Buddhist, though now predominantly Taoist approach to Chi Kung emphasizing the cultivation of both spirituality (human nature) and the physical body.

Shiou Chi: 修氣

Cultivate the Chi. Cultivate implies to protect, maintain, and refine. A Buddhist Chi Kung training.

Shiou Shenn: 修身

Cultivate the physical body. Cultivate implies to protect, maintain, and refine. A Buddhist Chi Kung training.

Shou Shyh Faan Ting: 收視返聽

Withdraw the sight and reverse listening. The first step in meditation, where you draw your attention inside you, away from the sensations of the outside world.

Shuang Shiou: 雙修

Double cultivation. A Chi Kung training method in which Chi is exchanged with a partner in order to balance the Chi in both people.

Shuu: 蜀

Szechuan province.

Shyr Yueh Hwai Tai: 十月懷胎

Ten months of pregnancy. A stage in Taoist Chi Kung when the spiritual embryo is nourished.

Shyuan Guan: 玄關

Tricky gates. The many key places in Chi Kung training.

Song Gang: 鬆肛

Relax the anus.

Su Wen: 素問

A very old medical book.

Syh Dah Jie Kong: 四大皆空

Four large are empty. A stage of Buddhist training where all of the four elements (earth, water, fire, and air) are absent from the mind so that one is completely indifferent to worldly temptations.

Tai Chi Chuan: 太極拳

Great ultimate fist. An internal martial art.

Tao Jia (Tao Jiaw): 道家 (道教)

The Tao family. Taoism. Created by Lao Tzyy during the Jou dynasty (1122-934 B.C.). In the Han dynasty (c. 58 A.D.), it was mixed with Buddhism to become the Taoist religion (Tao Jiaw).

Tao Te Ching: 道德經

Morality Classic. Written by Lao Tzyy.

Tao Wai Tsae Yaw: 道外採藥

To pick up the herb outside of the Tao. A Taoist Chi Kung training.

Tian Chyr: 天池

Heavenly pond. The place under the tongue where saliva is generated.

Tiea Bu Shan: 鐵布衫

Iron shirt. Kung Fu training which toughens the body externally and internally.

Tii Shyi: 體息

Body breathing, or skin breathing. In Chi Kung, the exchanging of Chi with the surrounding environment through the skin.

Tuei Na: 推拿

Literally: push and grab. A style of massage and manipulation for treatment of injuries and many illnesses.

Tyau Hsin: 調心

To regulate the emotional mind.

Tyau Shenn: 調身

To regulate the body.

Tyau Shyi: 調息

To regulate the breathing.

Tzai Jie Pay: 栽接派

Plant and Graft Division. A style of Taoist Chi Kung.

Tzy: 子

Midnight.

Tzy-Wuu: 子午

The time between midnight and noon.

Wai Dan: 外丹

External elixir. External Chi Kung exercises in which Chi is built up in the limbs and then led to the body.

Wai Juang: 外壯

External strength. Muscular strength, which can be seen externally.

Wey Chi: 衛氣

Guardian Chi. The Chi shield which wards off negative external influences.

Wuu: 午

Noon.

Wuu Chi Chaur Yuan: 五氣朝元

Five Chis toward their origins. A goal of Chi Kung wherein the Chi of the five Yin organs is kept at the right (original) level.

Wuu Hsin: 五心

Five centers. The face, the Laogong cavities in both palms, and the Yongquan cavities on the bottoms of both feet.

Wuu-Tzy: 午子

The time between noon and midnight.

Wuudang Mountain: 武當山

Located in Fubei province in China.

Yang: 陽

In Chinese philosophy, the active, positive, masculine polarity. In Chinese medicine, Yang means excessive, overactive, overheated.

Yangchiao Mei: 陽蹻脈

Yang Heel Vessel. One of the eight extraordinary vessels.

Yangwei Mei: 陽維脈

Yang Linking Vessel. One of the eight extraordinary vessels.

Yeang Shen: 養神

To refine and nurse the spirit.

Yi: 意

Mind. Specifically, the mind which is generated by clear thinking and judgement, and which is able to make you calm, peaceful, and wise.

Yi Chi Shiang Her: 意氣相合

Yi and Chi mutually combine.

Yi Gin Ching: 易筋經

Literally: Changing Muscle/Tendon Classic, usually called The Muscle/Tendon Changing Classic. Credited to Da Mo around 550 A.D., this work discusses Wai Dan Chi Kung training for strengthening the physical body.

Yii Yi Yiin Chi: 以意引氣

Use your Yi (wisdom mind) to lead your Chi.

Yin: 陰

In Chinese philosophy, the passive, negative, feminine polarity. In Chinese medicine, Yin means deficient. The Yin (internal) organs are the Heart, Lungs, Liver, Kidneys, Spleen, and Pericardium.

Yinchiao Mei: 陰蹻脈

Yin Heel Vessel. One of the eight extraordinary vessels.

Ying Chi: 營氣

Managing Chi. It manages the functioning of the organs and the body.

Yinwei Mei: 陰維脈

Yin Linking Vessel. One of the eight extraordinary vessels.

Yuan Chi: 元氣

Original Chi. Created from the Original Essence inherited from your parents.

Yuan Chiaw: 元竅

Original key point. Key points to the training.

Yuan Jieng: 元精

Original Essence. The fundamental, original substance inherited from your parents, it is converted into Original Chi.

Yuan Shen: 元神

Original Spirit. The spirit you already had when you were born.

Yuhjeen: 玉枕

Jade pillow. One of the three gates of Small Circulation training.

Appendix C

Translation of Chinese Terms

氣功 Chi Kung
楊欽銘 Yang Chin-Ming
李青雲 Li Ching-Yuen
清康熙 Ching Kang Shi
綦江縣 Chyi Jiang Hsien
四川 Szechuan
開縣 Kai Hsien
陳家場 Chen Jia Charng
乾隆 Chyan Long
岳鍾琪 Yeuh Jong-Chyi
楊森 Yang Sen
萬縣 Wann Hsien
Er Bae Wuu Shyr Suey
二百五十歲人瑞實記　Ren Ruey Shyr Jih
中外文庫 Jong Wai Wen Kuh
坎 Kan
離 Lii
陰 Yin
陽 Yang

ABOUT THE AUTHOR
楊俊敏 Yang Jwing-Ming
武術 Wushu
功夫 Kung Fu
少林 Shaolin
白鶴 Pai Huo
曾金灶 Cheng Gin-Gsao
擒拿 Chin Na
太極拳 Tai Chi Chuan
高濤 Kao Tao
淡江學院 Tamkang College
台北縣 Taipei Hsien
長拳 Chang Chuan

李茂清 Li Mao-Ching
國術 Kuoshu
國立台灣大學 National Taiwan University
勁 Jing
連步拳 Lien Bu Chuan
功力拳 Gung Li Chuan
少林擒拿 Shaolin Chin Na
外丹氣功 Wai Dan Chi Kung

PREFACE AND
CONTENTS
易筋 Yi Gin
洗髓 Shii Soei
梁 Liang
易筋經 Yi Gin Ching
洗髓經 Shii Soei Ching
推拿 Tuei Na
按摩 Ann Mo
點穴 Dien Shiuh
武當 Wuudang
峨嵋 Ermei
禪 Charn
忍 Zen
丹鼎道功 Dan Diing Tao Kung
密宗神功 Mih Tzong Shen Kung
達磨 Da Mo
外丹 Wai Dan
內丹 Nei Dan
外壯 Wai Juang
內壯 Nei Juang
練精化氣 Liann Jieng Huah Chi
練氣化神 Liann Chi Huah Shen
洗髓伐毛 Shii Soei Fa Mau

-282-

練神返虛 Liann Shen Faan Shiu
粉碎虛空 Feen Suory Shiu Kong

Chapter 1
骨髓 Guu Soei
腦髓 Nao Soei
神 Shen
練精 Liann Jieng
練氣 Liann Chi
練神 Liann Shen
任脈 Ren Mei
督脈 Du Mei
靈台 Lingtai
小九天 Sheau Jeau Tian
後天法 Hou Tian Faa
八卦 Ba Kua
形意 Hsing Yi
六合八法 Liu Ho Ba Fa
岳飛 Yeuh Fei
唐 Tarng
李世民 Li Shyh-Min
僧兵 Seng Bing
戚繼光 Chi Jih-Guang
明 Ming
真本易筋經 Jen Been Yi Gin Ching
蔣竹莊 Jiang Jwu-Juang
涵芬樓 Harn Fen Lou
中國神功 Jong Gwo Shen Kung
恭鑑老人 Gong Jiann Lao Ren
Jong Gwo Shii Soei Kung
中國洗髓功夫之真諦 Fu Jy Jen Dih
喬長虹 Chyau Charng-Horng

Chapter 2
商 Shang
漢 Han
臭皮囊 Chow Pyi Nang
張道陵 Chang Tao-Ling
道教 Tao Jiaw
老子 Lao Tzyy
李耳 Li Erh
道德經 Tao Te Ching
莊周 Juang Jou
莊子 Juang Tzyy
魏孝文帝 Wey Shiaw Wen Dih
少室 Shao Shyh
登峰縣 Deng Feng Hsien
河南 Henan
跛伱 Pao Jaco
彌勒佛 Mi Leh For
魏孝明帝 Wey Shiaw Ming Dih
孝昌 Shiaw Chang
梁武帝 Liang Wuu Dih
大同 Dah Torng
陸游 Lu Yu
禪宗 Charn Tzong
慧可 Huoy Kee

繼光 Jih Guang
僧璨 Seng Tsann
道信 Tao Sjinn
弘忍 Horng Zen
慈能 Huoy Neng
禪宗六祖 Charn Tzong Liow Tzuu
神會 Shen Huey
開元 Kai Yuan
禪宗七祖 Charn Tzong Chii Tzuu
佛道一家 For Tao Yi Jia
福建 Fujian
泉州 Chyuan Jou
河北 Hebei
紅龍 Horng Long
李靖 Li Jing
真觀 Jen Guan
太和 Tay Her
蜀 Shuu
般剌密諦 Ban Tsyh Mih Dih
四川 Szechuan
徐鴻 Shyu Horng
虹辭 Chyon Ran
炭敦 Horng Yih
紹興 Shaw Shing
徽 Huei
欽 Chin
鄂 Eh
金 Gin
揚子江 Yangtze River
少保 Shao Bao
湖北 Hubei
嵩山 Song Mountain
牛臯 Niou Gaw
湯陰 Tang Yin
鶴九臯撿峯 Heh Jeou Fuu
秦月 Chin Kua
張月峯 Chang Yeuh-Feng
長白山羌 Chang Bae Mountain
羌 Chiang
山東 Shandong
膠崂 Leau Lau
神勇戴 Shen Yeong
戴 Day
順治 Shuenn Tyh
岳武穆 Yeuh Wu Mu

Chapter 3
七情六慾 Chii Ching Liow Yuh
心 Hsin
四大皆空 Syh Dah Jie Kong
喇嘛 Laa Ma
密宗 Mih Tzong
精 Jieng
三花聚頂 San Huea Jiuh Diing
金丹大道 Gin Dan Dah Tao
雙修 Shuang Shiou

-283-

道外採藥 Tao Wai Tsae Yaw
栽接派 Tzai Jie Pay
元 Yuan
六祖説傳法 Liow Tzuu Shwo Chwan Faa
修身 Shiou Shenn
修氣 Shiou Chi
練身 Liann Shenn
調身 Tyau Shenn
調心 Tyau Hsin
調息 Tyau Shyi
凝神 Ning Shen
伏氣 Fwu Chi
攝精 Sher Jieng
開竅 Kai Chiaw
肉功 Nei Kung
悟真篇 Wuh Jen Pian
抱朴子 Baw Poh Tzyy
葛洪 Ger Horng
神交 Shen Jiau
漢書藝文誌 Han Shu Yih Wen Jyh
營氣 Ying Chi
衛氣 Wey Chi
神胎 Shen Tai
神嬰 Shen Ing
靈胎 Ling Tai

Chapter 4
意 Yi
勞宮 Laogong
湧泉 Yongquan
息 Shyi
神息相依 Shen Shyi Shiang Yi
會陰 Huiyin
仙骨 Shian Guu
百會 Baihui

Chapter 5
力 Li
子 Tzy
午 Wuu
子午 Tzy-Wuu
午子 Wuu-Tzy
泥丸宮 Ni Wan Gong
性命雙修 Shing Ming Shuang Shiou
氣數 Chi Shuu
精神 Jieng-Shen
三戈 San Tsair
五氣朝元 Wuu Chi Chaur Yuan
收視返聽 Shou Shyh Faan Ting
項羽 Shiang Yu
烏猥 Wu Huoh
劉邦 Liou Ban
達磨壯氣功 Da Mo Juang Chi Kung
散功 Sann Kung
孟子 Mencius
鐵布衫 Tiea Bu Shan
金鐘罩 Gin Jong Jaw

體息 Tii Shyi
膚息 Fu Shyi
經 Ching
絡 Lou
脈 Mei
元精 Yuan Jieng
氣海 Qihai

Chapter 6
意氣相合 Yi Chi Shiang Her
百日築基 Bae Ryh Jwu Ji
小週天 Sheau Jou Tian
磨礪 Mo Li
海底 Hai Dii
大週天 Da Jou Tian
崑崙 Kuen Luen
駕鶴西歸 Jiah Heh Shi Guei
返童 Faan Torng
起火 Chii Huoo
正呼吸 Jeng Hu Shi
反呼吸 Faan Hu Shi
尾閭 Weilu
鬆肛 Song Gang
閉肛 Bih Gang
三關 San Guan
長強 Changqiang
以意引氣 Yii Yi Yiin Chi
夾脊 Jargi
命門 Mingmen
玉枕 Yuhjeen
風府 Fengfu
搭搞 Da Chyau
天池 Tian Chyr
五心 Wuu Hsin
三年有成道人 San Nian Yeou Cherng
紫凝道人 Tzyy Ning Tao Ren

Chapter 7
奇經八脈 Chyi Ching Ba Mei
素問 Su Wen
衝脈 Chong Mei
元氣 Yuan Chi
帶脈 Dai Mei
陽蹻脈 Yangchiao Mei
陰蹻脈 Yinchiao Mei
陽維脈 Yangwei Mei
陰維脈 Yinwei Mei
玄關 Shyuan Guan
谷神 Guu Shen
神谷 Shen Guu
黃庭 Huang Ting
十月懷胎 Shyr Yueh Hwai Tai
三年哺乳 San Nian Buh Ruu
九年面壁 Jeou Nian Miann Bih
聖胎 Sheng Tai
玉環穴 Yuh Hwan Shiuh
Torng Ren Yu Shiuh Jen

-284-

INDEX